Dialectical Behavior Therapy
with Suicidal Adolescents

Dialectical Behavior Therapy
with Suicidal Adolescents

ALEC L. MILLER
JILL H. RATHUS
MARSHA M. LINEHAN

Foreword by Charles R. Swenson

THE GUILFORD PRESS
New York / London

Library of Congress Cataloging-in-Publication Data

Miller, Alec L.
    Dialectical behavior therapy with suicidal adolescents / by Alec L.
Miller, Jill H. Rathus, & Marsha M. Linehan.
        p. ; cm.
    Includes bibliographical references and index.
    ISBN-13: 978-1-59385-383-9 (alk. paper)
    ISBN-10: 1-59385-383-1 (alk. paper)
    1. Dialectical behavior therapy.   2. Teenagers—Suicidal
behavior.   3. Teenagers—Mental health.   4. Self-destructive
behavior.   I. Rathus, Jill H.   II. Linehan, Marsha.   III. Title.
    [DNLM: 1. Adolescent.   2. Suicide—prevention &
control.   3. Adolescent Psychology.   4. Behavior Therapy—
methods.   5. Self-Injurious Behavior—therapy.   WS 463 M6468d
2006]
    RC569.5.S45M552 2006
    616.89′142—dc22
                                                            2006022291

We dedicate this book to our clients and their families. They have taught us about resilience, compassion, perseverance, and courage. Their lives, and their work with us to develop a version of dialectical behavior therapy that is effective for them, have served as the inspiration for our book.

About the Authors

ALEC L. MILLER, PSYD, is Associate Professor of Psychiatry and Behavioral Sciences, Chief of Child and Adolescent Psychology, Director of the Adolescent Depression and Suicide Program, Director of Mental Health Services at P. S. 8 School-Based Health Program, and Associate Director of the Psychology Internship Training Program at Montefiore Medical Center/Albert Einstein College of Medicine, Bronx, New York. In addition, he is Cofounder of Cognitive and Behavioral Consultants of Westchester, Fellow of the American Psychological Association, President of the American Psychological Association's Society of Clinical Psychology Section on Clinical Emergencies and Crises, and past Chair of the International Society for the Improvement and Training of Dialectical Behavior Therapy. He is Associate Editor of *Cognitive and Behavioral Practice* and serves as a consultant to the U.S. Food and Drug Administration's Suicide Classification Project as well as to other organizations. Dr. Miller received his BA from the University of Michigan before earning his doctorate in clinical psychology from the Ferkauf Graduate School of Psychology of Yeshiva University, Bronx, New York. He has received federal, state, and private grant research funding, and he has published numerous peer-reviewed journal articles, book chapters, and books on topics including dialectical behavior therapy (DBT), adolescent suicide, childhood maltreatment, and borderline personality disorder. He has conducted over 200 lectures and workshops around the world, training thousands of mental health professionals in DBT.

JILL H. RATHUS, PHD, is Associate Professor of Psychology, Founder and Director of the Dialectical Behavior Therapy Program, and Director of the Specialty Concentration in Family Violence in the Clinical Psychology Doctoral Program at Long Island University/C.W. Post Campus in Brookville, New York. She has developed and conducted programs in DBT for adolescents and adults as well as males referred for intimate partner violence, and has received foundation and university funding to study, adapt, and develop assessment tools for DBT. She serves on grant review committees for the National Institute of Mental Health and as an ad hoc reviewer to several psychology journals, trains mental health professionals and graduate students in DBT, consults widely in research and treatment development, and maintains a private practice in Great Neck, New York. Dr. Rathus received her BA from Cornell University and her PhD in psychology from the State University of New York at Stony Brook. She has published numerous peer-reviewed articles and chapters on DBT, adolescent suicide, couple therapy, intimate partner violence, personality disorders, assessment, and anxiety disorders, and has written three prior books: *Marital Distress: Cognitive Behavioral Interventions for Couples*, *Assessment of Family Violence*, and *Assessment of Partner Violence*.

MARSHA M. LINEHAN, PHD, is Professor of Psychology and Adjunct Professor of Psychiatry and Behavioral Sciences at the University of Washington, Seattle, and Director of the Behavioral Research and Therapy Clinics there. She is founder of the Marie Institute of Behavioral Technology and the company Behavioral Tech, LLC. She is past President of the Association for Advancement of Behavior Therapy, Fellow and President-elect of the Society of Clinical Psychology (Division 12 of the American Psychological Association), and Fellow of the American Psychopathological Association. She has written three books, including two treatment manuals: *Cognitive-Behavioral Treatment for Borderline Personality Disorder* and *Skills Training Manual for Treating Borderline Personality Disorder*. Dr. Linehan has received several awards recognizing her clinical and research contributions, including the Louis I. Dublin Award for Lifetime Achievement in the Field of Suicide and the Distinguished Scientist Award from the Society for a Science of Clinical Psychology (Division 12, Section 3 of the American Psychological Association), as well as awards for Distinguished Research in Suicide (American Foundation for Suicide Prevention), Distinguished Contributions to the Practice of Psychology (American Association of Applied and Preventive Psychology), Distinguished Contributions for Clinical Activities (Association for Advancement of Behavior Therapy), Distinguished Scientific Contributions to Clinical Psychology (Society of Clinical Psychology), Lifetime Achievement Award (Society of Clinical Psychology Section on Clinical Emergencies and Crises), and Diplomate of the American Board of Behavioral Psychology.

Foreword

Alec Miller is a jazz pianist. A jazz musician holds tight to his fundamentals and improvises within the rules. That's exactly what it takes to adapt an evidence-based treatment to a new population.

Jill Rathus is a mother of twins. A parent of twins seeks balance and searches for truth in opposing perspectives. That's just what it takes to work dialectically with multiproblem, suicidal teens and their families.

Dialectical behavior therapy (DBT) evolved from Marsha Linehan's own application of standard cognitive-behavioral therapy (CBT) to individuals with suicidal and self-injurious behaviors. It did not work. The patients, typically of a highly sensitive and emotionally reactive nature, and having endured years feeling misunderstood and judged by those around them, felt "corrected" and invalidated by the direct focus on behavioral change. Weekly crises trumped problem-solving procedures. But guided by a steady focus on behavioral outcomes, Linehan stayed the course, improvising within the rules. She modified her use of CBT strategies to fit the individuals and the moment. She eliminated strategies that didn't seem to work. She experimented with interventions from other individual and family psychotherapy models, self-help programs, and spiritual practices, preserving those that met with success. Developed first from a straight, then slightly modified, behavioral model, DBT arrived on the scene as a synthesis of three paradigms: *behaviorism* as a means of changing behavior; *mindfulness* as a means of fostering awareness, acceptance, and compassion; and *dialectics* as a means of finding fluidity and balancing acceptance and change in the face of rigidity and impasse. The first draft of the treatment manual was completed in 1984 and tested in a randomized controlled trial that was published in the *Archives of General Psychiatry* in 1991. The psychotherapy manual and the skills training manual were both published in 1993. In the past 13 years DBT has been subjected to dozens of research trials, including eight published randomized controlled trials essentially confirming the initial findings.

Well acquainted from having been psychology interns together at Montefiore Medical Center several years earlier, Alec Miller and Jill Rathus found themselves working together again in 1995 at Montefiore's Adolescent Depression and Suicide Program, where Miller was appointed director of the program and Rathus director of research. Miller and Rathus began a search for empirically validated treatment approaches to depressed and suicidal adolescents. The very first time I met them was when they came to the New York Hospital–Cornell Medical Center in White Plains, New York, to learn first hand about my inpatient adaptation of DBT for individuals diagnosed with borderline personality disorder. Encouraged by what they saw, they wondered whether they could similarly adapt DBT to the treatment of suicidal youth. I urged them to try it. Even though at the time there were limited research data to support using a diagnosis of borderline personality disorder in patients younger than 18 years of age, the chronic dysfunctional behavioral patterns and skills deficits showed obvious overlap with those of our patients.

Having come up empty-handed in their search for an evidence-based treatment specifically developed for suicidal teens, they turned to the project of modifying DBT for their patients. But what would they need to change about DBT to fit it to teenagers and families? And how could they know which features of DBT to preserve; that is, which features were essential to the documented positive outcomes? There was simply no way to answer these questions, questions that arise every time someone adapts an evidence-based treatment to a new population or setting. The strategy chosen by Miller and Rathus was to do DBT "by the book" with their population, modifying it only when needed. Through a trial-and-error strategy similar to Linehan's on the road from CBT to DBT, they eventually developed their own treatment manual and subjected it to a pilot research trial. The results gleaned from this quasi-experimental design were impressive and have by now already had a far-reaching impact.

They wisely held tight to the strategy of adhering to the highest degree possible to standard DBT. But the modifications that eventually took hold and that appear in this book are terribly imaginative and will intuitively make sense to any clinician familiar with teens and families. Let me give you a small taste. To adjust to the adolescent's shorter time perspective (a 1-year commitment to treatment could seem a lifetime), Miller and Rathus shortened the duration of treatment to 16 weeks. To adjust to the shorter duration, they reduced the number of skills taught in the four standard skills training modules. After several rounds involving family members in DBT skills training, they designed a fifth module for patients and families called "Walking the Middle Path." To bring the skills package to both patients and families, they arrived at a multiple family skills group format followed by a graduate group for the teenagers without the families. Synthesizing principles of family therapy with principles and strategies of DBT, they developed a DBT family therapy approach that could be offered when individual family therapy seemed indicated. As they grew familiar with the typical transactional patterns among patients, families, and therapists that interfered with treatment progress, they described a set of dialectical dilemmas, thereby sharpening case formulations and treatment interventions. This book finally presents the comprehensive treatment package developed by Miller and Rathus, along with variations arrived at by others in adapting DBT to this population (e.g., some have not found it necessary to shorten the 1-year treatment duration in their adaptations for teens and families).

Adapting DBT for multiproblem suicidal adolescents and their families has been an enormous undertaking. For mental health practitioners now to learn, implement, practice, and research this treatment will require a significant, sustained effort by program administrators, clinicians, researchers, families, and patients. How can we justify a commitment of this magnitude? At the very least we need to consider the scope of the problem as documented in statistics and the unmistakable suffering and disruption that clinicians routinely see, alongside the absence of any treatment with demonstrated efficacy.

The scope of the problem of the suicidal teenager is substantial and has been increasing. As the authors note in the first chapter, suicide is the third leading cause of death in the United States in the age group from 10 to 19 years. For each completed suicide there are 100–200 suicide attempts; 16- to 18-year-olds make more suicide attempts than any other age group across the life span. In an average U.S. high school classroom, one boy and two girls have made suicide attempts in the previous year. The incidence of nonsuicidal self-injurious behavior in teens appears to be increasing. The more problem behaviors a teenager engages in (e.g., binge drinking, unsafe sex, cigarette smoking, violence, and disturbed eating behaviors), the more likely he or she is to make suicide attempts.

On a daily basis clinicians come face to face with chaos and hopelessness in the lives of multiproblem suicidal teens and their families. While the teenage patient spirals toward higher risk behaviors, the parents alternate between tightening their grasp, searching for help, and throwing up their hands. As exhaustion grows for those in the family and treatment systems, hospital admission looms again and again as the only relief in the moment. Suicide is in the air. Clinicians and some family members become painfully aware that they have no evidence-based (or even consensus) treatment to which to turn, a fact that itself heightens despair.

This picture is painfully familiar to me in private practice and in consultations to families, mental health programs, and schools. I have heard hundreds of variations on the same story for years in workshops across the United States, in Canada, and in Europe. If I had a dollar for each time a hopeful mental health practitioner asked me, with anticipatory excitement (and impatience), when the adolescent DBT book would be out, I could contribute a tidy sum toward a randomized controlled trial. And that is what we need next. This book lays the groundwork for that.

I applaud the authors for sticking to fundamentals, for improvising daringly within the rules, for finding synthesis and balance among differing perspectives, and for their painstaking insistence on getting it right in spite of growing pressures to get it done faster. Good jazz is not easy to come by.

CHARLES R. SWENSON, MD
University of Massachusetts School of Medicine, Worcester;
private practice, Northampton, Massachusetts

Acknowledgments

All three authors:

This book could not have been written if it were not for the guidance, input, and support of so many people during the past decade.

We cannot begin to describe the appreciation we feel toward Barbara Watkins, our editor at The Guilford Press, who served as our compass, our cowriter, and our cheerleader. Her endless patience sustained us, and her meticulous editing made the book what it is.

We wish to thank many other experts in adolescent treatments—those doing dialectical behavior therapy (DBT) mostly by the book, those also adapting it, and those integrating it into other forms of treatment. Alan Fruzzetti, Kelly Koerner, Dan Santisteban, Brad Beach, Tony Dubose, Nancy Gordon, Jennifer Sayrs, Soonie Kim, Shari Manning, and Linda Smith, to name a few, gave many helpful suggestions and ideas from their own work with adolescents and families.

Alec L. Miller and Jill H. Rathus:

We first want to thank Marsha Linehan, for her genius, inspiration, and mentorship, and for her encouragement to build upon and adapt her work. Her input at every stage has clarified and enhanced our thinking and writing, and has made us better clinicians and teachers in the process.

Back in 1995, it was Scott Wetzler who first suggested considering DBT as a possibly relevant evidence-based treatment for our multiproblem suicidal adolescent population at Montefiore Medical Center, and we thank him for this. We also thank Charles Swenson, whose passion for DBT and encouragement about our adaptation idea confirmed our decision to start our journey, and whose ongoing support and mentorship have been invaluable. We would like to honor the memory of Cindy Sanderson, who first trained us in DBT and inspired us with her talent and wit to become not only DBT therapists but also DBT trainers. Perry Hoffman provided the consultation for our program as it took off the ground and offered many helpful insights about working with families. We would like to acknowledge the American Foundation for Suicide Prevention for awarding Jill the original grant in 1995 that supported our intensive training in DBT. Marcia Landsman deserves enormous gratitude for contributing to the original Montefiore DBT program, serving as one of the first DBT therapists, eventually leading both the multifamily skills training group and the adolescent graduate group for several years, and sharing insights that helped inform our adaptation. Juliet Glinski, Kristen Woodberry, Aimee Mitchell, and Jay Indik all contributed to our thinking about synthesizing family therapy and DBT. Laura Silver McGuire deserves acknowledgment for helping us formulate our set of adolescent dialectical dilemmas and secondary treatment targets. Finally, we also appreciate Behavioral Tech and the group of DBT trainers and colleagues from around the world whose friendship and support have greatly influenced us personally and professionally.

Alec L. Miller:

I would like to thank Dale and Bruno Terilli, Ginny Gerbino, Jeff Atlas, Michael Quittman, Bill Arsenio, Scott Wetzler, and Bill Sanderson, all of whom have served as professional mentors to me in very different ways. Thanks also to T. Byram Karasu, Bruce Schwartz, George Como, and Judy Berenson, who have supported me and my clinical research program at Montefiore Medical Center since 1995. As a child psychiatry fellow, subsequent colleague, and friend, Laurence Katz went on to initiate an inpatient adaptation of adolescent DBT, and his curious intellect always forced me to clarify my own thinking about DBT theory and practice. Valerie Porr, an advocate, provider, and educator, has been another source of support to me during these years.

Thanks to my countless psychology interns, psychology externs, psychiatry residents, and fellows, whose inquisitive minds helped me to crystallize my thinking at nearly each therapist consultation meeting, supervisory session, and lecture. Some of my former trainees (not mentioned above) to whom I am particularly grateful for sharing ideas on my consultation team, treating adolescents and their families, coleading groups with me, and participating in various scholarly endeavors include Pam Straining, Catherine Monk, Sharon Wyman, Jonathan Huppert, Jordana Muhlmeister, Kim Halaby, Julie Nathan, David Markowitz, Marc Gurtman, Gabriella Johr, Lizz Dexter-Mazza, Arielle Goldkang, Carrie Spindel, Jennifer Muehlenkamp, Colleen McClain Jacobson, Maribel Rivera, Nira Golombeck, and Debbie Neft. I owe many thanks to my current and former staff and DBT colleagues at Montefiore who have supported me personally and professionally, many of whom were former trainees mentioned above. Jennifer Hartstein stands out in particular for her innumerable contributions over the past few years; others include Jill Emanuele, Elizabeth Wagner, Lori Greene, and Lisa Lyons. Special thanks to Madelyn Garcia, my assistant at Montefiore, who has continued to function as my right arm and often as my left brain. Without her, I would not have been able to carry out my various professional responsibilities and still write and rewrite this book.

I am very grateful to my friends and family, who empathically understood why deadlines for "the book" rendered me unable to attend myriad barbecues. In particular, I wish to thank my parents, who not only influenced my career choice by serving as role models themselves, but also have functioned as sources of unyielding support and encouragement ever since. My sister has provided me with good humor and helpful advice over these years. Finally, I am forever indebted to my wife for being my best friend, most invaluable sounding board, source of emotional support, and ultimate cheerleader, and for making her own sacrifices during this process. My wonderful children, Jenna and Ian, have taught me how amazingly rewarding and challenging it is to be a parent. In true "making lemonade out of lemons" fashion, these life lessons have made me a better DBT therapist by enhancing my capacity to validate the parents and children with whom I work.

Jill H. Rathus:

I want to thank my staff and colleagues at Long Island University, C.W. Post Campus. Cathy Kudlack helped me in innumerable ways and always greeted my clients in the Psychological Services Center with a smile. Dolores Burns is always friendly, supportive, and willing to lend a hand, and has helped me to become more computer-savvy. I also want to thank Robert Keisner, Eva Feindler, David Roll, Danielle Knafo, Marshall Silverstein, Geoff Goodman, Camilo Ortiz, and Joyce Roll. In addition, Laura Silver McGuire, the assistant clinic director, was my expert coleader in multifamily skills training groups during my first year of conducting DBT at Post.

Also at Post are many graduate students who helped with the completion of this project. I'd particularly like to thank Lauren Sher, Matthew Brightman, and Christine Cantner, who worked reliably and tirelessly over many long hours assisting me with research for the book. I would also like to thank the many excellent graduate student therapists and skills trainers (most of whom have since graduated) who participated with me on my DBT teams at Post over the years, including Nick Cavuoto, Vince Passarelli, Dan Wagner, Anthony Anzalone, Kristen Baker, Lauren Wisely, Martha Stroh, Danielle Kramer-Phelan, Alan Phelan, Wayne Zito, Mandy Habib, Ayme Turnbull, Dawn Cuglietto, Tinia Aperghi, Jacqueline Widmer, Koby Meydan, Peter Wigg, and Andrea Riskin.

In addition, I would like to acknowledge my Stony Brook faculty—particularly Daniel O'Leary, an inspiring mentor who set the bar high and whose influence continues to touch me strongly in my career, and Marvin Goldfried, who had himself worked with Marsha Linehan and first introduced me to DBT in his intervention class in 1988, years before her texts were published! I also want to thank another important early mentor, Bill Sanderson, for furthering my training in research and cognitive-behavioral therapy while I was on internship at Montefiore. Bill also invited me to write my first book, *Marital Distress*, as part of his edited series on empirically validated treatments, and continues to be a valued and trusted colleague. Other colleagues who contributed to the process of writing this book, whether through direct words of support and guidance or through their teaching and writing, include Zina Rutkin, Ruth DeRosa, David Pelcovitz, and Jon Kabat-Zinn.

Finally, I would like to thank my family. My parents have helped me keep my eye on the ball regarding the completion of this long project, and have been a tremendous source of guidance, support, and encouragement in general. My aunt, Rita Shawn (an accomplished social worker), has supported this work and shown a continued interest in it. I thank my husband, Lloyd, who has patiently tolerated the many busy years of this book-writing process without giving up on me! I appreciate the clarity of thinking and support he provides while he keeps me laughing. I also appreciate how he exemplifies a balance of the two DBT interaction styles: irreverence and reciprocal communication. My daughters, Lauren and Julia, provide me with daily inspiration and joy. They manage to keep me young while building my wisdom. They are wonderful teachers and continually challenge me to live in the moment, pay close attention, and keep my life in balance.

Marsha M. Linehan:

Alec Miller and Jill Rathus are experts in the treatments of suicidal and difficult-to-treat adolescents. This book is a reflection of their courage in taking on this population, as well as their willingness to take a complex treatment like DBT and make it not only their own but available to kids who have complex lives but little ability to understand a complex treatment. Believe it: They wrote most of this book. With marvelous good humor, they put up with having the original treatment developer hanging over their shoulders at practically every sentence, and certainly at every proposed modification, adaptation, or addition. I am intensely grateful that they allowed me to work with them on this book.

I would also like to thank the many DBT researchers, particularly the principal investigators who have managed the arduous task of conducting randomized clinical trials, all of whom are referenced in this book. Without their research, we would not have the evidence that DBT is indeed an effective treatment for suicidal behaviors. And without that evidence, there would be little need for this book.

I am especially appreciative of my executive assistant, Elaine Franks. Without her at my side—organizing, encouraging, reminding, and running interference—I could not have contributed what I did to this book. Katie Korslund took over the reins of our research clinic to free up my time to work on this book, and I could not have done it otherwise. The National Institute of Mental Health took a chance on me before I knew anything, and since 1980 has continuously funded my research on treating suicidal behaviors. Without that funding, the research that made this book possible would not have been done. Jane Pearson, a tireless advocate for research on suicidal behaviors, and James Breiling, an equally tireless advocate for research on borderline personality disorder (BPD), have supported our work with suicidal patients meeting criteria for BPD. Finally, I want to thank The Guilford Press and Seymour Weingarten. They too took a chance on me many years ago, and have never failed to support my work and the dissemination of DBT.

Contents

Dialectical Behavior Therapy
with Suicidal Adolescents

Introduction

In 1995 the first author of this book, Alec Miller, was given the exciting and challenging opportunity to direct an outpatient program for depressed and suicidal multiproblem adolescents, many of whom also engaged in nonsuicidal self-injurious behavior (NSIB). The second author, Jill Rathus, was research coordinator of this outpatient program at the time. In collaboration, the two of us surveyed the literature to identify effective psychosocial treatments for this population. Sadly, we were not able to find a single randomized treatment study for suicidal youth. The only established psychosocial treatment for suicidal individuals was dialectical behavior therapy (DBT) for women diagnosed with borderline personality disorder (BPD) (Linehan, 1993a, 1993b). Upon closer evaluation, we became convinced that DBT could be adapted to the needs of the suicidal multiproblem teens who were presenting to our program. We quickly sought out intensive training in DBT from the treatment developer and third author, Marsha Linehan. We then developed and began empirically evaluating our adaptation of DBT to our adolescent population, with promising though preliminary results (Miller, Rathus, Linehan, Wetzler, & Leigh, 1997; Rathus & Miller, 2002).

DBT has been found effective for older adolescents and adults diagnosed with BPD, in large part because it explicitly targets the internal and external risk factors for suicidal behavior and NSIB. Of those self-injuring teens referred to our outpatient program at Montefiore, 37% meet at least three Axis II diagnostic criteria for BPD (e.g., angry outbursts, confusion about self, and impulsive behaviors), and 26% meet full criteria (i.e., at least five out of nine) (Jacobson, Muehlenkamp, & Miller, 2006). We believe that this treatment is beneficial to those with subthreshold BPD (i.e., three or four features), as we consider DBT a prophalaxis against developing the more ingrained, refractory set of behavioral problems seen in BPD.

THE MULTIPROBLEM ADOLESCENT AND EMOTIONAL DYSREGULATION

Although many normal adolescents exhibit some degree of emotional dysregulation, the treatment described in this book is not intended for the prototypical teen exhibiting fairly benign mood lability, such as slamming a door or occasionally cursing at a family member in a fit of rage. Nor is DBT intended for an adolescent with a single episode of major depression who makes a first suicide attempt following an acute stressor. There are less comprehensive therapies that are likely to be effective and less time-intensive for these aforementioned youth.

We believe that DBT is most appropriate for those suicidal teens who exhibit a more chronic form of emotion dysregulation with numerous coexisting problems (some will meet criteria for BPD and others will not, as noted above). Miller and Taylor (2005) found, for example, that the more problem behaviors an adolescent has(such as violent behavior, binge

1

drinking, cigarette smoking, high-risk sexual behavior, disturbed eating behavior, or illicit drug use), the greater the risk of suicidal behavior. Compared to adolescents with zero problem behaviors, the odds of a medically treated suicide attempt increased exponentially with the addition of each new problem behavior, culminating in a 277.3 times greater risk when six problem behaviors were present.

Moreover, emotion dysregulation almost by definition results in multiple problems. As Chapter 3 explains, chronic emotion dysregulation results in cognitive and behavioral dysregulation. These in turn result in the "crisis-generating behavior" that therapists often observe in clients diagnosed with BPD (see Chapter 5)—that is, a vicious cycle of impulsive, self-destructive, or otherwise harmful behaviors. These behaviors are high-priority treatment targets in DBT, and they are viewed either as natural outgrowths of emotion dysregulation or as attempts to re-regulate painful, dysregulated emotions.

Thus this book focuses on treating those suicidal adolescents who exhibit multiple problem behaviors. In addition to borderline personality features and various problem behaviors as mentioned above, many of the teens referred to us for DBT present with at least two to three Axis I mental disorders. These include (but are not limited to) mood disorders, such as major depression or bipolar I or II disorder; anxiety disorders, such as panic disorder, generalized anxiety disorder, social phobia, or posttraumatic stress disorder (PTSD); substance use disorders, such as alcohol and cannabis abuse/dependence; eating disorders, such as bulimia nervosa; and disruptive behavior disorders, such as attention-deficit/hyperactivity disorder (ADHD), conduct disorder, or oppositional defiant disorder. The term "multiproblem" thus also applies to teens presenting with multiple mental disorders.

PROBLEMS IN DEFINING SUICIDAL BEHAVIORS

One of the challenges in writing a book on suicide is the lack of definitional clarity that exists in the field of suicidology. There is no consensus for defining suicide attempts or NSIB. Many suicidologists use different terminology to define the same behavior, such as "parasuicide," "deliberate self-harm," "self-injurious behavior," "suicidal gestures," or "suicide attempts." Linehan's (1993a) original text on DBT employed the commonly used term "parasuicide," as coined by Kreitman (1977), to inclusively characterize deliberate self-harm behaviors with or without intent to die. As per Linehan (1993a), using the term "parasuicide" still required clinicians to assess suicidal intent for each behavior; it was intended to reduce the pejorative language commonly associated with nonlethal deliberate self-harm (e.g., suicidal gestures, manipulative suicide attempts). In the meantime, the World Health Organization (WHO) has changed its suicide-related terminology (e.g., "parasuicide," "suicide attempt," "completed suicide") several times in the midst of its long-term WHO/EURO Multicentre Study (Bille-Brahe, Kerkhor, DeLeo, & Schmidke, 2004). At present, the WHO has chosen to use the term "suicide attempt" any time an individual does not die, regardless of the presence of suicidal intent (Bille-Brahe et al., 2004).

In an effort not to contribute further to the definitional confusion, we define our terms early in Chapter 1 and use them consistently throughout the book. We want the reader to understand what types of behaviors along the self-harm spectrum we are referring to. Although many young clients do engage in both suicidal behaviors and NSIB, some adolescents have engaged only in NSIB and have never experienced suicidal ideation or engaged in suicide attempts, while others have engaged only in suicidal behaviors and have never engaged in NSIB (Jacobson et al., 2006). Thus we choose to use the term "NSIB" to help distinguish those teens who deliberately harm themselves but have no intent to die from teens with suicidal intent.

Since 1995, we have gained considerable experience in employing our modified treatment with a broad range of adolescents from varied ethnic, cultural, and socioeconomic backgrounds and treatment settings. These settings include Montefiore Medical Center's Adolescent Depression and Suicide Program, an inner-city outpatient program for predominantly impoverished and underprivileged Hispanic and African American youth and their families in the Bronx; Long Island University, C. W. Post Campus Psychological Services Center (the graduate program's training clinic), which serves a largely white middle-class population; the University of Washington Behavioral Research and Therapy Clinic, which provides services for men and women of varied ethnicities and economic backgrounds who are 18 years of age and older and who are diagnosed with BPD; and, finally, private practice settings in White Plains, New York (Alec Miller) and Great Neck, New York (Jill Rathus), which primarily serve suburban middle- and upper-middle-class teens and families. In addition, we have learned a considerable amount by providing training and consultation in numerous outpatient, inpatient, day treatment, and residential settings employing DBT throughout the United States and around the world, including Canada, Germany, Sweden, Norway, and the United Kingdom. Thus we have developed a considerable amount of clinical wisdom, which has informed the direction of our therapy and research. We have written this book to share this clinical wisdom with the thousands of mental health professionals who, on a daily basis, are confronted with the challenging task of attempting to provide effective treatment for suicidal multiproblem adolescents.

ORGANIZATION OF THE BOOK

In this book we discuss the "why," the "how," and the "what" of DBT for multiproblem suicidal adolescents, and we offer clinical guidance from our experiences in implementing DBT for this population. In Chapter 1 we familiarize readers with the key distal and proximal risk factors for suicidal behavior in adolescents, drawn from the most recent research. A knowledge base of these risk factors is critically important for clinicians working with this population. We also discuss BPD (a diagnostic risk factor in and of itself), particularly the validity, reliability, and stability of this diagnosis among adolescents.

In Chapter 2 we briefly review the existing literature on treatment for suicidal individuals, while pointing out the dearth of research with suicidal adolescents. We have found very little support in the research for treating suicidal behaviors and NSIB indirectly by treating the associated mental disorder (e.g., major depression). The evidence points toward treating such behaviors directly, independently of the coexisting mental disorder, as the more promising approach. Direct treatment is the approach used in DBT.

Chapters 3–5 describe key aspects of DBT, with an emphasis on its application to adolescents and families. Chapter 3 gives an overview of DBT as a whole, including its theoretical basis, its hierarchy of behavioral treatment goals (with suicidal behaviors as primary targets), and the strategies used to achieve its goals. Chapter 4 focuses on the ways that DBT programs can be organized in order to fulfill five essential functions. This chapter also explores issues in setting up a DBT program for adolescents; these include defining the population, discussing who should be part of the treatment team, considering what modes will be implemented, and considering whether to make adaptations from standard DBT. We then describe specific adaptations we have made to the standard treatment. Chapter 5 describes in detail the patterns of alternating behavioral extremes that DBT calls "dialectical dilemmas." These patterns help sustain dysfunctional behaviors, and so the patterns themselves are considered secondary treatment targets in DBT. We discuss how the three dialectical dilemmas identified in standard DBT apply to adolescents. We then introduce three new patterns of oscillating extremes that we have identified as characteristic of emotionally dysregulated adolescents and their families.

Starting with Chapter 6, we show readers what the clinical assessment and treatment process can look like when DBT is applied to suicidal multiproblem adolescents. Chapter 6 focuses on assessment of suicide risk, diagnoses, and treatment feasibility. We make recommendations about which instruments may be most valuable in assessing for mental disorders as well as suicide risk factors. We also suggest how to determine whether a potential client is appropriate for a specific DBT program. This chapter introduces 15-year-old "Jessica" (a fictionalized composite) and her family. Through them we illustrate the nitty-gritty of applying DBT, starting here with the assessment process.

Orienting clients to DBT and obtaining their commitment to the treatment represent a crucial pretreatment stage in DBT. Chapter 7 reviews specific strategies for doing this with adolescents and families, and shows how this was done with Jessica and her family. Given the extremely high rate of treatment dropout among suicidal adolescents (Trautman, Stewart, & Morishima, 1993), it is imperative for clinicians to learn how to engage teens and their parents effectively in treatment. These strategies, used with teens and parents alike, are also used to establish and maintain commitment to the reduction of suicidal behavior and other relevant behaviors (such as drug use, school avoidance, and binge eating, to name a few).

Chapter 8 describes how to conduct DBT on an individual basis with adolescents. Using several examples with Jessica, we show how an individual therapist identifies and targets suicidal behaviors by using a variety of change and acceptance strategies. The chapter concludes with several transcripts of telephone coaching by the therapist with his suicidal client.

In Chapter 9 we discuss the rationale and the practicalities of including family members in treatment with suicidal adolescents. This is an important adaptation of DBT with adolescents. (As we discuss in detail in Chapter 10, families can also be included in skills training sessions.) Family therapy sessions are especially important when family interactions are contributing to an adolescent's self-injurious behaviors, or when parent behaviors interfere with the treatment or with other primary treatment targets and goals. This chapter describes a session with Jessica and her family, and illustrates the use of crisis strategies and discussion of dialectical dilemmas in family sessions.

Chapter 10 covers DBT skills training and its application to adolescents and their family members. We begin with practical issues, such as who should participate in skills training and who should conduct this modality of treatment. We then discuss skills training content and the typical schedule, highlighting possible adaptations for teens and parents. We also offer clinical tips for each module, and in general for teaching the skills to adolescents and family members. (In addition, Appendix A offers a collection of mindfulness exercises that we have found particularly engaging for adolescents.) Finally, Chapter 10 introduces a new module designed specifically for adolescents and family members: "Walking the Middle Path." (The complete module, consisting of lecture/discussion points and client handouts, can be found in Appendices B and C.)

Chapter 11 first addresses assessing treatment progress. This section emphasizes ongoing clinical indicators of treatment progress, focusing more on process than an outcome. Next we present options for running a graduate group and describe a particular model we have developed for such a group. Finally, we speak about terminating treatment. This topic includes both moving from one phase of DBT to the next, and terminating the treatment as a whole. Although this discussion reflects standard DBT practice, we highlight issues that are particular to transitions or termination with adolescents and their families.

Chapter 12 discusses program issues (i.e., issues that may challenge effective treatment delivery). We focus both on barriers to getting a program started and on challenges to carrying out effective treatment once a program is underway. The chapter presents common programmatic issues and obstacles, and provides recommendations for addressing them.

We hope that this book offers many useful ideas to those DBT practitioners who are already working with suicidal teens or considering such work. We also hope that this book introduces DBT to clinicians who may not yet be familiar with it. Note that further reading and training in DBT are essential to be qualified to practice it. Those interested should read the original DBT texts, *Cognitive-Behavioral Treatment of Borderline Personality Disorder* (Linehan, 1993a), and *Skills Training Manual for Treating Borderline Personality Disorder* (Linehan, 1993b). The treatment in its entirety is contained in these two texts; the present volume describes ways to adapt the treatment for an adolescent population. DBT workshops and other training opportunities are offered by numerous clinical psychology programs, in psychology and psychiatry residencies, and at international conferences for mental health professionals. In particular, we recommend the annual meeting of the International Society for the Improvement and Training of DBT, which meets with the Association for Behavioral and Cognitive Therapies; and Behavioral Tech, LLC, an international mental health training company wholly owned by the nonprofit Marie Institute of Behavioral Technology (see http://behavioraltech.org and http://marieinstitute.org).

Suicidal behaviors in adolescents are a prevalent problem and a leading reason for admission to inpatient psychiatric units in the United States and abroad. With shorter lengths of stay mandated by managed care companies, psychiatric hospitals have become revolving doors for highly troubled multiproblem youth. Given the number and complexity of the problems these adolescents present, treatment approaches need to be comprehensive yet flexible. To date, there is no known treatment with established efficacy for suicidal multiproblem adolescents. For this reason, we and other colleagues have been expanding upon DBT to include consumer-friendly adaptations for treating such adolescents. We believe that this multimodal treatment approach offers enormous hope for desperately needed effective interventions with this population.

CHAPTER 1

Suicidal Behaviors in Adolescents
Who Is Most at Risk?

THE EXTENT OF THE PROBLEM

Adolescent suicide is a major public health problem and accounts for at least 100,000 annual deaths in young people worldwide (WHO, 2002). In the United States, suicide accounts for more adolescent deaths than all natural causes combined, with more than 2,000 youth dying by suicide per year (Anderson, 2002). Suicide ranked as the third leading cause of death among the 10- to 14-year-old and 15- to 19-year-old age groups in the United States in 2000, preceded only by accidents and homicide (Anderson, 2002). Nearly 20 percent of adolescents in the middle school and high school age groups report having seriously considered attempting suicide during the past year (Grunbaum et al., 2002). In the United States, the Centers for Disease Control and Prevention's (CDC's) large Youth Risk Behavior Surveillance (YRBS) survey also found that nearly 15% of adolescents had made a specific plan to attempt suicide, and that 8.8% of adolescents reported a suicide attempt; this 8.8% represented over 1 million teenagers, of whom approximately 700,000 received medical attention for their attempts (Grunbaum et al., 2002). These results are consistent with those cited in other epidemiological studies in the United States (Gould, Wallenstein, Kleinman, O'Carroll, & Mercy, 1998; Reynolds & Mazza, 1992; Roberts, Chen, & Roberts, 1997; Wichstrom, 2000; Windle, Miller-Tutzauer, & Domenico, 1992).

Although suicide attempts are less common before adolescence, they increase significantly during adolescence, with a peak between 16 and 18 years of age (Lewinsohn, Rohde, & Seeley, 1996). After age 18, there is a marked decline in frequency of suicide attempts, especially for young women (Kessler, Borges, & Walters, 1999; Lewinsohn, Rohde, Seeley, & Baldwin, 2001). As a result, the highest prevalence rate of suicide attempts across the life span exists during adolescence. For each youth suicide, there are approximately 100–200 suicide attempts (American Association on Suicidology, 2003). Researchers have found that between 31% and 50% of adolescent suicide attempters reattempt suicide (Shaffer & Piacentini, 1994), with 27% (males) and 21% (females) reattempting within 3 months of their first attempt (Lewinsohn et al., 1996). These data have major treatment implications, including the need for rapid intervention following the first attempt, as well as the need for treatment that targets both the internal and external conditions contributing to multiple attempts.

As the research reviewed in this chapter will show, the adolescents most at risk for multiple suicide attempts have multiple problems and meet criteria for at least one mental disorder. In an analysis of the 1999 YRBS data, Miller and Taylor (2005) found that the more problem behaviors an adolescent has, the greater his or her risk of suicidal behavior. "Problem behaviors" were defined as including violent behavior, binge drinking, cigarette smoking, high-risk sexual behavior, disturbed eating behavior, and illicit drug use. Compared to adolescents with zero problem behaviors, the odds of a medically treated suicide attempt were 2.3 times greater among respondents with one, 8.8 with two, 18.3 with three, 30.8 with four, 50.0 with five, and 277.3 with six problem behaviors (Miller & Taylor, 2005).

In contrast to suicide attempts, what we are calling "nonsuicidal self-injurious behavior" (NSIB) involves intentionally injuring oneself in a manner that often results in damage to body tissue, but without any conscious suicidal intent. Incidence of NSIB is increasing, especially among adolescents (Hawton & Fagg, 1992; Hawton, Harriss, Simkin, Bale, & Bond, 2004). Although the prevalence estimates need to be interpreted with caution, due to the limited number of studies, adolescents in community studies are reporting that they engage in NSIB at extremely high rates—between 18% and 15.9% (Muehlenkamp & Gutierrez, 2004 and CDC, 2004). College student populations engage in NSIB at similar rates, ranging from 12% (Favazza, 1998) to 35% (Gratz, 2001). Youth who cut themselves, especially repeatedly, have a significant risk of suicide (Cooper et al., 2005).

In the next part of this chapter, we define adolescent suicidal behaviors in more detail. We then examine the existing research on risk factors, highlighting specific behavioral and environmental conditions that appear to increase suicidal risk in adolescents, and comparing those with risk factors for adults. In Chapter 2 we review the research on existing treatments, including preliminary findings on DBT adaptations for suicidal adolescents. We describe DBT, with those adaptations that we feel are most effective for multiproblem suicidal adolescents, in subsequent chapters.

DEFINING ADOLESCENT SUICIDAL BEHAVIORS

"Suicidal behaviors" include completed suicide, suicide attempts, and suicidal ideation. Because it can often be extremely difficult to assess the degree of suicide intent accompanying intentional self-injury, many suicidologists also consider NSIB as falling into the larger spectrum of adolescent suicidal behaviors, even though NSIB by definition involves no suicidal intent (Berman & Jobes, 1991; Brent et al., 1988; Lewinsohn et al., 1996; Reynolds & Mazza, 1994). We include NSIB within the general category of suicidal behaviors for a number of reasons. First, although some intentional self-injury is clearly without any suicide intent, intentional self-injury often occurs with enormous ambivalence or with swiftly changing intent, such that retrospective analyses of intent may be exceptionally difficult. Second, a behavior that starts as suicidal can evolve into a nonsuicidal act and vice versa. Third, intentional but nonsuicidal self-injury can itself be lethal. That is, it can unintentionally become a suicidal act. Some behaviors categorized as suicide may in fact have been nonsuicidal but none-the-less lethal self-injuries. Finally, and most important clinically, intentional self-injury even without suicide intent is a potent predictor of eventual suicide. It is a behavior with important overlapping characteristics. By excluding this behavior from the general category of suicidal behaviors it is extremely easy for both client and clinician to marginalize or trivialize the behavior. Indeed, many adolescent clients do engage in both suicide attempts and NSIB (Linehan, 1993a). Clearly, however, some youth engage only in NSIB and never in suicidal behavior, while others engage only in suicidal behavior and never in NSIB (Jacobson et al., 2006). Thus, the term "NSIB" helps distinguish not only those teens who deliberately self-injure with no intent to die from those who do have suicidal intent, but also the two types of self-injurious behavior in the same person. This can be critical when precipitants and consequences are very different for the two types of behavior. In this book, we define "completed suicide" as an intentional, self-inflicted death. A "suicide attempt" is self-injurious behavior with ambivalent or certain intent to die. "NSIB" is defined by the lack of an intent to die in the context of deliberate self-injury. "Suicidal ideation" consists of thoughts about being dead or killing oneself and can vary widely in clinical significance, depending on its qualities and context. To a large extent, these definitions hinge on the determination of an intent to die—but in the real world, intent is not always clear or easy to assess.

What Is a Suicide Attempt?

Suicidologists' disagreements about how to define a suicide attempt generally revolve around the degree of intent necessary for a behavior to be considered suicidal (Linehan & Shearin, 1988; Farmer, 1988; Bille-Brahe et al., 2004). Some investigators infer or assume intent rather than measure it, and label all intentional self-injurious behavior not resulting in death as "suicide attempt." Yet not all self-injury is intended to result in death. Brent, Perper, and Allman (1987) and Lewinsohn, Rohde, Seeley, and Klein (1997) reported that among adolescents who acted to self-inflict harm, approximately one-fourth reported no intent to die, and only about one-third of those seen in emergency rooms stated that they had wanted to die. Some investigators have attempted to provide a nomenclature for suicidal behavior that incorporates information about intent to die. O'Carroll et al. (1996), for example, classify a self-injurious behavior in which there is no intent to die but rather intent to communicate distress to someone else as "instrumental suicide-related behavior." As we have noted in the Introduction, the WHO currently uses the term "suicide attempt" any time an individual does not die, regardless of whether suicidal intent is present (Bille-Brahe et al., 2004).

In addition to the definitional confusion across research studies internationally, clinical assessment of suicidal intent in adolescents and adults remains a challenge because self-reports of suicidal ideation, intent, and behavior are unreliable. For example, one study using both pencil-and-paper questionnaires and a semistructured interview format to evaluate adolescents' self-reports of suicidality reported discrepancies between assessment modalities in 50% of the 48 adolescents (Velting, Rathus, & Asnis, 1998). Moreover, adolescents' reports of attempts often indicate ambivalence, further complicating their accurate assessment (King et al., 1995). However, when interviewers are reliably trained and use a structured interview format, they can be reliable judges of suicidal intent with older adolescents and adults (Linehan, Heard, & Armstrong, 1993b).

What Is NSIB?

In a recent review article on NSIB, Gratz (2003) offered the following definition: "Deliberate self-harm may be defined as the deliberate, direct destruction or alteration of body tissue, without conscious suicidal intent but resulting in injury severe enough for tissue damage to occur" (p. 192). NSIB has been associated with a number of mental disorders, including schizophrenia (Herpertz, 1995), trichotillomania, personality disorders, eating disorders, substance use disorders, PTSD, and intermittent explosive disorder (Favazza & Rosenthal, 1990; Zlotnick, Mattia, & Zimmerman, 1999), as well as mental retardation and a variety of neurological, developmental, and genetic disorders (Schroeder, Oster-Granite, & Thompson, 2002). In particular, these researchers and others have found impulsive NSIB to occur in up to 80% of clients with BPD, as compared to prevalence estimates of approximately 4% in the general population of mental health treatment seekers (Shearer, Peter, Quaytman, & Wadman, 1988). Among clients diagnosed with BPD, the onset is usually reported during early adolescence, whereas onset appears later during young adulthood among individuals without BPD (Symons, 2002).

There is growing evidence that suicidal behaviors and NSIB have different phenomenological pathways (Muehlenkamp & Gutierrez, 2004), functions (Brown, Comtois, & Linehan, 2002), and correlates (Boergers, Spirito, & Donaldson, 1998; Herpertz, 1995; Pattison & Kahan, 1983). As Groholt, Ekeberg, Wichstrom, and Haldorsen (2000) point out, suicidal acts pose greater risks and may require different interventions than repetitive NSIB. Furthermore, a client who repeatedly cuts one's arm to temporarily relieve anger may have difficulty developing a therapeutic alliance with a therapist who focuses primarily on reasons for living instead of alternative methods of managing anger. Therefore, assessing intent allows us to discriminate behaviors that are suicide attempts (i.e., self-injurious behavior with varying levels of intent to die) from self-harming acts that involve no intent to die.

While the evidence to support the relationship between impulsivity and NSIB is mixed, the empirical research suggests that childhood sexual and physical abuse and emotional neglect account for significant variance in the risk for NSIB in adulthood (Gratz, 2003). Moreover, the function of NSIB is commonly conceptualized as a means of regulating emotions (Linehan, 1993a). Both clinical and empirical research suggests that NSIB functions as a form of emotional avoidance and escape from unwanted emotions (Gratz, 2003).

Although suicidal behaviors and NSIB should be considered clinically distinct entities, it is also important to remember that individuals can engage in both types of behaviors at different points in their lives. Lipschitz et al. (1999) found that adolescents hospitalized for suicidal behaviors were more likely also to exhibit NSIB than adolescents hospitalized for other problems were. In one study of adults, 37% of those with self-injury had histories of suicide attempts (Herpertz, 1995). Other studies have found that 10–27% of self-injuring adults eventually die from suicide (Stanley, Gameroff, Michalsen, & Mann, 2001; Cowmeadow, 1995).

What Is Suicidal Ideation?

As with the other terms discussed here, researchers have been unable to reach a consensus on a definition of "suicidal ideation," and so comparing findings from different studies has been difficult (King, 1997). More recently, researchers have suggested conceptualizing suicidal ideation as occurring on a continuum of increasing clinical significance, and some have begun to operationalize definitions that help to overcome the difficulties (Lewinsohn et al., 1996; Roberts et al., 1997). Members of the Oregon Adolescent Depression Project (Lewinsohn et al., 1996) put forth the following categories to operationalize suicidal ideation, in order of increasing severity: "thoughts of death or dying," "wishing to be dead," "thought of hurting (or killing) self," and "suicidal plan."

Suicidal ideation most generally involves current thoughts of death, of killing oneself, or of being killed. Some adolescents may present with passive suicidal ideation (e.g., "I wish I were dead") but report having no plan or intent to kill themselves. For a subgroup of these adolescents, the idea of actively taking their own lives is unfathomable. In contrast, some adolescents report active suicidal ideation that is more alarming to the clinician (e.g., "I feel like killing myself"). When asked, these clients may report having a specific plan to kill themselves. A suicidal plan involves identifying a specific method, and possibly a given time frame, in which an adolescent plans to kill him- or herself. Once an adolescent reports having a plan, the clinician must assess for suicidal intent. "Intent" characterizes the adolescent's level of commitment in carrying out the plan. For some adolescents, suicidal intent may be clear and definite; however, many report ambivalence or minimal intent to die (Brent et al., 1993b; King et al., 1995). Hence adolescents may report having a specific plan but have no intent to die (e.g., "I thought about jumping off a bridge, but I would never do it"). Others may describe their intent as ambivalent (e.g., "I am thinking about taking an overdose, but I am not sure if I can go through with it"). Still others may have full intent to kill themselves (e.g., "I intend to shoot myself with my own gun this Sunday when my parents leave town"). Further complicating matters is the inconsistency across assessments in adolescents' reports of their own suicidal behavior, as noted earlier (Velting et al., 1998).

Suicidal ideation is a strong predictor, if not one of the best predictors, of suicide attempts (Andrews & Lewinsohn, 1992; Kienhorst, DeWilde, van den Bout, Diekstra, & Wolters, 1990). Lewinsohn et al. (1996) found in their prospective study that two dimensions of suicidal ideation were highly correlated: severity and duration. Specifically, adolescents who spent more time thinking about suicide also tended to have more serious thoughts about suicide. More importantly, adolescents who indicated a greater intensity of suicidal ideation (i.e., by endorsing a greater number of items during the past week) were more likely to attempt suicide (Lewinsohn et al., 1996). In sum, as suicidal ideation becomes more frequent and intense, the risk of suicide attempts increases. Researchers have discovered that suicidal ideation is commonly associated with an Axis I disorder in adolescents; it is most strongly associated with depression, but also occurs in anxiety, disruptive behavior, and substance use disorders (Lewinsohn et al., 1996).

CHALLENGES IN DETERMINING RISK FACTORS FOR ADOLESCENT SUICIDAL BEHAVIORS

One of the greatest frustrations for clinicians, researchers, and family members is the inability to predict in advance which individual adolescents will attempt or complete suicide. It is unlikely that the state of the art will improve dramatically in the near future. Research is limited by both ethical problems and recording errors in determining whether predictions are accurate. There is also the more general problem of predicting infrequent events. The best that can be done is to describe the characteristics of subpopulations in which rates of suicide are higher than in the general population. Such a description can then be used to determine whether or not a given adolescent is at high risk for suicide.

Suicidologists have worked vigorously to identify risk factors for adolescent suicidal behaviors. The research has clearly demonstrated that certain distal and proximal risk factors, when combined, increase the probability of suicidal behavior. The most important distal factors linked with adolescent vulnerability to suicide are prior suicidal behaviors, mental disorders, chronic family disturbance, gender, homosexual or bisexual orientation, and ethnicity. Important proximal risk factors are stressful life events, sexual and physical abuse, academic difficulties, functional impairment from physical disease or injury, suicide in the social milieu, and access to suicidal means. Suicide risk increases when proximal risk factors occur in the context of distal risk factors. Hence, for example, Lewinsohn et al. (1996) hasten to point out that stressful life events should be considered "red flags" for clinicians. By the same token, however, a young client's experiencing one or more stressful life events per se should not alarm the clinician, since many adolescents experience such events without suicide as a consequence. Thus Lewinsohn, Rohde, and Seeley (1994) make two important points for clinicians to remember:

1. A proximal risk factor in combination with one or more distal risk factors is what heightens the risk of suicide.
2. Past suicidal behaviors are stronger predictors of future suicidal behaviors than stressful life events or other proximal risk factors.

However, assessment of risk is complicated by the fact that some risk factors can be considered both distal and proximal. For example, social and environmental factors such as family conflict and parental psychopathology can function as proximal factors that cause or exacerbate existing mental disorders or psychological pain, which in turn increase the risk of suicide. Table 1.1 summarizes the key distal and proximal risk factors for suicide in adolescents that have been identified in the research. Below we review these risk factors in more detail.

DISTAL RISK FACTORS

Prior Suicidal Behaviors

The best predictors of future suicidal behaviors among adolescents and adults are past suicidal behaviors. In particular, it has become well established that a prior suicide attempt is one of the single most important predictors of completed suicide (Gould, Greenberg, Velting, & Shaffer, 2003; Shafii, Carrigan, Whittinghill, & Derrick, 1985), with a 30-fold increased risk for boys and a 3-fold increased risk for girls (Shaffer et al., 1996). Numerous "psychological autopsy" studies of adolescents who complete suicide have found high rates of previous suicide attempts, ranging between 10% and 44% (Brent et al., 1988; Marttunen, Aro, & Lönnqvist, 1992; Shafii et al., 1985).

Several prospective studies followed adolescents admitted to psychiatric inpatient units for suicidal behaviors from 4 to 15 years postadmission. Documented suicide rates of these clients ranged from 9% to 11.3% (Motto, 1984; Otto, 1972). In a follow-up study of adolescents evaluated in an emergency room after suicide attempts, researchers discovered that 8.7% of the males and 1.2% of the females committed suicide within 5 years (Kotila, 1992). Gender differences are consistent across studies.

Mental Disorders

Clinical researchers agree that suicidal behaviors among adolescents are clearly associated with diagnosable mental disorders (Andrews & Lewinsohn, 1992; Brent et al., 1988; Kovacs, Goldston, & Gatsonis, 1993; Lewinsohn et al., 1996; Rich, Young, & Fowler, 1986; Shaffer, Garland, Gould, Fisher, & Trautman, 1988; Shaffi et al., 1985). Psychological autopsy studies

TABLE 1.1. General Risk Factors for Adolescent Suicidal Behavior

Distal risk factors	Proximal risk factors
• Prior suicidal behaviors	• Stressful life events
• Mental disorders	• Childhood sexual and physical abuse
• Depression and anxiety	• Academic difficulties
• Substance use	• Functional impairment from physical disease and injury
• Impulsive, disruptive, and antisocial behaviors	• Suicide in the social milieu
• BPD	• Accessible means of suicide
• Comorbidity	
• Disturbed family context	
• Gender	
• Sexual orientation	
• Ethnicity	
• SES (less certain)	

have reported that over 90% of adolescents completing suicide had a mental illness at the time of their death, although younger adolescents completing suicide tend to have lower rates of mental illness, averaging around 60% (Beautrais, 2001; Brent, Baugher, Bridge, Chen, & Chiappetta, 1999a; Groholt, Ekeberg, Wichstrom, & Haldorsen, 1998; Shaffer et al., 1996). Although various mental disorders have been found among these adolescents, three classes of Axis I disorders characterize most attempted and completed suicides among adolescents internationally: depressive and anxiety disorders; impulsive, disruptive, and antisocial behavior disorder; and substance-related disorders (Andrews & Lewinsohn, 1992; Berman & Jobes, 1991; Brent et al., 1993b; Fergusson & Lynskey, 1995; Gould et al., 2003; Marttunen, Aro, Henriksson, & Lönngvist, 1991; Pfeffer, Newcorn, Kaplan, Mizruchi, & Plutchik, 1988; Shaffer et al., 1996; Sigurdson, Staley, Matas, Hildahl, & Squair, 1994). In addition, personality disorders (especially BPD) are increasingly being linked with adolescent suicidality, as is comorbidity of both Axis I and Axis II disorders.

Depression and Anxiety

Depressive disorders have been reported among adolescents attempting and completing suicide, at rates ranging from 49% to 64% (Brent et al., 1993; Marttunen et al., 1991; Rich et al., 1986; Shaffer et al., 1996), with the highest rates among psychiatric inpatients (Spirito, Brown, Overholser, & Fritz, 1989). In Finland, Marttunen et al. (1991) found depression to be the most prevalent diagnosis among their adolescents who completed suicide, with half of the boys and two-thirds of the girls meeting diagnostic criteria. Suicidal behaviors are common among adolescents with early-onset depressive disorders (Brent et al., 1993b; Kovacs et al., 1993; Pfeffer et al., 1991). Indeed, Kovacs et al. (1993) found a four- to fivefold increase in suicidal ideation and behavior among adolescents with depressive disorders as compared to adolescents with other mental disorders.

These statistics are noteworthy, since the risk of developing a depressive disorder increases as one gets older, but rises dramatically between the ages of 9 and 19 (King, 1997). At any one time, approximately 1 in 20 children and adolescents suffer from major depressive disorder (Essau & Dobson, 1999). Bipolar disorders, while less prevalent among adolescents, have been considered a significant risk factor in some studies (Brent et al., 1988, 1993) but not in others (Marttunen et al., 1991; Shaffer, Gould, & Hicks, 1994).

High rates of comorbidity between anxiety and depression have been documented in children and adolescents (Brady & Kendall, 1992). Among adults, there is increasing evidence not only that anxiety symptoms are associated with the severity of the depression, but that severe anxiety may be a risk factor for suicide, especially when it is associated with depression (Fawcett, 1997). Lewinsohn et al. (1996) identified anxiety disorders as a risk factor for suicidal behavior among adolescents. More recently, Goldston et al. (1999) reported trait anxiety to be predictive of posthospitalization suicide attempts, independent of mental disorder. In another study, investigators found that adolescents with a history of panic attacks were three times more likely to express suicidal ideation and two times more likely to report suicide attempts than those without a history of panic attacks (Pilowsky, Wu, & Anthony, 1999). These findings were true even after the investigators controlled for depression, drug and alcohol use, gender, and ethnicity/race. PTSD has also been associated with adolescent suicidal behavior (Giaconia et al., 1995; Mazza, 2000).

Other researchers have found evidence of anxiety and perfectionism among a subgroup of adolescents completing suicide (Shaffer et al., 1988). In two other studies of such adolescents, researchers found many of their sample characterized by withdrawn, lonely, supersensitive, and inhibited personality styles (Hoberman & Garfinkel, 1988; Shafii et al., 1985).

Impulsive, Disruptive, and Antisocial Behaviors

Several researchers have suggested that most completed suicides by adolescents are impulsive acts, with only about 25% providing evidence of planning (Hoberman & Garfinkel, 1988; Shaffer et al., 1988). Aggression with impulsivity has also been linked with suicidal behavior in both children and adolescents (Apter et al., 1995; Brent et al., 1994; Garfinkel, Froese, & Hood, 1982; Grosz et al., 1994; Inamdar, Lewis, Siomopoulos, Shanok, & Lamela, 1982; Pfeffer et al., 1988; Plutchik, van Praag, & Conte, 1989). In a study examining the prevalence of suicidal and violent behaviors in a sample of 51 hospitalized adolescents, Inamdar et al. (1982) found that 67% had been violent, 43% had been suicidal, and 28% had been both. Plutchik et al. (1989) have theorized that suicide risk is increased when aggressive impulses are triggered, then amplified by forces such as substance abuse, and not reduced by opposing forces such as appeasement from others. A study of suicidal adults suggested that a personality style marked by pronounced impulsivity and aggression characterized individuals at risk for suicide attempts, regardless of Axis I mental disorder (Mann, Waternauz, Haas, & Malone, 1999).

It should not then be a surprise that disruptive behavior disorders are common diagnoses found among suicidal adolescents (Kovacs et al., 1993; Marttunen, Aro, Henriksson, & Lönnqvist, 1994; Shafii et al., 1985), especially males (Brent et al., 1993; Shaffer et al., 1996). In a longitudinal study, Kovacs et al. (1993) found that 45% of youth diagnosed with conduct disorders, substance use disorders, and depressive disorders made suicide attempts, compared to only 22% of youth with depressive disorders only and 10% of youth with no depressive disorders. Other researchers have suggested that conduct disorders in adolescents may play a role equal to or even larger than that of depression in adolescent suicidal behaviors. Apter, Bleich, Plutchik, Mendelsohn, and Tyano (1988) found higher scale scores for suicidality on the Schedule for Affective Disorders and Schizophrenia for School-Age Children (K-SADS) for adolescents with conduct disorder than for those with major depressive disorder, even though those adolescents diagnosed with conduct disorder were less depressed. Apter et al. (1995) have suggested that aggression, a large component of conduct disorder, may be as important a risk factor as depression in some kinds of suicidal behavior. These researchers hypothesize two classes of suicidal behavior during adolescence: a wish to die (depression) and a wish not to be here for a time (poor impulse control). Apter and colleagues elaborate by stating that the first type of suicidal behavior characterizes disorders with prominent depression (such as major depressive disorder and anorexia nervosa), and that the second characterizes disorders of impulse control (such as conduct disorder).

Substance Use and Abuse

Substance use and abuse have been found with great frequency among adolescents attempting and completing suicide, and are therefore considered primary risk factors for adolescent suicidal behavior (Brent, Perper, & Allman, 1987; Crumley, 1979; Hoberman & Garfinkel, 1988; Marttunen et al., 1995; Rich et al., 1986; Shaffer et al., 1996; Shafii et al., 1985; Sigurdson et al., 1994). In studies of substance-using adolescents, suicide attempts occur at rates threefold those of non-substance-using adolescents, with the "wish to die" increasing dramatically after the onset of substance use (Berman & Schwartz, 1990).

In studies conducted internationally of *completed* suicide among adolescents and young adults, evidence of alcohol or other substance abuse was found in 28–54% of cases (Brent et al., 1987; Hawton, Fagg, & McKeown, 1989; Hoberman & Garfinkel, 1988; McKenry, Tishler, & Kelley, 1982; Shaffi et al., 1985; Marttunen et al., 1991; Rich et al., 1986). In a psychological autopsy study of 120 individuals under 20 years of age who completed suicide, Shaffer et al. (1996) reported drug and/or alcohol abuse as a risk factor for older adolescent males. Other studies to date have not highlighted such significant gender differences with regard to this risk factor. One recent study evaluated 89 consecutive admissions to a specialty outpatient clinic for depressed and suicidal inner-city teens. Of the 49 subjects with histories of self-injurious behavior, 18.4% met diagnostic criteria for cannabis abuse or dependence (Velting & Miller, 1999).

Personality Disorders

Due to the commonly held belief among mental health professionals that personality is still evolving during adolescence, there has been a reluctance to diagnose personality disorders among this age group. Yet, as we will discuss in more detail later, there is considerable overlap between the characteristics of those at high risk for suicidal behavior and those diagnosed with a personality disorder, especially BPD. Linehan, Rizvi, Welch, and Page (in press) reviewed diagnoses given to individuals who completed suicide over 14 research samples. They found personality disorder rates of 40–53% in these individuals, and concluded that these disorders are as great a risk factor for suicidal behaviors as major depression and schizophrenia are. In three out of four adolescent and youth suicide samples, they found similar high rates (see later discussion).

The relationship between suicidal behavior and personality disorders (particularly BPD) in adolescents has been recognized for over two decades (Brent et al., 1994; Clarkin, Friedman, Hurt, Corn, & Aronoff, 1984; Crumley, 1979; Marton et al., 1989; Marttunen et al., 1995; McManus, Lerner, Robbins, & Barbour, 1984; Pfeffer et al., 1988; Runeson & Beskow, 1991). Personality disorders and the tendency to engage in impulsive violence have become critical risk factors for completed suicide among adolescents (Brent et al., 1994). Brent et al. (1993a) compared adolescent inpatients who had attempted suicide with never-suicidal inpatient controls and found that the suicidal clients were more likely than the controls to have personality disorders or features of such disorders (81% vs. 58%, respectively), particularly those of the borderline type (32% vs. 10%). Those who had attempted suicide showed greater severity of borderline behavioral criteria even after suicidality was removed as a criterion. One report from Sweden described a similar rate of 33% for BPD among adolescents and young adults completing suicide (Runeson & Beskow, 1991). In a Finnish study of females ages 13–22 years who completed suicide, Marttunen et al. (1995) found that 26% of their 1,397 subjects met criteria for BPD. Velting, Rathus, and Miller (2000) found that American adolescents attempting suicide had higher levels of borderline behavioral criteria on the Millon Adolescent Clinical Inventory than nonsuicidal outpatient controls. As with other types of psychopathology, comorbidity of BPD with major depression and substance use among suicidal adolescents heightens the suicide risk (Marttunen et al., 1995; see "Comorbidity," below). It has been suggested that the co-occurrence of mood and personality disorders represents a particularly significant risk factor for suicidal behavior (Blumenthal & Kupfer, 1986).

Comorbidity

Comorbidity of mental disorders is the rule rather than the exception among adolescents (Volkmar & Woolstorn, 1997), and comorbid disorders are often present in adolescents who commit suicide (Rich et al., 1986; Shafii et al, 1988). Although suicidal adolescents may abuse substances in the absence of other Axis I disorders, substance-related disorders often coexist in the presence of depression and/or disruptive behavior disorders (Berman & Jobes, 1991;

Bukstein, Glancy, & Kaminer, 1992; Lewinsohn et al., 1996; Shaffer et al., 1996). Depression, conduct disorder, and substance abuse frequently present concurrently, with the frequency and lethality of attempts increasing with the degree of comorbidity (Frances & Blumenthal, 1989). Depression comorbid with alcohol/substance abuse, conduct problems, and/or BPD represents a particularly high-risk profile for completed suicide and other suicidal behaviors among teenagers (Brent et al., 1993b; Kovacs et al., 1993; Marttunen et al., 1995; Shafii et al., 1985).

Although most adolescents who make a suicide attempt have a diagnosable mental disorder, it is important to note that most adolescents with a mental disorder do not make a suicide attempt (Lewinsohn et al., 1996). Adolescents at highest risk for suicide tend to have high rates of comorbidity of both Axis I and Axis II disorders. As should be clear by now, suicidal behaviors span diagnostic categories. As we will show a bit later, assessing risk by identifying specific diagnostic categories is not as clinically helpful as looking for specific clusters of affective, cognitive, and behavioral characteristics across diagnostic categories. We continue now with our review of distal risk factors for adolescent suicidal behaviors.

Disturbed Family Context

Parents, by the nature of their roles, have direct and long-standing influences on the health of their children. When parents manifest their own serious problems, which may result in conflictual relations with their adolescents, the question becomes this: How and to what extent do parents (and other family members) affect adolescents' suicidal behavior? Various theories coupled with research data suggest that family functioning plays an important role in the etiology and maintenance of adolescent suicidal behavior (Adams, Overholser, & Lehnert, 1994; Berman & Jobes, 1991; King, Segal, Naylor, & Evans, 1993). Research has found that when family processes are disturbed, there is an increased risk of suicidal ideation and attempts among adolescents (Pfeffer, 1989).

A family history of suicidal behavior significantly increases the risk of completed suicide (Brent et al., 1988; Gould, Fisher, Flory, & Shaffer, 1996; Shafii et al., 1985) and attempted suicide (Bridge, Brent, Johnson, & Connolly, 1997; Johnson, Brent, Bridge, & Connolly, 1998). Agerbo, Nordentoft, and Mortensen's (2002) Danish Registry Study found youth suicide to be nearly five times more likely in the offspring of mothers who had completed suicide and twice as common in the offspring of fathers, even after adjustments for parental mental disorders.

Parental mental disorders, particularly depression and substance abuse, have been associated with suicidal ideation, attempts, and completed suicide in adolescents (Brent et al., 1988; Bukstein et al., 1993; Gould et al., 1996; Kashani, Goddard, & Reid, 1989). Impaired parent–child communication and low levels of emotional support and expressiveness are also associated with adolescent suicidal behavior (Campbell, Milling, Laughlin, & Bush, 1993; Garber, Little, Hilsman, & Weaver, 1998; Keitner et al., 1990; King et al., 1993; Martin & Waite, 1994; Pfeffer, 1989; Wagner, 1997).

Although some researchers suggest that a disproportionate number of adolescents attempting suicide do not live in stable, intact homes (Beautrais, 2001; Brent et al., 1993c; Groholt et al., 1998), the association between separation/divorce and suicide decreases when parental mental disorders are accounted for (Gould et al., 1996; King et al., 1993). King (1997) asserts that while these findings do not support the specific link to suicidal behavior, family loss and instability are important as risk factors for multiple poor outcomes. Interestingly, Lewinsohn et al. (1996) found higher rates of multiple suicide attempts among those adolescents who had a parent die before an adolescent was 12 years of age. These researchers suggest that parental loss may be an important yet underinvestigated suicide risk factor for predicting repeated suicide attempts in those with a history of one such attempt. Thus disturbances in family functioning appear to be important, but the extent to which disturbances in family functioning affect adolescent suicidal behavior remains unclear. Nevertheless, these findings support the need to evaluate and treat the suicidal adolescent within the context of his or her family system.

Gender

Over the past 30 years, the incidence of completed suicide and suicide attempts in older adolescents (i.e., ages 15–19) has shown significant gender and ethnic variations. Whereas suicidal ideation and attempts are more common among females in the United States (Gould et al., 1998; Grunbaum et al., 2002; Lewinsohn et al., 1996), completed suicide is five times more common among 15- to 19-year-old males (Anderson, 2002). While these gender differences are found to be similar in Western Europe, New Zealand, Australia, and North America, they are not consistent around the world. In fact, completed suicide rates for males and females are equal in some Asian countries and are higher among females in China (WHO, 2002).

Studies have consistently found gender differences among adolescents who attempt suicide as well (Gould et al., 2003). Approximately 10–20% of girls versus 4–10% of boys report having made a suicide attempt during their lifetime. Hence girls report attempting suicide two to four times as frequently as boys. In fact, King (1997) suggests that in a typical high school classroom, it is likely that two girls and one boy have made a suicide attempt during the past year.

Several factors may explain why females make more suicide attempts while males have a greater frequency of completed suicides. First, females have higher rates of mood disorders, which are associated with suicidal behavior (Brent et al., 1999a; Shaffer et al., 1996). Males have higher rates of aggressive behavior and substance abuse, which are often associated with completed suicide (Shaffer et al., 1994). Second, females in the United States choose less lethal methods, such as overdoses (females, 30%; males, 6.7%) (Anderson, 2002). Third, females often experience higher rates of sexual abuse, which is correlated with suicidal behavior as well (Friedman et al., 1982). Fourth, according to Linehan's (1973) study of American college students, older adolescents and young adults perceive nonfatal suicidal behavior as more "feminine" and less potent than killing oneself. Others have described nonfatal suicidal behavior as "feminine" because it is interpreted as a call for help—a behavior that is expected of women (Suter, 1976). In contrast, females who complete suicide are viewed more negatively and the behavior is perceived as more unacceptable than in males, since suicide involves a degree of self-determination that may be considered incompatible with femininity (Canetto, 1997b). In the United States, cultural scripts of gender and suicidal behavior are likely to influence adolescents' decisions about suicidal behavior (Canetto, 1997a). Adolescents are quite sensitive and responsive to cultural messages—even more so than adults, given that they are in the midst of defining their identities. Thus the influence of "gender-appropriate" ideas of suicidal behavior may be significant and requires further evaluation.

Sexual Orientation

Cross-sectional and longitudinal epidemiological studies have found homosexual adolescents of both sexes to be two to six times more likely to attempt suicide than their heterosexual peers (Blake et al., 2001; Garofolo, Wolf, Wissow, Woods, & Goodman, 1999; Harry, 1989; Remafedi, French, Story, Resnick, & Blum, 1998; Russell & Joyner, 2001). According to Harry's (1989) review, risk for attempts is typically heightened at about 18–19 years of age, when a teen is "coming out."

In a study of 137 gay and bisexual males between the ages of 14 and 21 (drawn from a nonclinical sample), nearly one-third of the subjects reported at least one suicide attempt, and almost half of them had repeatedly attempted suicide, with 54% of the attempts considered moderate to high in lethality risk (Remafedi, Farrow, & Deisher, 1993). One-third of the attempts occurred in the same years subjects identified themselves as homosexual or bisexual, yet "suicide attempts were not explained by experiences with discrimination, violence, loss of friendship, or current personal attitudes toward homosexuality" (Remafedi et al., 1993, p. 495). Rather, gender nonconformity and precocious psychosexual development were predictive of suicidal behavior: The younger these subjects were when they identified themselves as homosexual/bisexual, the more likely they were to report suicidal behavior. The authors suggested as a possible reason for this that early and middle adolescents may be less able to cope with the isolation and stigma associated with a homosexual identity than older adolescents, who may have better-developed coping skills.

Remafedi et al. (1998) examined the relationship between sexual orientation and suicide risk in a population-based sample of adolescents. They conducted a cross-sectional statewide survey of public school students in grades 7–12. Among the 394 students who described themselves as bisexual/homosexual and 336 gender-matched heterosexual students, suicide attempts were reported by 28.1% of bisexual/homosexual males, 20.5% of bisexual/homosexual females, 14.5% of heterosexual females, and 4.2% of heterosexual males. Thus for males, but not for females, bisexual/homosexual orientation was significantly associated with suicide attempts.

In another population-based sample of 3,365 public high school students in grades 9–12, Garofalo et al. (1999) found that self-identified gay, lesbian, and "not-sure" youth were 3.41 times more likely to report a suicide attempt than their peers. Similar to Remafedi et al.'s (1998) results, Garofalo et al. (1999) found sexual orientation to have an independent association with suicide attempts for males. For females, the association of sexual orientation with suicidality may be mediated by drug use and violence/victimization behaviors. It may also be lesbians are less likely to be identified by others as gay during adolescence, and therefore their sexual orientation may not be independently associated with suicidal behavior (Downey, 1994).

Ethnicity

In the United States, youth suicide is most common among Native Americans (Anderson, 2002; Middlebrook, LeMaster, Beals, Novins, & Manson, 2001). White youth have higher rates than African American youth, with Asians/Pacific Islanders having the lowest rates. Based on a significant increase in suicide among African American males between 1986 and 1994, the long-standing difference between African Americans and white has declined. Importantly, since the mid-1990s, there has been a gradual decline in suicide rates among both white and African American males and females (Gould et al., 2003). There are no clear explanations for this decline during the past decade. Hispanics have a relatively low suicide completion rate, but are significantly more likely than either white or African American adolescents to report suicidal ideation and to have made a suicide attempt (Kann, Kinchen, Williams, & Ross, 2000; Reynolds & Mazza, 1992; Tortolero & Roberts, 2001).

In one study of suicidal behavior among inner-city Hispanic adolescent females, researchers compared 33 subjects and their mothers with a matched nonsuicidal control group, to begin to generate a set of hypotheses to explain this behavior (Razin et al., 1991). The findings were as follows: Attempts were nearly always impulsive and nonlethal, though often with a stated wish to die. Nearly all were overdoses, and were precipitated by conflicts with mothers or boyfriends. Attempting girls' parents were less often born in the United States; their mothers seemed medically less healthy; and their extended families were more often supported by public assistance and had higher rates of criminal and mental problems. School performance was poorer among attempting girls, who often had suffered more and earlier losses—especially of biological fathers, with whom few had ongoing relationships. They had also recently lost friends and expressed a mistrustful stance toward friendships. Similarly, their mothers had fewer friends and more often expressed a mistrustful stance. Relationships with mothers seemed more intense, desperate, and even violent, and attempting girls were much more "parentified" (i.e., mothering their mothers). Although knowledge of suicidal models was common in both groups, the mothers of attempting girls knew even more models among family, friends, and neighbors than did their daughters or the nonsuicidal subjects or their mothers. More of the suicidal girls' mothers had themselves made attempts. Families of most attempting girls were usually mobilized by the attempts. This list of findings serves as an initial profile of risk factors for suicidal behavior among inner-city Hispanic adolescent females. However, given the small sample size and the fact that some reported findings did not reach statistical significance, the study's conclusiveness is limited.

Socioeconomic Status

The data are mixed regarding the effect of SES and suicide. Several studies have found youth attempting suicide to have lower SES than community controls, even after other social and mental health risk factors are controlled for (Beautrais, Joyce, & Mulder, 1996; Fergusson, Woodward, & Horwood, 2000; Wunderlich, Bronish, & Wiichen, 1998). Interestingly, Gould et al. (1996) reported that African American youth who had completed suicide had significantly higher SES than their general population counterparts, but no such effect was found among white or Hispanic youth completing suicide. Other studies have found little effect of low SES on suicide completion generally, after controlling for family history of mental illness or suicide (Agerbo et al., 2002; Brent et al., 1988).

PROXIMAL RISK FACTORS

In most cases, a distal risk factor is not sufficient in itself to precipitate suicidal behavior. Most adolescent suicidal behavior is triggered when a proximal risk factor, such as a stressful life event, is combined with a distal risk factor (Lewinsohn et al., 1996; Shaffer et al., 1988). Below we review some of the common proximal risk factors associated with adolescent suicidal behavior.

Stressful Life Events

Historically, interpersonal conflicts and separations are considered the most common precipitants to adolescent suicide (Marttunen, Aro, & Lönngvist, 1993; Spirito et al., 1989). Breakup of a romantic relationship, disciplinary crises or legal problems, humiliation, and arguments are some of the stressful life events identified in attempted and completed suicides of youth around the world, even after controlling for psychopathology, family, and personality factors (Beautrais, 2001; Brent et al., 1993c; Gould et al., 1996; Lewinsohn et al., 1996; Marttunen et al., 1993; Runeson, Beskow, & Waern, 1996; Shaffer et al., 1988). Specific stressors may vary with age. For example, romantic difficulties are more common precipitants among older adolescents, while parent–child conflicts are more common among younger adolescents (Brent et al., 1999).

Sexual and Physical Abuse

Researchers have found that both childhood sexual abuse and physical abuse are also associated with suicidal behavior in adolescents, even after controlling for a variety of potentially confounding variables, including an adolescent's psychopathology, parental psychopathology, and demographics (Brent et al., 1993c, 1999; Fergusson, Horwood, & Lynskey, 1996; Gould et al., 2003; Johnson et al, 2002).

Academic Difficulties

School difficulties, not working or attending school, and dropping out of high school (without attempting to earn a general equivalency diploma go on to college), have been identified as risk factors for attempted and completed suicide in several countries, even after controlling for psychopathology and social risk factors (Beautrais et al., 1996; Gould et al., 1996; Wunderlich et al., 1998).

Functional Impairment from Physical Disease and Injury

Physical diseases and injuries, to the extent that they result in functional impairment, have also been found to increase the risk of future suicide attempts in adolescents (Lewinsohn et al., 1996). Being diagnosed as having AIDS or as being HIV-positive, while considered a more definitive risk factor among adults, has not received adequate empirical study among adolescents. Prior studies of adults diagnosed with AIDS report a 7- to 36-fold increased risk of suicide (Kizer, Green, Perkins, Coebbert, & Hughes, 1988; Cote, Biggar, & Dannengerg, 1992). To date, no studies have examined this question among adolescents diagnosed with AIDS. Although suicidal ideation and other types of psychiatric morbidity in HIV-infected people have been described in several reports (Lyketsos & Federman, 1995; McKegney & O'Dowd, 1992), few definitive data exist examining the risk of suicide among individuals found positive for the HIV infection. One of the few studies examining this question among 4,147 HIV-seropositive military service applicants, including older adolescents and adults, reported no significant increased risk of death by suicide in the months following HIV screening (Dannenberg, McNeil, Brundage, & Brookmeyer, 1996). These investigators point out that because suicide risk is reported to be greatly increased after symptomatic HIV disease is present, clinicians should carefully assess persons with HIV infection for suicidal risk factors during initial counseling and subsequent counseling and medical care.

Suicide in the Social Milieu

Exposure to the suicidal behavior of others can precipitate imitative suicidal behavior, at least in some individuals (Velting & Gould, 1997). Adolescents are highly susceptible to suggestion and imitative behavior, as these are primary modes of social learning and identity formation. Velting and Gould (1997) propose that modeling cues through personal acquaintance, community exposures, and exposure to media coverage may all play a role in imitative suicidal behavior. Numerous studies have found that significantly more peers, friends, and/or family members had attempted or completed suicide in the social networks or families of persons with suicide ideation, attempts, and completions than in control groups (Brent, Bridge, Johnson, & Connolly, 1996a; Brent, Moritz, Bridge, Perper, & Canobbio, 1996b; Garfinkel et al., 1982; Gould et al., 1996; Harkavy-Friedman, Asnis, Boeck, & Difiore, 1987; Shafii et al., 1985; Smith & Crawford, 1986). In addition to increased rates of suicidal behaviors in these relatives and friends, suicidologists have examined suicide clusters and the influence of the media on adolescents.

A "suicide cluster" may be defined as a group of suicide attempts that occur closer together in time and space than would normally be expected in a given community (CDC, 1988). In a review of the literature on suicide clusters, Velting and Gould (1997) argue that suicide contagion is a real effect, even though it appears to be a less potent risk factor than other psychiatric and psychosocial risk factors for suicide. Of all age groups, adolescents are at highest risk for clustering of attempted and completed suicides, with only minimal effects beyond 24 years of age (Brent et al., 1989; Gould et al., 1990, 1996); therefore, this age group should be allotted the greatest amount of resources for prevention and postvention work (Velting & Gould, 1997).

Regarding media influence, there has been a marked increase in studies examining the impact on suicide rates around the world of media-covered nonfictional and fictional suicides. Studies have begun to emphasize characteristics such as age, gender, and performance as important to the modeling effect, since perceived similarity between observer and model appears to facilitate imitation. In an example from a fictional 6-week TV serial broadcast in Germany, a 19-year-old male was portrayed as committing suicide by jumping in front of a train (Schmidtke & Hafner, 1988). Results revealed a subsequent 86% increase in the number of railway-related suicides among 15- to 29-year-old males, and a 147% increase among 15- to 19-year-old males. Although this example involved a fictional suicide, research has shown that real suicides covered in the media result even more clearly in subsequent suicides (especially for teenagers), and that the magnitude of the suicide increase is proportional to the amount, duration, and prominence of media coverage (Gould, 2001; Velting & Gould, 1997).

Accessible Means of Suicide

Accessibility to the means of suicide (e.g., firearms) is a significant proximal risk factor. The most common method of suicide in the United States, regardless of age, race, or gender, is the use of firearms. According to the National Center for Health Statistics (1996), 67.5% of the total number (3,344) of young persons committing suicide in 1994 used firearms. The probability of suicide increases fivefold when a firearm is kept in the home (Brent et al., 1991; Rosenberg, Mercy, & Houk, 1991). One study has found that the availability of guns in the home contributes more heavily to the population attributable risk percentage for suicide among adolescents under the age of 16 than does psychopathology (Brent, 1999). Other common methods used by males for completed suicides in the United States include jumping, hanging, and carbon monoxide poisoning. For females, the next most frequent methods include overdosing on pills or ingesting solid and liquid poisons (Minino, Arias, Kochanek, Murphy, & Smith, 2002).

Worldwide, however, hanging is the most common method of suicide. For example, in New Zealand and Australia, 54% and 36%, respectively, of youth suicides were accounted for by hanging (Berman, Jobes, & Silverman, 2006). In other countries with large agrarian societies, the use of pesticides is the most common method of suicide (Eddleston & Phillips, 2004).

The overwhelming majority of adolescent suicide *attempts* in the United States and the United Kingdom involve intentional overdose (Berman et al., 2006). In one large community study in the United States, ingestion and cutting accounted for 86% of the suicide attempts reported by girls and 45% of those reported by boys (Lewinsohn et al., 1996). In addition to ingestion (20%) and self-cutting (25%), Lewinsohn et al. (1996) found that other common methods used in attempts by boys were firearms (15%), hanging (11%), and "other" (22%), which included activities such as shooting air into one's veins and running into traffic. When overdosing, adolescents most often use analgesics and prescribed medications (for themselves or their parents), such as antidepressants and tranquilizers (Worden, 1989).

Berman and Jobes (1991) highlight a number of factors that have been identified to explain the choice of method used:

1) Availability and accessibility (i.e., ease to obtain)
2) Sociocultural acceptance (i.e., normative use)
3) Knowledgeability (i.e., familiarity with use)
4) Social or behavior suggestion (e.g., modeling)
5) Saliency (e.g., suggested by publicity)
6) Personal, symbolic meaning of act or setting (e.g., a landmark jumping site such as the Golden Gate Bridge)
7) Intentionality and rescue-ability (i.e., if intent is high, methods of choice will be those most lethal, most efficient, and least likely to be interfered with). (p. 105)

Given the high number of impulsive suicides among adolescents, clinicians must take into account in their assessments the aforementioned factors, especially availability and accessibility. In addition, substance use at the time of suicidal behavior has been found to be related to the lethality of the method used (Brent et al., 1987).

Medical lethality of method and suicide intent have been found to be highly correlated, although they are certainly not synonymous. Robbins and Alessi (1985) found a high correlation between adolescent inpatients' suicidal intent and the medical lethality of their suicide attempts. In contrast to these results, however, other researchers have discovered that the medical lethality of the chosen method does not always match the adolescents' intent to die. For example, Harris and Myers (1997) found that adolescents who overdosed without intent to die (i.e., their intent was to cause drowsiness or unconsciousness) seriously underestimated the dangerousness of their actions. Specifically, 42% of an adolescent sample underestimated the dose of acetaminophen that could cause harm, and 50% underestimated the dose that could cause death. Thus many adolescents seriously underestimate the dangerousness of acetaminophen in overdose and lack knowledge regarding side effects of overdose, including toxicity. These findings indicate that a clinician must assess suicidal intent apart from medical lethality when ascertaining the seriousness of an attempt.

THE ADOLESCENTS AT HIGHEST RISK FOR SUICIDAL BEHAVIOR

Table 1.2 presents a detailed list of the evidence-based risk factors for suicidal attempts and completions. Many of these behaviors apply to both suicidal adolescents and adults; each factor specific to adolescents has been marked with an asterisk (*). The same demographic and environmental risk factors appear in both Tables 1.1 and 1.2. The second table, however, offers a more detailed picture of personal, environmental, and behavioral characteristics. Those adolescents at high risk tend to have multiple problems across cognitive, emotional, interpersonal, and behavioral domains of functioning. It's important to note that the factors putting adolescents most at risk for suicidal behaviors overlap significantly with the behavioral criteria for BPD (see the next section). The multiple risk factors for suicide found in these youth also

TABLE 1.2. Specific Risk Factors for Suicide Attempts and Completed Suicides in Adults and Adolescents

	Suicide attempts	Completed suicides
Personal characteristics		
Demographic		
1. Gender	Females > males	Males > females
2. Age	Increases with age (during adolescence)*	Increases with age (during adolescence)*
3. Race	Hispanic (females) > white > African American*	Native American > white > African American > Hispanic
4. Nationality	—	Chinese females > males
5. Sexual orientation	Bisexual/homosexual orientation (males > females); younger > older adolescents; risk when "coming out."*	
History	Childhood sexual and physical abuse, neglect	Childhood sexual and physical abuse
	Family history of suicidal behavior	Family history of suicidal behavior
Genetic/biochemical		
1. CSF 5-HIAA[a]	—	Low in adults; not demonstrated in adolescents
2. Family history	High in biological relatives	High in biological relatives
Environmental characteristics		
Life changes/negative life events	Losses (particularly interpersonal—e.g., breakup of romantic relationship, relative or friend died, disciplinary crisis, humiliation, arguments)*	Losses (particularly interpersonal—e.g., breakup of romantic relationship, relative or friend died, disciplinary crisis, humiliation, arguments)*
	Arrested or has legal problems; jail	Arrested or has legal problems; jail
	Friend attempted/completed suicide	Friend attempted/completed suicide
	Academic difficulties; high school dropout, no college	Academic difficulties; high school dropout, no college
Family context	Parental mental disorders (depressive/substance-related)	Parental mental disorders (depressive/substance-related)
	Aggression, abuse, neglect toward child	Aggression, abuse, neglect toward child
	Poor parent–child communication; adolescent perceives parent(s) as uncaring and/or overprotective	Poor parent–child communication

(*cont.*)

TABLE 1.2 (*cont.*)

	Suicide attempts	Completed suicides
Social support	Socially isolated	Socially isolated
Models	Modeling by peers,* community exposure,* media coverage*	Suicide contagion/clusters* Modeling by peers*, community exposure*, media coverage*
Method availability	Available	Available
Behavioral characteristics		
Cognitive		
1. Style	Impulsive	Impulsive, perfectionistic
2. Content	Poor interpersonal problem solving	Poor interpersonal problem solving
	Low reasons for living	Low reasons for living
		Negative self-concept
Physiological/emotional/mental disorder		
1. Affective	Anxious, depressed, angry	Depressed, angry
2. Somatic	Low frustration tolerance	Uncomfortable with people
		Poor health
		Insomnia
3. Mental disorder	Axis I: MDD,[b] bipolar, substance use, conduct disorder,* anxiety	Axis I: MDD, bipolar, substance use, conduct disorder,* schizophrenia
	Axis II: BPD, ASPD[c]	Axis II: BPD, ASPD
Action/overt motor		
1. Interpersonal	Interpersonal conflicts	Low social involvement
		Interpersonal conflicts
2. Dysfunctional patterns a. Previous suicide attempt	30–50%; 21–27% will reattempt within 3 months of first attempt*	
b. Intent		50–88% give some indication in the weeks prior to death that they are in distress

Note. An asterisk (*) indicates an adolescent-specific risk factor. Data from Linehan (1993a).
[a]CSF 5-HIAA, cerebrospinal fluid 5-hydroxyindoleacetic acid (a metabolite of serotonin).
[b]MDD, major depressive disorder.
[c]ASPD, antisocial personality disorder.

include substance-related and other Axis I mental disorders, comorbid psychopathology, and familial dysfunction, to name a few. These persistent difficulties impair social, school, and occupational functioning, and such impairment in turn increases the likelihood of future suicide attempts. Follow-up studies indicate that about 10–50% of adolescents who attempt suicide make future attempts (Spirito et al., 1989), and that up to about 11% of attempting adolescents eventually die by suicide (Shaffer & Piacentini, 1994). Thus the high rate of continued psychological disturbance exhibited by adolescents who attempt suicide indicates the pressing need for effective psychological interventions for this group. Studies with adults who attempt suicide suggest that treatment may reduce repeated attempts and enhance social adjustment (Linehan, Armstrong, Suarez, Allmon, & Heard, 1991; Shaffer & Piacentini, 1994). Yet as many as 50% of adolescents who attempt suicide fail to receive any follow-up mental health treatment (Spirito et al., 1989), and of those who do receive such treatment, up to 77% do not attend therapy appointments or fail to complete treatment (Trautman et al., 1993). These high rates of noncompliance with treatment further hinder efforts to develop and evaluate psychological interventions for this group. In the next chapter we turn to the treatment outcome research for suicidal behaviors.

THE OVERLAP BETWEEN SUICIDAL BEHAVIORS AND BPD IN ADOLESCENTS

As noted earlier, the diagnosis of BPD in adolescents has historically been a controversial issue. In the recent empirical literature, however, there appears to be initial support for the existence of BPD in adolescents. According to the *Diagnostic and Statistical Manual of Mental Disorders*, fourth edition, text revision (DSM-IV-TR), "recurrent suicidal behavior . . . or self-mutilating behavior" (American Psychiatric Association, [APA], 2000, p. 710) is the fifth diagnostic criterion for BPD. Completed suicides occur in 8–10% of persons diagnosed with BPD, and self-mutilative acts and suicide threats and attempts are extremely common (APA, 2000).

In reviewing four studies of adolescents and young adults who completed suicide, Linehan et al. (in press) found that with one exception (Rich & Runeson, 1992), the results were remarkably consistent in indicating high rates of personality disorders among these young persons when compared to matched-pair community control groups (Brent et al., 1994; Lesage et al., 1994) and to a sample of adults over 30 years of age who completed suicide (Rich et al., 1986). As noted earlier, it has been suggested that the co-occurrence of mood and personality disorders represents a particularly significant risk factor for suicidal behaviors (Blumenthal & Kupfer, 1986).

Numerous studies suggest that BPD can be validly and reliably diagnosed in adolescents (Bernstein et al., 1993; Marton et al., 1989; Chanen et al., 2004; Bradley, Jenei, & Weston, 2005). In fact, in a large epidemiological study still underway, Zanarini (2003) reports that 3.3% of 10,000 children age 11 assessed in Great Britain met full diagnostic criteria for BPD. These numbers are higher than the estimated 2% prevalence rate for BPD in adults in the general population (APA, 2000); they thus imply the potential for some children and adolescents to "mature out" of the BPD diagnosis within adulthood, especially if treatment is sought. Unfortunately, however, some researchers suggest that for a subgroup of adolescents, the BPD diagnosis is stable.

Crawford, Cohen, and Brook (2001) examined the dimensional stability of behavioral criteria for DSM-IV Cluster B personality disorders over an 8-year period in a sample of 408 community adolescents who were not receiving treatment. The results indicated that these criteria had moderate stability (.63 for boys, .69 for girls) across time. Interestingly, the stability estimates for Cluster B behavioral criteria were drastically reduced when assessed as categorical diagnoses; this suggests that the stability of personality dysfunction in adolescents may be better detected via a dimensional approach, due to the fact that adolescence is a fluid developmental period. Chanen et al. (2004) assessed the stability of personality disorder diagnoses among adolescent outpatients ($n = 101$) over 2 years; they used the Structured Clinical Interview for DSM-IV Axis II Personality Disorders (SCID-II; First, Gibbon, Spitzer, Williams, & Benjamin, 1997) which allows for both categorical and dimensional assessment of personality disorders, in general and BPD more specifically. Eleven of 101 participants met criteria for BPD at baseline, and 12 of 96 participants met criteria for BPD at follow-up. Consistent with Crawford et al.'s work, Cluster B behavioral criteria showed moderate stability across time (intraclass correlation coefficient = .61, r = .63).

Researchers exploring the validity of BPD in adolescents point to the consistent relationships found between BPD and associated areas of dysfunction and distress as evidence of diagnostic validity. Levy et al. (1999) investigated both the concurrent and predictive validity of personality disorder diagnoses in adolescents via baseline and 2-year follow-up assessments of 142 inpatient adolescents on various clinician-rated and self-rated measures of distress and dysfunction. From the total sample, 86 participants were diagnosed with a personality disorder; 71 (89%) of these were diagnosed with BPD, so we assume that the results pertain most closely to a diagnosis of BPD. Consistent with other research, support was found for the concurrent validity of a personality disorder diagnosis in adolescent inpatients. In other words, at baseline, adolescents with a personality disorder (most often BPD) were more functionally impaired as measured by Global Assessment of Functioning Scale scores than those without a personality disorder. In addition, adolescents with a personality disorder scored significantly higher on 10 of the 12 Symptom Checklist-90—Revised (SCL-90-R; Derogatis, 1994) subscales, indicating that such a diagnosis is associated with functional impairments. Lastly, those with a personality disorder showed significantly greater dysfunction in the areas of drug use and further psychiatric hospitalizations at the 2-year follow-up than those without personality disorder (Levy et al., 1999). Kasen, Cohen, Skodol, Johnson, and Brook (1999) found that the odds of a personality disorder in young adulthood increased, given a personality disorder during adolescence in the same cluster. Hence, these patients are at high risk for ongoing problems in multiple domains of functioning. In sum, the presence of a BPD diagnosis in adolescence is associated with significant functional impairment and poor prognosis.

In a recent study examining gender differences among adolescents diagnosed with BPD, Bradley et al. (2005) found that the behavioral criteria and phenomenology of adolescent girls with BPD were similar to those of adults. In contrast, adolescent boys meeting BPD criteria had a more aggressive, disruptive, antisocial presentation. These results require further investigation.

However, personality disorders tend not to be diagnosed in multiproblem suicidal adolescents. Reasons that clinicians may not apply the diagnosis to teens include, but are not limited to, the following:

1. Reasons of training (many child and adolescent mental health professionals are not trained to assess personality disorders in adolescents, due to the general belief that they do not exist that early).
2. Questions regarding the reliability and the validity of the diagnosis in adolescents.
3. Reasons of perceived competence (many mental health professionals do not believe that they are competent to treat personality disorders in any age group).

4. The wish to maintain a sense of hope about a young person's prognosis (since personality disorders have historically been recalcitrant to standard therapies).
5. Concerns about stigmatizing an adolescent with a personality disorder diagnosis.
6. Fiscal reasons (insurance companies often will not reimburse treatment for personality disorders).
7. The belief that the DSM-IV-TR system is nondevelopmental and thereby does not take into account childhood traits and behavior problems that are continuous with adult personality disorders (Kernberg, Weiner, & Bardenstein, 2000; Miller, Muehlenkamp, & Jacobson, 2006).

Despite all these doubts and beliefs, the pattern of results in the empirical literature indicates that the prevalence, reliability, and validity of BPD in adolescent samples are largely comparable to those found among adults with BPD (Miller et al., 2006). This comparability in and of itself suggests that BPD appears to operate in a similar fashion and has a similar course, regardless of age and developmental period. Studies also clearly indicate that while there is a legitimate subgroup of severely affected adolescents for whom the diagnosis remains stable over time, there appears to be a less severely affected subgroup that moves in and out of the diagnosis. Hence there is clinical relevance in identifing those for whom the diagnosis is stable, so as to provide appropriate treatments. Regardless of the presence of a full-fledged disorder, BPD *behavioral criteria* in an adolescent (even if fewer than five are present) may indeed accurately reflect significant distress and dysfunction (e.g., suicidality, self-cutting, identity disturbance, academic failure, social dysfunction, disturbed eating, and substance abuse) that require intervention. If more clinicians asess for and consider the diagnosis of BPD, many more adolescents will be appropriately assessed and treated for their BPD behavioral criteria; as a result, fewer will develop an ingrained and refractory pattern of dysfunctional behaviors, and fewer will be at heightened risk for suicidal behaviors and NSIB (Miller et al., 2006).

With the emerging empirically supported treatment for BPD (Lieb, Zanarini, Schmal, Lineban, & Bohus, 2004), coupled with the findings from longitudinal studies that BPD remits in large numbers of treated adults (Paris & Zweig-Frank, 2001; Zanarini, Frankenburg, Hennen, & Silk, 2003), the BPD diagnosis should no longer be considered "hopeless." Furthermore, insurance is increasingly reimbursing for DBT as treatment for a BPD diagnosis in adults. Given the current situation, lack of appropriate diagnosis can function as a substantial barrier to effective treatment. At the same time, more research is indicated to further clarify the issues pertaining to the diagnosis of BPD in adolescents.

CONCLUSION

The factors that put adolescents most at risk for suicidal behaviors significantly overlap with the behavioral criteria for BPD. The multiple risk factors for suicide found in these youth have been reviewed in this chapter. The next chapter reviews the existing treatments for multi-problem suicidal adolescents.

CHAPTER 2

What Do We Know about Effective Treatments for Suicidal Adolescents?

All treatments attempt to change or ameliorate the factors that are presumed to underlie or control clients' problems. How this is done, however, can vary widely. There are two basic strategies for treating suicidal behaviors in clinical populations. The first strategy assumes that such behaviors are effects of some other underlying mental disorder. Treatment time and focus are allocated to treating the mental disorder, in the belief that its cure will in turn reduce the behaviors. Except to maintain life, no special modifications are made in the treatment of the underlying disorder. Reductions in suicidal behaviors are an indirect benefit of therapy. This approach is the model underlying most psychodynamic and biological approaches to treatment. The second strategy is to focus directly on the reduction of suicidal behaviors. In these treatments, reduction of these behaviors is an explicit treatment goal, and the specific behaviors are targets of intervention. When this strategy is pursued, therapy sessions focus on engaging the client in a discussion of current and immediately past suicidal behaviors (including suicidal ideation, threats, and communication), as well as of NSIB episodes. Explicit connections are then made to presumed underlying or controlling factors. This second model underlies most behavioral and cognitive-behavioral approaches to treatment. In this chapter we review the research on various treatments' effectiveness for suicidal behaviors in both adolescents and adults. We group these approaches in the first two sections of the chapter by their strategy—indirect or direct targeting of the suicidal behaviors.

TREATING SUICIDAL BEHAVIORS INDIRECTLY BY TREATING ASSOCIATED DISORDERS

Unfortunately, data are very sparse regarding which treatments for primary mental disorders actually reduce the risk of completed suicide, suicide attempts, or suicidal ideation. The exclusion of highly suicidal individuals from most studies notwithstanding, investigators frequently include measures of suicidal behaviors in their outcome batteries, especially in studies of pharmacotherapy.

While lithium treatment has been correlated with reduced rates of suicide attempts and fatalities in adults diagnosed with bipolar disorders (Baldessarini & Jamison, 1999), and clozapine has been shown to reduce suicidal ideation and behavior among adults diagnosed with schizophrenia and schizoaffective disorder (Meltzer & Okayli, 1995), pharmacotherapy researchers have focused most of their attention on depressive disorders. Since mood disorders are the most common diagnoses related to suicide, researchers hypothesize that effective treatment of depression will reduce the incidence of suicide. Although this assumption makes intuitive sense, there are actually few or no empirical data to back up the assumption. Pharmacotherapy regimens that are more effective than placebo for reducing depression may or may not be more effective in reducing suicidal ideation or other suicidal behaviors (e.g., Beasley et al., 1992; Smith & Glaudin, 1992). To date, although there are many randomized clinical trials indicating that antidepressant medications reduce depression, there are no data from these trials suggesting that antidepressants reduce the incidence of either suicide attempts or completed suicide. For example, Buchholtz-Hansen, Wang, and Kragh-Sorensen (1993) followed 219 depressed inpatients who had previously been participants in multicenter trials of psychopharmacology. Not only were suicide rates higher than expected at follow-up, but there was no association between response to the antidepressant treatment and the suicide risk during the first 3 years of observation. Meta-analyses of pooled data from 17 double-blind clinical trials comparing fluoxetine ($n = 1,765$) with a tricyclic antidepressant ($n = 731$), a placebo ($n = 569$), or both in the treatment of individuals with major depression showed no significant reductions in suicidal acts as a result of taking antidepressants (Beasley, Sayler, Bosomworth, & Wernicke, 1991; Beasley et al., 1992).

In studies where actively suicidal individuals were not enrolled, the failure to find significant treatment effects may be attributable to the low base rate of suicidal acts in a nonsuicidal population. That is, the treatment may not be powerful enough to make a large difference, or our present statistics may not be powerful enough to detect a small difference. However, the findings reported by Beasley et al. (1991) of a pooled incidence of suicidal acts of 0.3% for fluoxetine, 0.2% for placebo, and 0.4% for tricyclic antidepressants suggest that power may not be the problem. The general lack of follow-up, however, may be an important factor. In the studies analyzed by Beasley et al., results were reported for only the 5–6 weeks that individuals were active in the treatment protocol; no follow-up data were reported. Even if reducing depression does reduce risk of suicidal behavior, it is unlikely that effects would show up so quickly. An absence of significant effects could also be due to equivalent efficacy across many interventions with low-risk clients. That is, any active treatment may be equally effective at suicide prevention within a population at low initial risk for suicide.

Looking at the relationship of reducing depression to reducing suicidal behavior from the reverse direction, Linehan and colleagues (Linehan, Armstrong, Suarez, Allmon, & Heard, 1991; Linehan et al., 2006b) showed that DBT resulted in a significant reduction in suicide attempts and other intentional self-injury, compared to either treatment as usual (TAU) or community treatment by experts, did so despite being no more effective in reducing depression than the control conditions. (Depression improved in all treatments.) Similarly, Sakinofsky, Roberts, Brown, Cumming, and James (1990) found that improvement in depression, hostility, locus of control, powerlessness, self-esteem, sensitivity to criticism, and social adjustment was not related to reduced risk for repeated intentional self-injury over the next 3 months.

Recently the U.S. Food and Drug Administration ordered a "black box" label to be placed on all antidepressant medications, to indicate the potential for increased suicidal ideation and other suicidal behaviors among children and adolescents using these medications (Delate, Gelenberg, Simmons, & Motheral, 2004). These concerns have led many families of depressed and suicidal youth to pursue nonpharmacological interventions. Despite preliminary findings from the Treatment for Adolescents with Depression Study (TADS) that for *non-suicidal* depressed youth, the combination of fluoxetine and CBT was more effective at reducing depression than fluoxetine alone, CBT alone, or a placebo (TADS Team, 2004), concerns remain about prescribing antidepressant medications for depressed adolescents. Clinicians are divided as to whether antidepressants should be recommended as a primary intervention for suicidal multiproblem youth. Thus there is a glaring need for effective behavioral interventions for these youth.

TREATING SUICIDAL BEHAVIORS DIRECTLY

Despite the incidence of completed suicide, suicide attempts, and suicidal ideation, there is remarkably little research on whether therapeutic interventions aimed directly at reducing suicide risk and associated behaviors are effective in achieving these aims. There are many books, articles, professional workshops, and legal precedents concerning treatment of suicidal behaviors, but very few of the recommended or required interventions have been subjected to controlled clinical trials. Thus, although there are standards of care for intervening with individuals at high risk for suicidal acts, there are few or no empirical data confirming that these standards of care are effective in preventing suicide or reducing the frequency or medical severity of suicide attempts.

Evaluations of Standards of Care

Emergency inpatient admission for suicidal individuals has been examined in only two studies; neither found the inpatient admission to be more beneficial than outpatient treatment (Waterhouse & Platt, 1990; Huey et al., 2004). Among inpatient programs, no differences have been found between behavioral and insight-oriented treatments (Liberman & Eckman, 1981), or among cognitive therapy, problem-solving therapy, and supportive treatment (Patsiokas & Clum, 1985). A number of studies have examined whether access to emergency treatment without requiring current suicidal behaviors might be effective. No beneficial effects were found for adolescents ages 12–16 years who were given access to emergency inpatient admission (Cotgrove, Zirinsky, Black, & Weston, 1995), or for adults who were given access to on-call psychiatrists (Morgan, Jones, & Owen, 1993; Evans, Morgan, Hayward, & Gunnell, 1999).

Three studies evaluated the coordination of care following inpatient admission for self-inflicted injury, with negative results. Two (Möller, 1992; Torhorst et al., 1987) examined the impact of continuing with the same clinician from inpatient to outpatient treatment compared to TAU. Contrary to predictions, in both studies the proportion of repeated self-inflicted injuries was higher in the continuity condition. A third study examined coordination of care with a patient's general practitioner. This involved sending a letter following emergency care for self-inflicted injury to notify the general practitioner of this emergency care; enclosed in this notification were expert consensus guidelines for appropriate follow-up, as well as a letter to send to the patient asking him or her to schedule an appointment. This was compared to a TAU condition. There were no differences in the rates of repeated self-injury.

Evaluations of Clinical Outreach

Studies comparing clinical TAU to clinical outreach efforts have had mixed results. Three out of four studies have found in-person outreach effective in reducing repeated self-injury (van Heeringen et al., 1995; Termansen & Bywater, 1975; Welu, 1977; Chowdhury, Hicks, & Kreitman, 1973). Two studies found no beneficial effect of telephone outreach, whether this consisted of a simple "befriending" call (Wold & Litman, 1976[3]) or a call to motivate suicidal individuals to attend or stay in treatment (Cedereke, Monti, & Öjehagen, 2002). Meta-analyses of intensive treatments plus outreach also did not find them to be effective (Hawton et al., 1998; van der Sande, Buskens, Allart, van der Graaf, & van Engeland, 1997).

The one exception to this conclusion is a very important intervention developed by Motto (1976), which consisted of sending nondemanding letters to 320 individuals who did not enter follow-up care after a hospitalization for depressive or suicidal states. Each letter was signed by the staff member who had interviewed the patient in the hospital; it consisted of a simple expression of concern, and invited a response if the patient wished to send one. Subsequent letters were individualized and included responses to comments previously received. Results showed that for the first 2 years, when contact with the participants was greatest, there was a lower percentage of suicides in the contact group than in the no-contact group; over the full 5 years of the study, the difference was not significant. It is important, however, that this difference was significant during the first 2 years following hospitalization, which is when suicides are most likely to occur (Motto & Bostrom, 2001). To date, this is the only intervention ever shown in a controlled trial to have a significant effect on completed suicide.

Evaluations of CBT

Various forms of CBT have been examined in randomized clinical trials. Two brief CBT interventions have been found more effective than TAU in reducing subsequent self-injury: 5 sessions of problem-solving CBT (Salkovskis, Atha, & Storer, 1990) and 10 sessions of CBT plus case management (Brown et al., 2005). However, a manual-assisted version of CBT, consisting of a brief CBT self-help manual plus up to 7 in-person sessions, was not more effective than TAU in reducing repeated self-inflicted injury (Evans et al., 1999; Tyrer et al., 2003). Only 60% of the individuals had at least 1 in-person session, however. Finally, no differences were found in two studies comparing skills training therapies to problem-solving therapy (McLeavey, Daly, Ludgate, & Murray, 1994) and to supportive therapy (Donaldson, Spirito, & Esposito-Smythers, 2005). Several trials have evaluated various forms of brief crisis-oriented problem-focused treatments, which share many similarities with CBT. These approaches have not been found more effective than TAU (Hawton et al., 1981, 1987; van der Sande, van Rooijen, et al., 1997; Gibbons, Butler, Urwin, & Gibbons, 1978).

DBT is the only treatment to date with more than one clinical trial demonstrating effectiveness in reducing suicide attempts and NSIB. When compared to TAU for suicidal women meeting criteria for BPD, the proportion of clients in DBT who made suicide attempts and engaged in NSIB in the following year and a 1-year follow-up was lower than for those in the TAU condition (Linehan et al., 1991) and (Linehan, Heard, & Armstrong, 1993a). A replication trial (Linehan et al., 2006b) found that among chronically suicidal women meeting criteria for BPD, the proportion of individuals with a suicide attempt during the 1 year of treatment and 1 year of follow-up was half that of individuals randomly assigned to nonbehavioral community expert psychotherapy. In addition, the medical risk of those suicide attempts and NSIB that did occur were lower in DBT than in TAU or in treatment by experts. Emergency room and inpatient admissions for suicidal behaviors were also lower in DBT than in treatment by experts. Similar outcomes were found in a third 12-month randomized clinical trial in the Netherlands evaluating DBT for women with BPD, compared with TAU (Verheul et al., 2003). Reductions in suicide attempts and self-injury were found in four other randomized clinical trials conducted by three different research groups (van den Bosch, Koeter, Stijnen, Verheul, van den Brink, 2005; Koons et al., 2001; Turner, 2000; Verheul et al., 2003).

Two meta-analyses across all CBT trials have reached different conclusions about the efficacy of CBT for suicidal individuals. One meta-analysis (Hawton et al., 1998) included crisis intervention but not DBT as a problem-solving therapy and did not find that therapy to be effective. In contrast, a second meta-analysis separated crisis interventions from CBT and included DBT in the CBT category. This meta-analysis found CBT, but not psychosocial crisis intervention, to be effective (van der Sande, Buskins, et al., 1997).

Evaluations of Integrative and Non-CBT Treatments

Six clinical trials have evaluated the effectiveness of psychotherapies other than CBT. Bateman and Fonagy (1999) demonstrated that an 18-month psychodynamically oriented partial hospitalization program for adults diagnosed with BPD was more effective than TAU at reducing suicide attempts and self-mutilation. These results, however, have not yet been replicated in a second trial or tested by an independent research team (Lieb et al., 2004).

Four sessions of interpersonal therapy provided in the home (Guthrie et al., 2001), and a "developmental group therapy" for adolescents (based on CBT, DBT, and psychodynamic therapies; Wood, Trainor, Rothwell, Moore, & Harrington, 2001), have been found to be more effective than TAU in reducing deliberate self-harm. It is unclear whether any of these "deliberate self-harm" behaviors were actually suicidal, however. Treatments not found to be more effective than TAU include 18 sessions of psychotherapy (including one home visit; Allard, Marshall, & Plante, 1992), four sessions of home-based family therapy for adolescents following self-injury (Harrington et al., 1998) and unspecified long-term therapy (i.e., one session per month for 12 months) (Torhorst, Möller, & Schmid-Bode, 1988).

Evaluations of Treatments for Suicidal and Nonsuicidal Self-Injurious Adolescents

Only four randomized treatment studies have explicitly focused on adolescent samples (Cotgrove et al., 1995; Harrington et al., 1998; Wood et al., 2001; and Huey et al., 2004). In the Cotgrove et al. (1995) study of adolescents age 15 and older, the investigators found no significant differences between the experimental (who were given access on request to inpatient care) and control (TAU) groups on measures of repeated self-injurious behavior.

In the second study, Harrington et al. (1998) randomly assigned subjects age 16 and greater to TAU or to TAU plus a short-term, action-oriented, home-based family intervention for adolescents who deliberately poisoned themselves. Investigators found that this intervention did not significantly reduce self-injurious behaviors. Thus brief family therapy alone for suicidal teens and families seems inadequate as a stand-alone intervention.

In a study of 63 adolescents ages 12–16 years, Wood et al. (2001) randomly assigned subjects either to "developmental group therapy" (containing components of CBT, DBT, and psychodynamic group psychotherapy) plus TAU or to TAU alone. These investigators employed Hawton and Catalan's (1982), definition of deliberate self-harm: "any intentional self-inflicted injury, irrespective of the apparent purpose of the act" (Wood et al., 2001, p. 1247). The interesting finding here was that adolescents who participated in the experimental group therapy were less likely to be "repeaters" of self-harm at the end of the study than adolescents who received TAU alone (2/32 vs. 10/31; odds ratio = 6.3). Interestingly, those adolescents who participated in the experimental group were also less likely to use TAU, had better school attendance, and had a lower rate of behavioral disorders than adolescents given TAU alone. More sessions of the group therapy were associated with a better outcome, whereas more sessions of TAU were associated with a worse outcome. Hence more of the "right" type of treatment may sometimes be better. Lastly, the interventions did not differ in terms of their effects on depression, suicidal ideation, or global outcome.

In the fourth study, Huey et al. (2004) evaluated whether an intensive family- and community-based treatment called "multisystemic therapy" (MST; Henggeler, Schoenwald,

Rowland, & Cunningham, 2002) could serve as a safe and effective outpatient intervention, compared to inpatient hospitalization of adolescents presenting with mental health emergencies. Participants were 156 males and females 10–17 years of age who were approved for psychiatric hospitalization because of suicidal ideation/planning or attempted suicide, homicidal ideation or behavior, psychosis, or other threat of harm to self or others. Subjects were randomly assigned to either the MST or inpatient psychiatric hospital condition. MST was delivered in each family's natural environment, including the home, the school, and the community, by intensively trained therapists.

The study compared group differences from pretreatment to posttreatment and at a 1-year follow-up. Relative to inpatient psychiatric hospitalization, MST was efficacious at reducing the frequency of attempted suicide, although it did not seem to have a greater impact on suicidal ideation, hopelessness, and depressive affect. As the investigators point out, it is possible that the superior effects of MST may reflect a regression to the mean, since the group receiving MST had significantly higher rates of attempted suicide at pretreatment. In addition, two limitations of this study should be noted here. First, it appears as though the "attempted suicide" measure included NSIB; if so, this would call into question the interpretation of the results. Second, 44% of the MST-treated youth were also admitted for psychiatric hospitalization during the course of treatment, because of behavioral emergencies that could not be managed in a community setting. Hence nearly half of those in the MST condition additionally received the comparison treatment, which ultimately confounds the results. The investigators did not report the results after controlling for those subjects who received both treatments.

CONCLUSIONS FROM RESEARCH FINDINGS

The results of controlled studies as a whole indicate that outpatient psychosocial treatments targeting suicidal behaviors directly, particularly CBT interventions, are effective in reducing the risk of future such behaviors in individuals identified as at high risk for them. However, only DBT has been replicated to date, as mentioned earlier in this chapter. In a previous review, Linehan, (1998) noted that 45% of clinical trials for self-inflicted injury excluded high-risk individuals. However, among the trials reported here that did not exclude such individuals, a significant reduction in self-injurious behavior was found. This finding highlights that individuals at high risk for suicidal behaviors and NSIB are able to benefit from outpatient treatments. In contrast, there are no data suggesting that inpatient treatments are effective at reducing suicidal behaviors and NSIB. Our review further suggests that the existing treatment research does not seem to support the premise of targeting suicidal behaviors indirectly by treating associated disorders. Rather, the treatment of suicidal behaviors and NSIB must be direct, although it must take into account the complexity and severity of co-occurring disorders in the patient.

TRIALS OF DBT WITH HIGH-RISK SUICIDAL ADOLESCENTS

DBT was originally developed specifically for chronically suicidal patients. These are patients who are unremittingly high in suicidal ideation, frequently threaten suicide or talk about taking their own lives, have difficulty articulating any reasons for living or staying alive, and may attempt suicide or engage in NSIB on multiple occasions. Although the treatment manuals describing DBT (Linehan, 1993a, 1993b) label it as a treatment for BPD, in fact the first drafts of these manuals never even mentioned BPD. The treatment and its theoretical underpinnings were originally developed to apply to suicidal individuals. The metamorphosis of the treatment into one aimed at BPD was due almost entirely to the substantial overlap between BPD and suicidal behavior (see Chapter 1).

DBT clinical trials have typically included older adolescents; however, to date there have been no analyses of treatment outcomes for adolescents alone. The success of DBT in reducing suicidal behaviors in adults diagnosed with BPD has led many clinicians to use it with adolescents who are also at high risk for such behaviors. As one of the few treatments to date showing efficacy for suicidal behaviors, the use of DBT for adolescents—either in its standard form or with adaptations for adolescents specifically—is widespread (Miller et al., 1997; Miller, Rathus, Dubose, Dexter-Mazza, & Goldklang, in press). However, promising preliminary research exists, and clinical experience is accumulating for implementing DBT with suicidal adolescents.

Two of us (Rathus & Miller, 2002) studied a version of DBT modified specifically for adolescents. Initial outcome data on our 12-week DBT program yielded promising results. In this quasi-experimental pilot investigation of suicidal adolescent outpatients with borderline personality features, we compared DBT ($n = 29$) to TAU ($n = 82$). The pilot sample was composed primarily of an ethnic minority (largely Hispanic) population. This is important, given the general dearth of behavior therapy and research with culturally diverse populations, as well as Hispanic adolescents' status of having a higher suicide attempt rate than adolescents from other ethnic groups. Results indicated significant differences between groups: 13% of adolescents receiving TAU versus 0% receiving DBT were psychiatrically hospitalized during treatment, and 40% of those receiving TAU versus 62% receiving DBT completed treatment. There were no significant differences between groups in number of suicide attempts (9% for those receiving TAU and 3% for those receiving DBT). However, because the group receiving DBT was initially classified as more impulsive, was diagnosed with a greater number of Axis I disorders, and had a greater number of prior hospitalizations than the group receiving TAU, it is possible that the adolescents receiving DBT were actually at higher risk for suicidality. Thus the fact that they were no more suicidal than the control group during treatment is noteworthy. Unfortunately, we did not formally measure NSIB at that time. When we examined pre–post change within the DBT group, there were significant reductions in suicidal ideation and Axis I and II symptomatology.

H. Fellows (personal communication, December 11, 1998) employed an adaptation of DBT for adolescents similar to ours (Rathus & Miller, 2002). This adaptation resulted in significant reductions in adolescents' use of costly treatment services. For example, prior to treatment the group had 539 inpatient psychiatric days, compared to 40 days during DBT treatment and 11 days during the 6-month posttreatment period.

Katz and colleagues (Katz & Cox, 2002; Katz, Gunasekara, Cox, & Miller, 2004) and Trupin and colleagues (2000) have begun adapting and evaluating DBT for adolescents in different settings, including inpatient and forensic programs. Preliminary results appear promising, although none of the DBT programs modified for adolescents have yet established efficacy through randomized controlled trials. It is clear that such trials are indicated to establish with full certainty whether DBT with adolescents is more effective than TAU. But in the meantime, we believe that DBT with appropriate modifications is highly promising for helping these adolescent clients.

Given the empirical evidence of DBT's efficacy with adults, applying it to high-risk suicidal adolescents makes sense, as long as attention is paid to the developmental issues pertaining to this age group. Regardless of diagnosis, DBT skills directly target significant problems in emotion regulation and behavioral control. These are the same problems that characterize high-risk suicidal youth who are typically referred to emergency rooms and inpatient units.

HOW DBT CONCEPTUALIZES SUICIDAL BEHAVIORS

As we discuss in greater detail in Chapter 3, DBT views suicidal behaviors as learned methods of coping with acute emotional suffering when no other coping options are available. The emotional picture of suicidal individuals is one of chronic, aversive emotion dysregulation. Those individuals who commit suicide are characterized by extreme dysphoria, often combined with high anxiety and panic (Fawcett, 1990). Generally, suicidal individuals are unlikely to have the ability to ameliorate or tolerate the emotional, interpersonal, and behavioral stresses in their lives. The cognitive difficulties found in studies of suicidal (primarily suicide-attempting) individuals include cognitive rigidity (Levenson & Neuringer, 1972; Neuringer, 1964; Patsiokas, Clum, & Luscomb, 1979; Vinoda, 1966), dichotomous thinking (Neuringer, 1961), and poor abstract and interpersonal problem solving (Goodstein, 1982; Levenson & Neuringer, 1971; Schotte & Clum, 1982). Impairments in problem solving may be related to deficits in specific (as compared to general) episodic memory capabilities (Williams, 1991), which have been found to characterize suicidal versus nonsuicidal individuals with mental disorders. In work at the University of Washington, we found that individuals with self-inflicted injuries exhibited a more passive (or dependent) interpersonal problem-solving style (Linehan, Camper, Chiles, Strosahl, & Shearin, 1987). Hopelessness is a strong predictor of both attempted suicide and eventual suicide (see Weishaar & Beck, 1992, for a review of this literature). Those who complete suicide are further characterized as indecisive and as having difficulties concentrating (Fawcett, 1990).

Suicidal behaviors can be viewed as problem-solving behaviors that function to remediate negative emotional arousal and distress either directly (e.g., by ending life [and presumably pain], putting an individual to sleep, or distracting him or her from emotional stimuli), or indirectly (e.g., by eliciting help from the environment), or as "inevitable" outcomes of unregulated and uncontrollable negative emotions. Although suicidal behaviors are not logically inevitable outcomes, paradigms of escape conditioning suggest that strong urges to escape or actual escape behaviors can be learned so completely that they become automatic for some individuals when faced with extreme and uncontrollable physical or emotional pain. Suicide, of course, is the ultimate escape from problems in one's life.

Suicidal behaviors, from a DBT perspective, are a result of two interacting conditions: (1) Individuals lack important interpersonal, self-regulation (including emotion regulation), and distress tolerance skills and capabilities; and (2) personal and environmental factors inhibit the use of those behavioral skills the individuals may already have. These personal and environmental factors also interfere with the development of new skills and capacities, in addition to reinforcing the inappropriate self-injurious behaviors.

DBT directly addresses these conditions by (1) teaching suicidal clients specific skills for interpersonal effectiveness, self-regulation (including emotion regulation) and distress tolerance; (2) structuring the treatment environment to motivate, reinforce, and individualize appropriate use of the skills; (3) identifying and breaking up learned behavioral sequences that precede clients' dysfunctional behaviors, and removing reinforcers for these behaviors; (4) providing treatment mechanisms to encourage the generalization of new skill capabilities from therapy to the life situations where they are needed; and (5) providing support for therapists treating high-risk suicidal individuals.

WHY EMPLOY DBT WITH SUICIDAL MULTIPROBLEM ADOLESCENTS?

As we will see in the chapters that follow, DBT flexibly addresses multiple problems and suicide risk factors concurrently (see Table 2.1). Most other empirically supported treatments de-

TABLE 2.1. BPD Characteristics, Suicide Risk Characteristics in Adolescents, and Corresponding DBT Skills Training Modules

BPD characteristics	Adolescent suicide risk	DBT skills module
Emotion dysregulation		
Emotional lability, angry outbursts	Depression, anger, anxiety, humiliation, guilt	Emotion Regulation
Interpersonal dysregulation		
Unstable relationships	Relationship breakup, interpersonal conflicts, chronic family disturbance, abuse and neglect, parental psychopathology	Interpersonal Effectiveness
Efforts to avoid loss	Social isolation, interpersonal loss, romantic breakups	
Behavioral dysregulation		
Suicide threats, parasuicidal behaviors	Suicide threats, parasuicidal behaviors	Distress Tolerance
Impulsive behaviors (e.g., drug and alcohol abuse, aggressive behaviors)	Impulsive behaviors (e.g., drug and alcohol abuse, aggressive behaviors)	
Significant functional impairment	Arrests, legal problems, jail, social and academic difficulties	
Cognitive dysregulation		
Poor problem solving	Poor problem solving, rigid thinking	Walking the Middle Path
Paranoid ideation	Academic difficulties	
Black-and-white thinking and acting	Poor parent–adolescent communication	
	Poor judgment, resulting in extreme risk taking	
Self dysregulation		
Identity confusion	Suicide contagion, media coverage	Core Mindfulness
Sense of emptiness	Unawareness of emotions	
Dissociation		

veloped for adolescents (e.g., other forms of CBT, interpersonal therapy) only deal with one major problem at a time (e.g., depression, school avoidance, interpersonal problems); in fact, they typically exclude teens who present with suicidality or multiple problems (Miller et al., 1997). DBT focuses on adolescents who have comorbid mental disorders (often excluded from treatment research studies) and who are currently suicidal (often excluded from outpatient treatment programs). DBT with adolescents employs multiple modes—concurrent individual therapy, multifamily skills training groups, family therapy as needed, between-session telephone consultations (with both teens and parents), and consultation to therapists—to achieve its numerous functions. These include increasing clients' motivation, skill acquisition, and skill generalization, and providing support and skill enhancement for therapists (to name a few). Also, DBT employs a target hierarchy; that is, the treatment is structured to address target behaviors according to their priority within each treatment mode, while at the same time allowing for flexibility within each session. For example, the therapist may begin the session by targeting a client's serious threats to commit suicide during the past week, and simultaneously addressing the binge-drinking episode related to the threats. Later in the same session, as time permits, the therapist and client may then target mood lability and episodic hopelessness. Clearly, this treatment can address a multitude of suicide risk factors for adolescents.

DBT also targets treatment noncompliance—a substantial problem with suicidal adolescents. In one study, Trautman et al. (1993) reported that 77% of adolescents who attempted suicide and presented to an emergency room subsequently failed to attend or complete traditional outpatient treatment. Other researchers have found that the average number of outpatient visits attended by adolescents who have attempted suicide is about five (Spirito et al., 1989). In addition to high treatment dropout rates, other forms of treatment noncompliance are rampant. Some adolescents attend sessions late; some are erratic with their therapy homework compliance; and some become noncollaborative during sessions, replying to all questions with "I don't know" or "I don't care." DBT is unique in its attention to such "therapy-interfering behaviors," ensuring that a therapist and client cannot overlook these behaviors when they arise.

As we will discuss later, DBT for adolescents can be adapted to target family dysfunction in addition to adolescents' individual difficulties. Many family members of suicidal multiproblem adolescents have their own problems. At a minimum, communication problems exist between parents and teens. Outpatient adolescent DBT teaches skills to family members in multifamily skills training groups or in family skills training sessions. Family therapy sessions can also be woven throughout the treatment. These often include family behavioral analyses, and they target invalidation, ineffective use of contingency management, and skills deficits (particularly in the interpersonal realm) (Miller, Glinski, Woodberry, Mitchell, & Indik, 2002; Woodberry, Miller, Glinski, Indik, & Mitchell, 2002).

DBT is a cost-effective outpatient treatment, since clients receiving this treatment typically require fewer psychiatric hospitalizations and emergency room visits (H. Fellows, personal communication, December 11, 1998; Linehan & Heard, 1999; Miller et al., 2002; Potenza, 1998). Inpatient settings that previously exhausted numerous resources on suicidal clients with BPD, because they had little to no guiding treatment philosophy, find DBT feasible and useful in providing a principle-driven treatment that offers the necessary structure (Katz et al., 2004).

Relatedly, DBT helps providers maintain a compassionate stance toward their adolescent clients and their families by employing a biosocial theory to explain the etiology and maintenance of BPD. This theoretical framework has far-reaching implications for clients and staff alike. First, inpatient milieu staff members employing this framework approach adolescents in a less judgmental manner, which inevitably provides a more therapeutic context for the adolescents' treatment. Moreover, the staff members interact more positively among themselves, which fosters a more positive work environment. Some adolescent programs indicate that they have had reductions in staff burnout after implementing DBT (Katz et al., 2004).

In sum, DBT with multiproblem suicidal adolescents makes sense, in the absence of established efficacy for any one treatment for this population. In the next chapter and throughout the rest of this book, we explain DBT and discuss its applications to work with multiproblem suicidal adolescents in a range of settings under a range of conditions.

CHAPTER 3

Dialectical Behavior Therapy
Treatment Stages, Primary Targets, and Strategies

DBT began as an application of the standard behavior therapy of the 1970s to treat suicidal individuals (Linehan, 1987a, 1987b). The basic premise of treatment was that individuals who wanted to be dead did not have the requisite skills to build a life worth living. However, in the process of developing the treatment, it quickly became apparent that a focus solely on change would not work. Many clients who attempted suicide were extremely sensitive to criticism and prone to emotion dysregulation. Efforts at helping such clients change led quickly to increased and at times overwhelming arousal. The result was often that the clients emotionally shut down—or, more rarely, stormed out of sessions or attacked their therapists. Dropping the emphasis on change, however, had equally problematic consequences. Clients interpreted this as their therapists' ignoring their palpable suffering or treating it as of little consequence. Either extreme hopelessness or rage at the therapists for apparent insensitivity often occurred. From either therapeutic stance (i.e., an exclusive focus on change or on acceptance), clients experienced their therapists as invalidating not only specific behaviors but also themselves as a whole. Research by Swann, Stein-Seroussi, and Giesler (1992) may explain how such perceived invalidation leads to problematic behavior in therapy. Their research revealed that when an individual's basic self-constructs are not verified, the individual's arousal increases. The increased arousal then leads to cognitive dysregulation and the failure to process new information.

To keep both a client and a therapist in the room working effectively on the problems at hand, the therapist had to figure out how to hold both acceptance and change in the therapy simultaneously. This synthesis, when found, could engender both new client change and new acceptance. The wish to change every painful experience had to be balanced with a corresponding effort at learning to accept life's inevitable pain. It was impossible to work on changing one set of problems if the client could not at least temporarily tolerate the pain of other problems. Without tolerance, at least for a short time, all problems converged and threatened to overwhelm both the client and the therapy. The inability to accept one's own behavior prohibits any ability to change, because it leads either to withdrawal and avoidance, or to emotional responses such as rage or intense shame. Both interfere with the observation and self-understanding necessary for effective change. Therefore, it became clear that it was as necessary for the client to hold the synthesis of acceptance and change as it was for the therapist. Although treatment of severe disorders requires the synthesis of many dialectical polarities,

This chapter is adapted from Linehan, Cochran, and Kehrer (2001). Copyright 2001 by The Guilford Press. Adapted by permission.

that of acceptance and change is the most fundamental. It was the necessity of this synthesis that led to use of the term "dialectical" as a descriptor of the standard behavior therapy applied in the treatment.

WHAT IS DBT?

A dialectical framework considers reality as continuous, dynamic, and holistic. Reality, from this perspective, is simultaneously both whole and consisting of bipolar opposites (e.g., an atom consisting of opposing positive and negative charges). Dialectical truth emerges through the combination (or "synthesis") of elements from both opposing positions (the "thesis" and "antithesis"). The tension between the thesis and antithesis within each system—positive and negative, good and bad, children and parents, client and therapist, person and environment, and so forth—and their subsequent integration are what produce change. The new state following change through synthesis however, also consists of polar forces; thus change is continuous and constitutes the essential nature of life. A very important dialectical idea is that all propositions contain within them their own oppositions. As Goldberg (1980, pp. 295–296) put it, "I assume that truth is paradoxical, that each article of wisdom contains within it its own contradictions, that truths stand side by side. Contradictory truths do not necessarily cancel each other out or dominate each other, but stand side by side, inviting participation and experimentation."

From the point of view of therapeutic dialogue and relationship, "dialectics" refers to change by persuasion and by making use of the oppositions inherent in the therapeutic relationship, rather than by formal impersonal logic. Through the therapeutic opposition of contradictory positions, both client and therapist can arrive at new meanings within old meanings, moving closer to the essence of the subject under consideration. The spirit of a dialectic point of view is never to accept a proposition as a final truth or an undisputable fact. Thus the question addressed by both client and therapist is "What is being left out of our understanding?" Dialectics as persuasion is represented in the specific dialectical strategies described a bit later in the chapter.

Dialectical Case Conceptualization

Dialectical assumptions influence case conceptualization in DBT in a number of ways. First, dialectics suggests that psychological disorders are best conceptualized as systemic dysfunctions. A systemic dysfunction is characterized by (1) defining disorder with respect to normal functioning, (2) assuming continuity between health and disorder, and (3) assuming that disorder results from multiple rather than single causes. Linehan's biosocial theory of BPD, presented below, assumes that BPD represents a breakdown in normal functioning, and that this disorder is best conceptualized as a systemic dysfunction of the emotion regulation system. The biosocial theory proposes that the pathogenesis of BPD results from numerous factors; some of these are constitutional predispositions that create individual differences in susceptibility to emotion dysregulation, while others result from the individual's interaction with the environment. Assuming a systemic view has the advantage of compelling the theorist to integrate work from a variety of fields and disciplines.

A second dialectical assumption underlying Linehan's biosocial theory of BPD is that the relationship between the individual and the environment is a transactional process, the outcome of which at any given moment depends on the nature of the transaction. Within social learning theory, this is known as the principle of "reciprocal determinism." Besides focusing on reciprocal influence, a transactional view also highlights the constant state of flux and change of the individual–environment system. Millon (1987) has made much the same point in discussing the etiology of BPD and the futility of locating the "cause" of the disorder in any single event or time period.

Both transactional and interactive models, such as the diathesis–stress model of psychopathology, call attention to the role of dysfunctional environments in bringing about disorder in the vulnerable individual. A transactional model, however, highlights a number of points that are easy to overlook in an interactive, diathesis–stress model. For example, a person (Person A) might act in a manner stressful to another individual (Person B) only because of the stress Person B is putting on Person A. For example, Person B could be a child who, due to an accident, requires most of the parents' free time just to meet survival needs—or an inpatient who, due to the need for constant suicide precautions, uses up much of the unit's nursing resources. Both of these environments are stretched in their ability to respond well to further stress. Both may invalidate Person B or temporarily "blame the victim" if any further demand on the system is made. Although the system (in these examples, the family and the therapeutic milieu) may have been predisposed to respond dysfunctionally in any case, such responses may have been avoided in the absence of exposure to the stress of that particular individual. A transactional, or dialectical, account of psychopathology may allow greater compassion because it is incompatible with the assignment of blame. This is particularly relevant with a label as stigmatized among mental health professionals as "borderline" (for examples of the misuse of the diagnosis, see Reiser & Levenson, 1984).

Theoretical Orientation to Treatment

Thus DBT's theoretical orientation to treatment is a blending of three theoretical positions: behavioral science, dialectical philosophy, and Zen practice. Behavioral science, the technology of behavior change, is countered by acceptance and tolerance of the client (with practices drawn both from Zen and from Western contemplative practice); these poles are balanced within the framework of a dialectical position. Although the term "dialectics" was first adopted as a description of this emphasis on balance, dialectics soon took on the status of guiding principles that have advanced the therapy in directions not originally anticipated. DBT is based within a consistent behaviorist theoretical position. However, the actual procedures and strategies overlap considerably with those of various alternative therapy orientations, including psychodynamic, client-centered, strategic, and cognitive therapies.

Core Elements of DBT

Core elements of DBT include the following:

1. Delineation of the functions that treatment must serve, and treatment modes to fulfill those functions (see Chapter 4, especially Table 4.1).
2. A biosocial theory of disorder that emphasizes reciprocal transactions over time between the individual and the individual's environment.
3. A developmental framework of one pretreatment and four treatment stages, with Stage 1 designed for clients with the most severe and complex problems, and subsequent stages designed for progressively less troubled clients (see Table 3.1, below).
4. Within each stage, a hierarchical prioritizing of behavioral treatment targets (see Table 3.2, below).

5. Sets of acceptance strategies, change strategies, and dialectical strategies used to achieve the behavioral targets (see Figures 3.1 and 3.2, below).
6. A dialectical framework of therapy, which emphasizes the transactional influence of client and therapist upon each other, and the importance of balancing the influence of the client on the therapist with a corresponding influence of the treatment team on the therapist (DBT is a community of therapists treating a community of clients).

A comprehensive description of each of these aspects of the treatment can be found in the original DBT treatment manuals (Linehan, 1993a, 1993b). In this chapter we discuss each of these elements with attention to their application to adolescents. To begin, it is helpful to have an overview of how standard DBT is structured. This in turn is tied to the first core element above—a delineation of treatment functions and modes.

AN OVERVIEW OF DBT PROGRAM STRUCTURE: FUNCTIONS AND MODES

The overall program structure of DBT is dictated by five essential functions that a comprehensive treatment program must fulfill: improving client motivation to change; enhancing client capabilities; generalization of new behaviors; structuring the environment; and enhancing therapist capability and motivation. The responsibility for fulfilling these functions is spread among various treatment modes, with focus and attention varying according to the mode. DBT has typically used four modes: individual therapy, group skills training, telephone consultation, and therapist consultation meetings. It is important to realize that it is not a mode itself that is critical, but its ability to address a particular function. For example, ensuring that new capabilities are generalized from therapy to a client's everyday life might be accomplished in various ways, depending on the setting. In a milieu setting, the entire staff might be taught to model, coach, and reinforce use of skills; in an outpatient setting, generalization usually occurs through telephone coaching. The individual therapist (who is always the primary therapist in DBT), together with the client, is responsible for organizing the treatment so that all functions are met. For a full discussion of functions and modes, see Chapter 4.

DBT'S BIOSOCIAL THEORY

DBT theorizes that the behaviors of suicidal/self-injurious clients with BPD and multiple other problems stem from a combination of biological and environmental factors. Specifically, these factors are emotion dysregulation (which is most likely biological in origin), and invalidating environments (where inadequate emotion regulation coaching and dysfunctional learning take place)—hence the term "biosocial" theory. This theory appears highly relevant to adolescents who may not meet full criteria for BPD but have borderline features, who engage in suicidal behaviors, and who suffer from numerous other problems.

Emotion Dysregulation

Linehan's biosocial theory suggests that BPD criterion behaviors, and suicidal behaviors in particular, are primarily due to pervasive dysfunctions in the emotion regulation system. Although the mechanisms of the initial vulnerability to dysregulation remain unclear, it is probable that biological factors play a primary role. The etiology of this initial vulnerability may range from genetic influences, to prenatal factors, to traumatic childhood events affecting development of the brain and nervous system.

Borderline behavioral patterns are functionally related to, or are unavoidable consequences of, this fundamental dysregulation across several (perhaps all) emotions, including both positive and negative emotions. From the perspective of DBT, this emotional dysfunction is the core pathology, and thus is neither simply symptomatic or definitional. This systemic dysregulation is produced by emotional vulnerability combined with difficulties in modulating emotional reactions. "Emotional vulnerability" is conceptualized as high sensitivity to emotional stimuli, intense emotional responses, and a slow return to emotional baseline. Deficits in emotion modulation include difficulties in (1) inhibiting mood-dependent dysfunctional behaviors; (2) organizing behavior in the service of goals, independent of current mood; (3) increasing or decreasing physiological arousal as needed; (4) distracting attention from emotionally evocative stimuli; and/or (5) experiencing emotion without either immediately withdrawing or producing an extreme secondary negative emotion (for further discussion, see Linehan, 1993a; Lynch, Chapman, Rosenthal, Kuo, & Linehan, 2006).

Invalidating Environments

Most individuals with an initial temperamental vulnerability to intense emotionality do not develop BPD. Thus the theory further suggests that particular developmental environments are necessary. The crucial developmental circumstances in Linehan's theory are "invalidating environments" (Linehan, 1987a, 1987b, 1989, 1993a). An invalidating environment is defined by the tendency to negate and/or respond erratically and inappropriately to private experiences, particularly to private experiences not accompanied by easily interpreted public accompaniments (e.g., feeling sick without having a high temperature). Private experiences, and especially emotional experiences and interpretations of events, are often not taken as valid responses to events; are punished, trivialized, dismissed, or disregarded; and/or are attributed to socially unacceptable characteristics, such as overreactivity, inability to see things realistically, lack of motivation, motivation to harm or manipulate, lack of discipline, or failure to adopt a positive (or, conversely, discriminating) attitude. Clients' verbal descriptions are often viewed as inaccurate descriptions of their private experiences (e.g., "You are so angry but won't admit it"). Invalidating environments emphasize controlling emotional expressiveness, oversimplify the ease of solving problems, and are intolerant of displays of negative affect. Emotional pain is attributed to lack of motivation, discipline, or effort. Individuals in an invalidating environment also tend to use punishment in their efforts to control behavior. Such a scenario exacerbates the emotional vulnerability and consequent emotion dysregulation of multiproblem individuals with BPD or borderline features, and their behavioral responses reciprocally influence their invalidating environments.

High rates of childhood abuse and trauma are reported among this population (Grilo, Sanislow, Fehon, Marino, & McGlashan, 1999; Sabo, 1997; Paris, 1997), suggesting that abuse, including sexual abuse, may be a prototypical invalidating experience for children. (Note also that research suggests a direct effect of early abusive experiences on emotion dysregulation, suggesting an additional pathway from childhood trauma to borderline personality features; see, e.g., Teicher, 2002.) More recent research, however, suggests that negative affect intensity/reactivity may be a stronger predictor of BPD symptoms than childhood sexual abuse, and that higher thought suppression may mediate the relationship between BPD symptoms and childhood sexual abuse (Rosenthal, Lynch, & Linehan, 2005). The transactional nature of the biosocial theory implies that individuals may develop borderline patterns of behavior via very different routes. Despite only moderate vulnerability to emotion dysregulation, a sufficiently invalidating environment may produce BPD patterns; conversely, even a "normal" level of invalidation may be sufficient to create BPD patterns for those who are highly vulnerable to emotion dysregulation (Koerner, & Linehan, 1997). Thus the relationship of early sexual abuse to BPD is still open to various interpretations (see, e.g., Silk, Lee, Hill, & Lohr, 1995; Fossati, Madeddu, & Maffei, 1999).

Although invalidating environments clearly prove maladaptive for children with extreme emotional sensitivity, it is noteworthy that such environments may arise despite the perfectly benign intentions of family members, or may even be present outside the family. Many factors can lead to invalidating family environments. For example, excessive and chronic stress on a family may simply tax the emotional resources of parents and leave them with little patience for attending to and seeking to understand a highly emotional child. Relatedly, the reciprocal interplay of biology and environment is continually operating, such that having a highly emotionally sensitive and reactive child in itself can place formidable stress on a "normal" family system, perhaps causing a "typically stressed" family to become "overstressed." Another scenario is the "perfect family," where children not only control their emotions effectively but also fit the mold of their parents' expectations vis-à-vis behavioral styles, skills, interests, and gender role identity. When one of the children in such a setting breaks this mold and demonstrates unique interests, talents, temperament, or needs, otherwise well-meaning parents may become invalidating out of confusion, lack of understanding, or simply an effort to redirect the child onto the "proper" path. Yet another scenario involves parents who themselves received severe invalidation from caretakers and thus simply never learned to validate or even tolerate emotional displays. Such parents, though again perhaps well-meaning, often themselves lack the skills repertoire to help children modulate emotions effectively. Finally, there is the chaotic family: Parents themselves may misuse substances; experience severe depression or anxiety; engage in self-harming or suicidal behaviors; sexually abuse their children; and/or be unable to work, maintain adequate housing, or protect their children from abuse by others. The ability of such a family to provide the nurturing and learning environment an emotionally vulnerable child needs is compromised in the extreme. Understanding the manifold potential sources of invalidation is particularly important in DBT with adolescents and their family members, so that the therapist can hold onto the nonjudgmental assumption that all clients are doing their best and can avoid maligning the parents.

In addition, a pervasively invalidating environment can occur outside the family context. For example, characteristics of a school or neighborhood setting may prove a strong mismatch for the temperament of an emotionally sensitive child. Difficulties with acculturation may also play a role, as new immigrants or children of immigrants strive to adapt to a new cultural environment and community.

Regardless of its source, the overall results of the transactional pattern between emotion dysregulation and the invalidating environment are the emotional and behavioral patterns exhibited by the adult with BPD or borderline characteristics. Such an individual has never learned how to label and regulate emotional arousal, how to tolerate emotional distress, or when to trust his or her own emotional responses as reflections of valid interpretations of events (Linehan, 1993a). In more optimal environments, public validation of a person's private, internal experiences results in the development of a stable identity. In an invalidating environment, however, an individual's private experiences are responded to erratically and with insensitivity. The individual thus learns to mistrust his or her internal states, and instead scans the environment for cues about how to act, think, or feel. This general reliance on others results in the individual's failure to develop a coherent sense of self. Emotion dysregulation also interferes with the development and maintenance of stable interpersonal relationships, which depend on both a stable sense of self and a capacity to self-regulate emotions. Moreover, the invalidating environment's tendency to trivialize or ignore the expression of negative emotion shapes an expressive style later seen in the adult with BPD or borderline features—a style that vacillates between inhibition and suppression of emotional experience and extreme behavioral displays. Behaviors such as overdosing, cutting, and burning have important affect-regulating properties and are additionally quite effective in eliciting helping behaviors from an environment that otherwise ignores efforts to ameliorate intense emotional pain. From this perspective, the dysfunctional behaviors characteristic of BPD can be viewed as maladaptive solutions to overwhelming, intensely painful negative affect.

Linehan (1993a) has described behavioral patterns that often interfere with effective therapy as falling on three bipolar dimensions. Vacillation between the opposing extremes of these behavioral dimensions is commonly observed in therapy, often as a result of changes in emotional intensity. Suicidal behaviors can be understood at either end of these continua—reflecting, for example, self-directed hostility at one end or an escape from extreme despair at the other end. DBT defines these behavior patterns as "dialectical dilemmas" and identifies them as secondary targets of treatment (Linehan, 1993a). DBT seeks to move clients away from these behavioral extremes and toward more balanced, synthesized behavior. The three behavioral dimensions expressed as dialectical dilemmas are (1) unrelenting crisis versus inhibited grieving, (2) emotional vulnerability versus self-invalidation, and (3) active passivity versus apparent competence. These dialectical dilemmas can be seen as a framework within which the primary therapy targets (discussed next) are achieved. In Chapter 5 we discuss how these three behavioral patterns appear in therapy with adolescents. We also then describe three new dialectical dilemmas specific to adolescents and their families.

Linehan, and behaviorists in general, take "behavior" to mean anything an organism does involving action and responding to stimulation (*Webster's New Universal Unabridged Dictionary*, 1983, p. 100). Conventionally, behaviorists categorize behavior as motor, cognitive/verbal, and physiological, all of which may be either public or private. There are several points to make here. First, the division of behavior into these three categories is arbitrary and is done here for conceptual clarity, rather than in response to evidence that these response modes actually are functionally separate systems. This point is especially relevant to understanding emotion regulation, given that basic research on emotions demonstrates that these response systems often overlap; they are somewhat, but definitely not wholly, independent. A related point here is that in contrast to biological and cognitive theories of BPD, biosocial theory suggests that there is no a priori reason for favoring explanations emphasizing one mode of behavior as intrinsically more important or compelling than others. Rather, from a biosocial perspective, the crucial question is under what conditions a given behavior–environment, behavior–behavior, or response system–response system relationship does hold, and under what conditions such a relationship enters causal pathways for the etiology and maintenance of BPD.

DBT'S STAGES OF THERAPY AND TREATMENT GOALS

DBT is conceptualized as occurring in four stages that match levels of severity and complexity of problems. An additional pretreatment stage prepares the client and therapist for work together and elicits a commitment from each to work toward the various treatment goals. Stage 1 of therapy is designed for an individual at the most severe and complex levels of BPD. Its primary focus is on stabilizing the client and achieving behavioral control. The major studies of DBT for BPD to date have focused on the severely and multiply disordered client who enters treatment at Stage 1, and this book also focuses on Stage 1 treatment. As clients become more and more functional, DBT increasingly resembles standard behavior therapy. DBT Stages 2–4 have the following treatment goals: to replace "quiet desperation" with non-traumatic emotional experiencing (Stage 2); to achieve "ordinary" happiness and unhappiness, and reduce ongoing disorders and problems in living (Stage 3); and to resolve a sense of incompleteness and achieve freedom and capacity for joy (Stage 4) (see Table 3.1). In sum, the orientation of the treatment is first toward getting the client's actions under control, then toward helping the client to feel better and to resolve problems in living, and finally toward helping the client to find joy and perhaps even a sense of transcendence.

The criteria for putting a client in Stage 1 are a high level of current disorder and the inability to realistically accomplish other goals before behavior and functioning come under better control. Level of disorder is determined by the severity and pervasiveness of problems, the disability or dysfunction that problems cause in daily activities, and the threat they pose to life (see Linehan, 1999). Individuals with both severe and pervasive problems that are either disabling (e.g., ones that keep the individuals out of school or necessary work; result in homelessness, loss of friends, and/or loss of close family members; and/or lead to treatment in emergency departments or inpatient units) or life-threatening (e.g., recent or current suicidality, life-threatening aggression toward others) are considered in need of Stage 1 treatment. Stage 1 DBT targets the reduction of out-of-control behavior patterns associated with severe and pervasive disorders, particularly behaviors associated with high risk of death. As Mintz (1968) suggested in discussing treatment of the suicidal client, all forms of psychotherapy are ineffective with a dead client. The same can be said of the individual who drops out of treatment. The adaptation of DBT for adolescents described in this book focuses primarily on Stage 1 targets.

Pretreatment Stage Targets: Orientation and Commitment to Treatment

In DBT, the specific tasks of the pretreatment stage are twofold. First, the client and therapist must arrive at a mutually informed decision to work together. Typically, the first session (or

---

TABLE 3.1. Hierarchy of Standard DBT Stages and Stage Targets

Pretreatment stage

Targets: Orientation and commitment to treatment
        Agreement on goals

Stage 1

Targets: 1. Decreasing life-threatening behaviors
        2. Decreasing therapy-interfering behaviors
        3. Decreasing quality-of-life interfering behaviors
        4. Increasing behavioral skills

Stage 2

Target: 5. Decreasing posttraumatic stress

Stage 3

Targets: 6. Increasing respect for self
        7. Achieving individual goals

Stage 4

Targets: 8. Resolving a sense of incompleteness
        9. Finding freedom and joy

Note. Adapted by permission from Linehan (1993a). Copyright 1993 by The Guilford Press. Adapted by permission.

more if needed) is presented as an opportunity for the client and therapist to explore this possibility. Diagnostic interviewing, history taking, and formal behavioral analyses of high-priority targeted behaviors can be woven into these initial therapy sessions or conducted separately. Second, the client and therapist must negotiate a common set of expectancies to guide the initial steps of therapy.

Agreements outlining specifically what client and therapist can expect from each other are discussed and agreed to. If the client has dysfunctional beliefs regarding the process of therapy, the therapist attempts to modify these. Issues addressed include the goals of treatment and general treatment procedures, how long therapy may last, what outcomes can reasonably be expected, and various myths the client may have about the process of therapy in general. A dialectical/biosocial view of the client's primary disorder is also presented.

Orientation covers several additional points. First, DBT is presented as a supportive therapy requiring a strong collaborative relationship between client and therapist. DBT is presented as a life enhancement program, where client and therapist function as a team to create a life worth living, rather than as a suicide prevention program. Second, DBT is described as a form of CBT with a primary emphasis on analyzing and replacing problematic behaviors with skillful behaviors. Third, the client is told that DBT is a skills-oriented therapy, with special emphasis on behavioral skill training. The commitment and orienting strategies, balanced by validation strategies (described later), are the most important strategies during this phase of treatment. In Chapter 7 we provide a detailed discussion of applying the pretreatment orientation and commitment strategies to adolescents and families. These pretreatment targets are an important part of DBT for adolescents.

Stage 1 Treatment Targets: Attaining Basic Capacities

The focus of Stage 1 of DBT is on attaining a life pattern that is reasonably functional and stable. In order for the client to attain such a life pattern, the therapist and client work toward four primary behavioral targets. "Targets" in DBT consist of making changes in sets of behaviors that are explicitly identified as needing such changes, typically through collaboration of therapist and client. These behaviors are prioritized for addressing in session, and are approached hierarchically and recursively as higher-priority behaviors reappear. Listed in order of importance, the four Stage 1 targets are (1) decreasing life-threatening behaviors, (2) decreasing therapy-interfering behaviors, (3) decreasing quality-of-life interfering behaviors, and (4) increasing behavioral skills.

DBT defines the four kinds of primary target behaviors very specifically. Clients are asked to monitor and record any occurrence of these primary target behaviors on DBT "diary cards," and to bring the cards with them to individual and skills training sessions. Routine review of diary cards helps keep both client and therapist focused on the primary targets. The discussion that follows reviews the primary target behaviors in detail, and examines what those behaviors typically look like in adolescents. Table 3.2 provides an overview list of DBT pretreatment and Stage 1 goals with adolescent-oriented specifics.

Decreasing Life-Threatening Behaviors

Many adolescents with BPD or borderline personality features make repeated suicide attempts, engage in other behaviors that may pose a risk to life (e.g., participating in gang violence; failing to take essential life-sustaining medications), engage in repeated NSIB, communicate suicidal ideation, or report suicide-related expectancies or affect. A smaller subgroup may also engage in homicidal ideation and behavior. Everything discussed below regarding

TABLE 3.2. Pretreatment and Stage 1 Treatment Targets Applied to Adolescents

Pretreatment stage

Targets: Informing adolescent about, and orienting adolescent to, DBT
         Informing adolescent's family about, and orienting family to, DBT
         Securing adolescent's commitment to treatment
         Securing adolescent's family's commitment to treatment
         Securing therapist's commitment to treatment

Stage 1

Targets: Decreasing life-threatening behaviors
- Suicidal/homicidal crisis behaviors
- Suicide attempts
- Attempted murder
- NSIB
- Suicidal ideation or communication
- Suicide-related expectancies
- Homicide-related expectancies
- Suicide-related affect
- Homicide-related affect

Decreasing therapy-interfering behaviors
- By the adolescent
- By the therapist
- By participating family members

Decreasing behaviors that interfere with quality of life
- High-risk, impulsive behaviors (e.g., driving fast or while drunk, HIV-related behaviors)
- Dysfunctional interpersonal interactions
- Substance-abuse-related behaviors
- School problems (e.g., nonattendance, school failure)
- Antisocial behaviors
- Impulsive behaviors
- Problems maintaining physical health

Increasing behavioral skills
- Interpersonal skills
- Distress tolerance skills
- Emotion regulation skills
- Core mindfulness skills
- Walking the middle path skills

---

decreasing life-threatening behaviors is equally applicable to homicidality as it is to suicidality. As mentioned above, DBT targets specific categories of suicidal behavior that include both certain and ambivalent suicide attempts, NSIB, suicidal ideation and communication, or other cognitions and emotions related to suicide. Although not all life-threatening behaviors are accompanied by intent to die, they are nevertheless included in the category of life-threatening behaviors for reasons given below. In-depth discussions of the rationale for each of these categories appear in Linehan (1993a).

Suicide Crisis Behaviors

Suicide crisis behaviors are those behaviors that suggest imminent danger to the client. These include, but are not limited to, threats of imminent suicidal intent, attaining lethal means (e.g., access to a gun or large supply of medications), preparations for suicide (e.g., leaving a note, giving away possessions, saying goodbye to people), or indirect messages about suicidal intention (e.g., statements such as "I won't be here then"). With new clients in particular, the therapist should always err on the conservative side in assessing and acting upon suicidal crisis behaviors. And with adolescents in particular, the therapist must remain vigilant to such signs—as teens sometimes have not brought themselves in for treatment, may not initially view their suicidal behaviors as a treatment target, and may not be forthright with this information.

Self-Injurious Behaviors

The central reason for including all self-injurious acts under the category of life-threatening behaviors, even in the absence of suicidal intent, is that self-injury is one of the best predictors of eventual suicide. Risk of suicide increases 50–100 times within the first 12 months after an episode of self-injury, compared to the general population risk (Cooper et al., 2005). Approximately one-half of persons who die by suicide have a history of self-injury, and this proportion increases to two-thirds in younger age groups (Appleby et al., 1999).

Other reasons for targeting NSIB include the fact that any act of deliberate self-injury is simply antithetical to the most basic goal of *any* psychotherapy, which is to work toward helping rather than injuring the client. It would be hard for a therapist to convey true caring and compassion if the therapist is sending the message that acts of intentional self-injury need not be addressed. Finally, self-injurious acts such as self-cutting often leave the body permanently scarred and pose a risk of accidental death.

We have found at times that it is difficult to get commitment from adolescents to work on reducing self-injurious behaviors. Not only are many wedded to NSIB because of its functions (e.g., it is often negatively reinforcing by reducing emotional pain); we have also seen clients, particularly in our suburban middle-class population, who are embedded in a high school subculture in which various forms of self-mutilation are normative and even prized. For example, some teens who scar themselves with razors also get tattoos and have multiple body piercings. They may have friends who share these behaviors and thus become accustomed to practically wearing their scars as badges of honor, representing suffering, pain (or perhaps tolerance of pain), and bravery. One high school senior believed that her scars from self-cutting legitimized her emotional pain to her friends—proving that she was not just a crybaby or a whiner, but in the "big leagues" of sufferers. This same teen repeatedly begged her mother for a tattoo, which she believed would further mark her as belonging to a certain group of "cool" but long-suffering youth (she finally got herself a tattoo upon turning 18). At an age where peer approval is critically important, we have seen adolescents who are clearly reinforced for their self-injurious behavior with the acceptance, sympathy, or "oohs and ahs" of their friends. Thus, as part of behavioral analysis, it is crucial for the therapist to assess peer-related antecedents and consequences.

Suicidal Ideation or Communication

DBT also targets clients' thoughts of suicide or communications about suicide, as these are reported either on the diary card, in session, on the telephone, or to friends, family members, or personnel. Suicidal thoughts might be related to planning, imagining, or expecting to commit suicide. Some clients have waxing and waning urges to die or to hurt themselves. These urges generally tend to be linked to the belief that these actions will supply a way out of their misery. Many threaten suicide repeatedly. Planning to commit, fantasizing about committing, expecting to commit, expressing the urge to commit, and threatening to commit suicide are all targeted directly by conducting behavioral analyses (see Chapter 8). Some teens may express extreme angst through listening to music that has self-harming, depressive, or apocalyptic themes. Thus adolescent self-report or parent report of such behavior must be taken seriously and assessed for its significance to the adolescent. (Fortunately, there is a recent trend for lyrics to attempt to alleviate adolescents' alienation and despair, as in the hit song "Hold On" by the band Good Charlotte; see Azerrad, 2004.)

Suicidal ideation may or may not be targeted as a life-threatening behavior. When it is associated with suicidal intent or planning, when it increases or is new, when it relates to engaging in self-injurious behaviors, or when it inhibits adaptive coping, it is addressed directly. However, at times suicidal ideation becomes a habitual way of thinking, is low-level and stable, and is not linked to any self-injury or other risk behaviors or states of mind. If the adolescent experiences this type of suicidal ideation, it does not get treated as a primary target unless there is a significant increase from an ongoing stable pattern. Note that making such a determination necessitates ongoing assessment of suicidality, as well as familiarity with a client's characteristic ideation regarding suicide and the triggers that commonly elicit suicidal ideation. Early in treatment, the therapist should err on the side of targeting such ideation directly.

Suicide-Related Expectancies

Suicide-related expectancies are the beliefs clients hold about what suicide or self-injurious acts will do for them. Such expectancies often relate to escaping misery or eliminating one's perceived role of being a burden to others. They also often involve notions about relief from intensely painful emotional states through distraction from chronic or transient difficult life circumstances; attaining temporary solace (e.g., going to sleep after overdosing); achieving desired responsiveness from others; hurting, upsetting, or "showing" others; being taken seriously by others; or gaining a desired admission to a hospital. Adolescents may be socially isolated and believe that a suicidal act will gain the attention of peers, or may be feeling rejected by a peer group or boyfriend/girlfriend and believe that suicide will gain the attention of these others or teach them a lesson.

As with suicidal ideation and communication, the therapist targets suicide-related expectancies when they relate to suicidal risk behaviors or impede skillful problem solving. Useful areas to assess include the client's expectancies about *positive and negative* outcomes of suicide or self-injury, as well as beliefs about the utility of alternative, adaptive coping options. For example, one intermittently suicidal adolescent expressed the belief that killing herself would devastate important people in her life (her parents, boyfriend, and certain close friends). In contrast to adolescents for whom upsetting others is a motivating factor in suicide, this girl believed that the extent of pain she would inflict on others by killing herself was reason enough not to do it. Thus focusing on these relationships became an important strategy in coping with her suicidal thinking.

Suicide-Related Affect

Like suicidal thoughts, communications, and expectancies, suicide-related affect is targeted directly only when it intensifies or when it is linked to suicidal crisis behaviors, self-injurious behaviors, or impairment in effective problem solving. Affective states are generally linked to suicidal behaviors/NSIB in one of two ways. First, acts of self-injury (or even plans to commit or images of committing such acts) often bring relief or escape from painful emotions, such as anger, depression, shame, or anxiety. Second, NSIB may be accompanied by positive affective states, such as feelings of calm, relaxation, eager anticipation, and pleasure. Such affective links to NSIB thus serve as one mechanism by which such acts get negatively or positively reinforced.

Decreasing Therapy-Interfering Behaviors

Suicidal adolescents with BPD or borderline characteristics share with their adult counterparts a tendency to experience repeated therapy failures, mostly because of their tendency to drop out of treatment prematurely (Trautman et al., 1993). Dropout, noncompliance, and other treatment-interfering behaviors by clients are seen often in the beginning stages of therapy with teens, as often they are brought in unwillingly by parents rather than having decided themselves to initiate therapy. In addition, they may be reluctant to share their therapy with family members (inclusion of family members is important in treating adolescents; we discuss it in detail later). Treatment-interfering behaviors also include motivational difficulties that impede progress; relational or other behavioral difficulties that burn out the therapist or the client and reduce the therapist's motivation to treat or the client's motivation to participate in therapy; a client's acting in ways that punish effective therapist behaviors and reinforce ineffective therapist behaviors; or a therapist's acting in ways that punish effective client behaviors and reinforce ineffective client behaviors.

Thus, second only to life-threatening behaviors, DBT places paramount emphasis on client and therapist behaviors that interfere with the success or continuation of therapy. (In DBT for adolescents, family members' therapy-interfering behaviors are also targeted as necessary; see below.) The target of decreasing therapy-interfering behaviors supersedes targets related to the client's quality of life, since if therapy is failing or on the brink of termination, discussion of these other issues becomes irrelevant. Put simply, a client who is not receiving therapy can obviously no longer benefit from therapy.

Client Therapy-Interfering Behaviors

Client behaviors that interfere with therapy include (1) behaviors that interfere with receiving therapy, (2) behaviors that interfere with other clients, and (3) behaviors that burn out the therapist.

Client behaviors that interfere with receiving therapy include behaviors that interfere with *attending* therapy, behaviors that interfere with *being attentive in the therapy session,* *noncollaborative* behaviors, and *noncompliant* behaviors. Examples of behaviors that interfere with attending therapy include repeated or prolonged hospitalizations (this also constitutes a quality-of-life-interfering behavior), canceling sessions, experiencing crises that disrupt therapy, or arriving to sessions late or leaving early. With adolescents, behaviors that interfere with therapy attendance can be complicated by parental factors. For example, some adolescents may need to come late, leave early, or miss sessions altogether because of parents' busy schedules or unreliability. Yet it is important to remember that, regardless of what caused a therapy-interfering behavior, it is still therapy-interfering behavior. Thus, in cases in which family or caregiver factors played a role, adolescents are neither blamed nor "let off the hook." Instead, problem-solving strategies are applied that emphasize ways to get to therapy even if a family member is unavailable. That is, part of coping effectively, particularly for adolescents living in chaotic home environments, entails flexible and advanced planning for attending therapy sessions. This might involve coaching an adolescent on effectively communicating to a parent about the importance of arriving to therapy on time, developing alternative transportation plans, or knowing when not to rely on an unreliable caretaker.

Examples of behaviors that interfere with being attentive in the therapy session include coming to a session under the influence of drugs or alcohol, being excessively tired in session, dissociating in session, or experiencing a panic attack or other extreme emotional states that interfere with participating in the session. We have noticed that adolescents in particular display behaviors that interfere with being attentive during group skills training sessions. Teenagers are highly distractible; easily engage with rather than ignore disruptive peer behaviors; and are prone to passing notes, doodling, giggling, flirting, and impulsively shouting out comments. Such behaviors are typically handled by skills trainers, but if they persist, they can also be addressed with a behavioral analysis by the primary therapist in the individual session. Chapter 10 details these issues.

Noncollaborative behaviors also interfere with receiving therapy; these involve breaches in the agreement on the goals, strategies, or procedures of therapy. They include such behaviors as not working or talking in therapy, arguing with or challenging the therapist repeatedly, failing to stick to the therapy targets, lying to the therapist, minimizing ratings on the diary card, or giving repeatedly vague or evasive answers to therapist questions. Adolescents who repeatedly respond with "I don't know," "I don't care," or "You got me" fall into this last category. Client behaviors that interfere with receiving therapy also include *noncompliant* behaviors. These include not bringing in or filling out diary cards, not completing homework assignments, not keeping agreements with the therapist, not engaging in session or group activities (e.g., role-playing new skills), or otherwise not participating in the treatment process. A common example is not calling the therapist before engaging in self-injurious behavior or not calling the therapist at times scheduled for phone consultation contacts.

Behaviors that interfere with other clients also fall under the rubric of client therapy-interfering behaviors. These behaviors may occur in connection with either individual or group sessions. In the context of an individual session, they may include engaging in behaviors that keep other clients from beginning their sessions on time, behaving loudly or explosively in session so that other clients hear the disturbance, or behaving in or around the clinic in ways that disturb other clients (e.g., some of our more rambunctious adolescents have been known to run down the clinic hallway shrieking and laughing loudly on their way out for their break). Such behaviors may also occur in group. These may involve threatening other group members or making hostile remarks to them; being disrespectful or openly judgmental of group members as they participate in group; inducing other clients to engage in destructive behaviors or behaviors incompatible with DBT agreements; or otherwise interfering with other clients' sense of comfort in, progress in, or compliance with therapy. The issue of inducing other clients to engage in destructive or non-DBT behaviors applies particularly to adolescents, who respond strongly to peer pressure. For example, the adolescents in our suburban population typically disperse during break time to use the restroom, get snacks, or smoke cigarettes just outside the clinic door. One evening the adolescents were nowhere to be found at the end of the group break. When one therapist went to search for them, she found them in the clinic parking lot—crowded into the car of one of the adolescents, blasting music, and smoking. The adolescent who drove the car had encouraged the others to spend the break there, which violated two agreements: (1) where the adolescents were expected to spend their break (i.e., in safe proximity to the group room), and (2) when they were supposed to return. As a therapy-interfering behavior, such a digression would typically be handled in two ways. The first would be for the skills trainers to address it immediately, by clarifying expectations about how and where to spend break, and obtaining a commitment to abide by these expectations. Depending on the overall context, group leaders might also skillfully express their feelings about the problematic behavior and make a request for specific behavior change (modeling interpersonal effectiveness skills taught in the skills group), or they might conduct a miniature behavioral analysis of the digression, with a rapid move to generating solutions and obtaining commitment. The second way would be for it to be addressed as a therapy-interfering behavior by a behavioral analysis within the next individual therapy session, provided that there was no target higher on the hierarchy to address during that session (the individual therapist would be informed of the problem during team consultation; see Chapter 8 on conducting a behavioral analysis).

Finally, behaviors that burn out the therapist are addressed within the category of client therapy-interfering behaviors. These include behaviors that exceed the therapist's personal limits (e.g., calling too frequently, repeatedly demanding extra session time); behaviors that push organizational limits (e.g., behaviors that threaten the program's existence in a particular setting); behaviors that decrease the therapist's motivation (e.g., hostile insults to the therapist, lack of progress toward goals); and behaviors that reduce milieu staff members' or group members' motivation (i.e., behaviors that reduce the motivation of others in the client's environment to care for the client).

Family Therapy-Interfering Behaviors

When working with adolescents, we include family members in treatment (see Chapter 9). Thus situations sometimes arise in which family members themselves engage in therapy-interfering behaviors. This provides a challenge, since the parents are not the clients per se and do not have the ongoing individual therapy format in which this might be addressed. The remaining chapters have woven through them discussions of how to handle family members' therapy-interfering behaviors as they pertain to orientation and commitment, individual therapy and family sessions, skills training sessions, and crisis situations. As a general rule, however, when a family member's therapy-interfering behavior also becomes therapy-interfering for the adolescent (e.g., not driving the teen to session, not permitting the teen to use the phone for *in vivo* coaching), the behavior also becomes a target for the adolescent's own session. This is because regardless of the fact that the adolescent may not have caused the behavior, problem solving must nevertheless occur to preserve the adolescent's participation in effective therapy.

Therapist Therapy-Interfering Behaviors

Therapist behaviors that interfere with therapy are just as important as client behaviors that interfere with therapy. The two main classes of therapist behaviors that can impede therapy are becoming nondialectical and engaging in behaviors that convey a lack of respect for the client. Examples of becoming nondialectical involve becoming imbalanced, such as being too acceptance- or too change-focused, or being too flexible or too rigid. Examples of showing disrespect to adolescents are talking in a condescending manner (e.g., using a formal or authoritarian "doctor-to-client" air), or releasing information and getting the "necessary" consent from parent but not "sufficient" consent from the adolescent.

Usually, becoming imbalanced or failing to convey respect to the client results from understandable conditions within the therapy or within the therapist's life outside the therapy. It is the role of the therapist consultation team to validate and support the therapist while helping him or her problem-solve to regain the balance needed for DBT. In DBT, clients are encouraged to bring up in session any behaviors on the part of the therapist that they experience as therapy-interfering. For adolescents, granting such permission is especially empowering and rewarding, and conveys a level of respect that they may perceive as rarely coming from adults.

Decreasing Behaviors that Interfere with Quality of Life

Suicidal clients often engage in a host of behaviors that, although not directly life-threatening, relate to maintaining a life of misery and interfere with building a life worth living. For adolescents, these behaviors may include the following: dysfunctional interpersonal relationship interactions (e.g., staying in abusive relationships, alienating caregivers); school- or work-related dysfunctional behaviors (e.g., cutting classes, failing exams or courses, being fired from an after-school job); impulsive behaviors (e.g., anger outbursts, promiscuous or unprotected sex); substance-abuse-related behaviors (e.g., driving while intoxicated); antisocial behaviors (e.g., violence, gang membership); mental-health-related dysfunctional behaviors (e.g., repeated hospitalizations, emergency room visits); other Axis I or Axis II diagnostic features (e.g., depression, social phobia); problems in maintaining physical health (e.g., not following medication regimens, such as insulin for clients with diabetes); and behaviors that interfere with long-term goals (e.g., extreme behavioral passivity, dropping out of high school, getting pregnant).

For a therapist working with an adolescent, targeting quality-of-life-interfering behaviors often requires a judgment call. For example, marijuana or alcohol use can clearly interfere with a teen's quality of life and relate to a pattern of risk behavior or other dysfunction. On the other hand, it is developmentally normative for adolescents to experiment with drugs and alcohol (see Chapter 5). Thus, with ambiguous behavior patterns, the therapist will need to assess whether the behavior seems extreme (e.g., addiction to heroin and selling drugs in high school to support the habit, as opposed to trying marijuana at a party); whether it relates to other risk patterns (e.g., getting drunk and then driving); whether it interferes with therapy (e.g., causing the teen to miss many therapy sessions in a row); or whether it threatens life (e.g., predictably precipitating a suicide attempt). Thus the therapist's task becomes both determining whether a behavior merits analysis as a target or not, and determining where in the hierarchy of targets a behavior falls. For example, a therapist might target a high-risk sexual practice (e.g., sex without using a condom, sex with multiple partners) as a behavior that threatens quality of life (e.g., it may result in an unwanted pregnancy or contraction of a nonfatal sexually transmitted disease), or may be tempted to target it as a behavior that threatens life itself (e.g., it may lead to contracting HIV). Note, however, that generally the classification of life-threatening behaviors is limited to those risk behaviors that involve *intentional* self-injury or that have realistic, *imminent* threat to life (thus behavior with risk of contracting HIV would not qualify).

Therefore, even though behaviors such as drunk driving and promiscuous sex could prove fatal, they would usually still be categorized under quality-of-life-interfering behaviors. In work with adolescents, therapists sometimes tend to move up the priority of such targets in response to the parents' urgings to do so. In addition, the therapist's own values will inevitably have some influence on the degree to which he or she will address certain behaviors, and may influence where he or she will place certain behaviors within the target hierarchy. It will be beneficial for the therapist to try to be aware of the role his or her values are playing in identifying behavioral targets, and to attempt to find the middle way between an overly lax and an overly conservative position. When in doubt, the therapist should bring these questions to the therapist consultation group. In addition, for ambiguous behavior patterns, the therapist will want to work collaboratively with the client to determine where these behaviors should be placed on the hierarchy. In general, the therapist will need to remember to assess carefully whether the behavior in question actually interferes with the adolescent's life quality, interferes with therapy, or threatens life, rather than blithely making assumptions. Behaviors deemed less harmful or serious (e.g., ordinary relationship conflict, ambivalence over career choice) are treated in later stages of DBT.

Increasing Behavioral Skills

As part of the aim of building a life worth living by reducing the aforementioned target behaviors, DBT simultaneously targets increasing behavioral skills. The skills training group provides the main forum for the acquisition and strengthening of these skills, while individual therapy helps clients to generalize the skills to the situations they encounter in their lives.

The skills taught in DBT correspond directly to the DBT conceptualization of the DSM-IV-TR BPD criteria. According to this conceptualization, these criteria fall into areas of dysregulation across several domains. DBT for adolescents maintains this conceptualization, even if an adolescent does not meet full criteria for BPD. The areas of dysregulation and the corresponding skills modules follow:

1. Interpersonal dysregulation: Interpersonal Effectiveness Skills
2. Behavioral and cognitive dysregulation: Distress Tolerance Skills
3. Emotion dysregulation: Emotion Regulation Skills
4. Self dysregulation: Core Mindfulness Skills

For adolescents and their families, in addition to these specific skills, we have developed a fifth module (Walking the Middle Path Skills) to address unbalanced thinking and behaviors. (This is discussed in Chapter 10; see also Appendices B and C.)

In the Chapter 4 we take a more detailed look at each treatment mode, including skills training, and discuss how it addresses Stage 1 treatment targets. As we will see, each mode addresses Stage 1 targets, but the hierarchy of those targets shifts according to the mode's function. The following section describes the various treatment strategies employed in DBT.

DBT TREATMENT STRATEGIES

"Treatment strategies" in DBT are coordinated sets of procedures used to achieve specific treatment goals. Although DBT strategies usually consist of a number of steps, use of a strategy does not necessarily require the application of every step. It is considerably more important that the therapist apply the intent of the strategy, rather than inflexibly leading the client through a series of prescribed maneuvers.

DBT employs five sets of treatment strategies to achieve the previously described behavioral targets: (1) dialectical strategies, (2) validation strategies, and (3) problem-solving strategies; (4) stylistic strategies; and (5) case management strategies. DBT strategies are illustrated in Figure 3.1. Within an individual session and with a given client, certain strategies may be used more than others, and not all strategies may be necessary or appropriate. Validation and problem-solving strategies, together with dialectical strategies, make up the core of DBT and form the heart of the treatment. DBT core strategies are listed in Figure 3.2. An abbreviated discussion of the DBT treatment strategies follows. For greater detail, the reader is referred to the treatment manual (Linehan, 1993a).

Dialectical Strategies

Dialectical strategies permeate the entire therapy. There are three types of dialectical strategies. The first has to do with how the therapist structures interactions within the therapy relationship; the second involves how the therapist defines skillful behaviors; and the third consists of certain specific strategies used during the conduct of treatment.

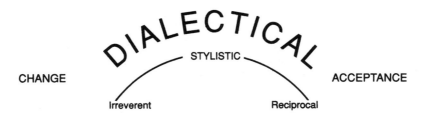

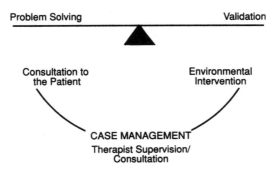

FIGURE 3.1. *Treatment strategies in DBT.*

From Linehan (1993a). Copyright 1993 by The Guilford Press. Reprinted by permission.

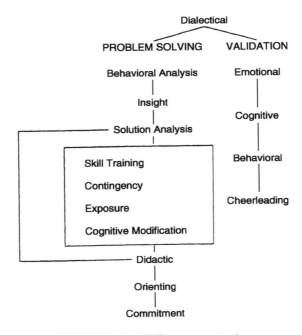

FIGURE 3.2. *DBT core strategies.*

From Linehan, Cochran, and Kehrer (2001). Copyright 2001 by The Guilford Press. Reprinted by permission.

Dialectics of the Relationship: Balancing Treatment Strategies

Dialectical strategies in the most general sense of the word have to do with how the therapist balances the dialectical tensions within the therapy relationship. As noted above, the fundamental dialectic within any psychotherapy, including that with clients who have BPD, is between acceptance and change. A dialectical therapeutic position is one of constantly combining acceptance with change, flexibility with stability, nurturing with challenging, and a focus on capabilities with a focus on deficits. The goal is to bring out the opposites, both in therapy and the client's life, and to provide conditions for syntheses. The presumption is that change may be facilitated by emphasizing acceptance, and acceptance by emphasizing change. The emphasis upon opposites sometimes takes place over time (i.e., over the whole of an interaction), rather than simultaneously or in each part of an interaction. Although many if not all psychotherapies, including cognitive and behavioral treatment, attend to these issues of balance, placing the concept of balance at the center of the treatment assures that the therapist remains attentive to its importance.

Strategies emphasizing acceptance are very similar to (or in some cases identical to) strategies used in client-centered therapy, as well as the case management outreach strategies emphasized in community psychiatry. Those emphasizing change are drawn primarily from cognitive and behavioral therapies. The categorization is artificial, however, since in many ways every strategy comprises both acceptance and change. Indeed, the best strategies are those that combine acceptance and change in one move. The overall emphasis on balance (both within and outside of therapy) is similar to that in gestalt and systems therapies.

Teaching Dialectical Behaviors

Behavioral extremes and rigidity—whether these are cognitive, emotional, or overtly behavioral—are signals that synthesis has not been achieved, and thus can be considered nondialectical. Instead, a middle path similar to that advocated in Zen Buddhism is advocated and modeled. "The middle way is not halfway between extremes, but a completely new path" (Aitken, 2003). This emphasis on balance is similar to the approach advocated in the relapse prevention model proposed by Marlatt and his colleagues (e.g., Marlatt & Donovan, 2005) for treating addictive behaviors. Thus the therapist helps the client move from "either–or" to "both–and." The key here is not to invalidate the first idea or polarity when asserting the second.

Specific Dialectical Strategies

here are eight specific dialectical treatment strategies: (1) entering the paradox, (2) using metaphor, (3) playing the devil's advocate, (4) extending, (5) activating the client's "wise mind," (6) making lemonade out of lemons (turning negatives into positives), (7) allowing natural change (and inconsistencies even within the therapeutic milieu), and (8) assessing dialectically by always asking the question "What is being left out here?" We describe a selection of these strategies below. For a complete review, the interested reader is referred to the DBT treatment manual (Linehan, 1993a).

Entering the Paradox

Entering the paradox is a powerful strategy because it contains the element of surprise. The therapist presents the paradox without explaining it and highlights the paradoxical contradictions within the behavior, the therapeutic process, and reality in general. The essence of the strategy is the therapist's refusal to step in with rational explanation; the client's attempts at logic are met with silence, a question, or a story designed to shed a small amount of light on the puzzle to be solved. The client is pushed to achieve understanding, move towards synthesis of the polarities, and resolve the dilemma him- or herself.

Linehan (1993a) has highlighted a number of typical paradoxes and their corresponding dialectical tensions encountered over the course of therapy. For example, clients are free to choose their own behavior, but can't stay in therapy if they do not work at changing their behavior. Clients are taught to achieve greater independence by becoming more skilled at asking for help from others. Clients have a right to kill themselves, but if they ever convince the therapist that suicide is imminent, they may be locked up. Clients are not responsible for being the way they are, but they are responsible for what they become. In highlighting these paradoxical realities, both client and therapist struggle with confronting and letting go of rigid patterns of thought, emotion, and behavior, so that more spontaneous and flexible patterns may emerge.

Using Metaphor: Parable, Myth, Analogy, and Story Telling

The use of metaphor, stories, parables, and myth is extremely important in DBT and provides an alternative means of teaching dialectical thinking. Stories are usually more interesting than didactic teaching approaches, are easier to remember, and encourage the search for different meanings of events under scrutiny. In general, the idea of metaphor is to take something the client does understand, and compare it to something the client does not understand. Used creatively, metaphors can aid understanding, suggest solutions to problems, and reframe both the problems of clients and those of the therapeutic process.

Playing Devil's Advocate

The devil's advocate strategy is quite similar to the argumentative approach used in rational–emotive and cognitive restructuring therapies as a method of addressing a client's dysfunctional beliefs or problematic rules. In this strategy, the therapist presents a propositional statement that is an extreme version of one of the client's own dysfunctional beliefs, and then plays the role of devil's advocate to counter the client's attempts to disprove the extreme statement or rule. For example, a client may state, "Because I'm overweight, I'd be better off dead." The therapist argues in favor of the dysfunctional belief, perhaps by suggesting that since this is true for her, the client, it must be true for others as well; hence all overweight people would be better off dead. The therapist might continue along these lines as follows: "And since the definition of what constitutes being overweight varies so much among individuals, there must be an awful lot of people who would be considered overweight by someone. That must mean they'd all be better off dead!" And "Gosh, I'm about 5 pounds overweight. I guess that means I'd be better off dead, too." Any reservations the client proposes can be countered by further exaggeration until the self-defeating nature of the belief becomes apparent.

The therapist often plays devil's advocate the first several sessions to elicit a strong commitment from the client. When the strategy is used in this manner, the therapist argues that since the therapy will be painful and difficult, it is not clear how making such a commitment (and therefore being accepted into treatment) could possibly be a good idea. This usually has the effect of moving the client to take the opposite position in favor of therapeutic change. For this use of the strategy to be successful, it is important that the therapist's argument seem reasonable enough to invite counterargument by the client, and that the argument be delivered with a straight face, in a naive but offbeat manner.

Extending

The term "extending" has been borrowed from aikido, a Japanese form of self-defense. In that context, extending occurs when the aikido practitioner waits for a challenger's movements to reach their natural completion, and then extends their endpoint slightly further than what would naturally occur, leaving the challenger vulnerable and off balance. In DBT, extending occurs when the therapist takes the severity or gravity of what the client is communicating more seriously than the client intends, or responds to a part of the client's communication that is not the part the client intends to be taken seriously. This strategy is the emotional equivalent of the devil's advocate strategy. It is particularly effective when the client is threatening dire consequences of an event or problem. Take the following interaction with a client, who is threatening suicide if an extra appointment time for the next day is not scheduled. The interchange occurs after attempts to find a mutually acceptable time have failed.

> CLIENT: I've got to see you tomorrow, or I'm sure I will end up killing myself. I just can't keep it together by myself any longer.
>
> THERAPIST: Hmm, I didn't realize you were so upset! We've got to do something immediately if you are so distressed that you might kill yourself. What about hospitalization? Maybe that is needed. Should I call your parents?
>
> CLIENT: I'm *not* going to the hospital! And you *can't* call my parents. Why won't you just give me an appointment?
>
> THERAPIST: How can we discuss such a mundane topic as session scheduling when your life is in danger? How are you planning to kill yourself?
>
> CLIENT: You know how. Why can't you cancel someone or move an appointment around? You could put an appointment with one of your students off until another time. *I can't stand it any more.*
>
> THERAPIST: I'm really concerned about you. Do you think I should call an ambulance?

The aspect of the communication that the therapist takes seriously (suicide as a possible consequence of not getting an appointment) is not the aspect (needing an extra appointment the next day) that the client wants taken seriously. The therapist takes the consequences seriously and extends the seriousness even further. The client wants the problem taken seriously, and indeed is extending the seriousness of the problem. What typically occurs when the therapist uses this strategy is that the client then deescalates the extreme communication (e.g., "No, don't bother calling an ambulance—I'm not going to do anything. I just really want to see you tomorrow!") The therapist can then attend directly to problem solving in regard to the client's request, thereby reinforcing the deescalated and direct communication (minus the threat) about the problem.

Making Lemonade out of Lemons

Making lemonade out of lemons is similar to the notion in psychodynamic therapy of utilizing a client's resistances; therapeutic problems are seen as opportunities for the therapist to help the client. The strategy involves taking something that is apparently problematic and turning it into an asset. Problems become opportunities to practice skills; suffering allows others to express empathy; weaknesses become strengths. The danger in using this strategy is that it is easily confused with the invalidating refrains repeatedly heard by clients with BPD or borderline features. The therapist should avoid the tendency to oversimplify the client's problems, and refrain from implying that the lemons in his or her life are really lemonade. While recognizing that the cloud is indeed black, the therapist assists the client in finding the positive characteristics of a situation and thus the silver lining.

Validation Strategies

As noted earlier, validation and problem-solving strategies, along with dialectical strategies, constitute the core of DBT and the heart of the treatment. Validation strategies are the most obvious acceptance strategies, while problem-solving strategies are the most obvious change strategies. Both validation and problem-solving strategies are used in every interaction with the client, although the relative frequency of each depends on the particular client and the current situation and vulnerabilities of that client. Many treatment impasses are due to an imbalance of one strategy over the other.

Clients with BPD or borderline features present themselves clinically as individuals in extreme emotional pain. They plead, and at times demand, that the therapist do something to change this state of affairs. It is very tempting to focus the energy of therapy on changing the client by modifying irrational thoughts, assumptions, or schemas; critiquing interpersonal behaviors or motives contributing to interpersonal problems; giving medication to change abnormal biology; reducing emotional overreactivity and intensity; and so on. In many respects, this focus recapitulates the invalidating environment by confirming the client's worst fears: The client is the problem, and indeed cannot trust his or her own reactions to events. Mistrust and invalidation of a person's response to events, however, is extremely aversive and can elicit intense fear, anger, shame, or a combination of all three. Thus the entire focus of change-based therapy can be aversive, since by necessity the focus contributes to and elicits self-invalidation.

"Validation" (according to the online version of the *Oxford English Dictionary*; Simpson & Weiner, 1989) means "a strengthening, reinforcement, confirming; an establishing or ratifying." It includes activities such as confirming, corroborating, substantiating, verifying, and authenticating. The act of validating is "to support or corroborate on a sound or authoritative basis . . . to attest to the truth or validity of something." To communicate that a response is valid is to say that it is "well-grounded or justifiable: being at once relevant and meaningful . . . logically correct . . . appropriate to the end in view [or effective] . . . having such force as to compel serious attention and [usually] acceptance." These are precisely the meanings associated with the term when used in the context of psychotherapy in DBT.

> The essence of validation is this: The therapist communicates to the client that her [*sic*] responses make sense and are understandable within her [*sic*] *current* life context or situation. The therapist actively accepts the client and communicates this acceptance to the client. The therapist takes the client's responses seriously and does not discount or trivialize them. Validation strategies require the therapist to search for, recognize, and reflect to the client the validity inherent in her [*sic*] response to events. With unruly children, parents have to catch them while they're good in order to reinforce their behavior; similarly, the therapist has to uncover the validity within the client's response, sometimes amplify it, and then reinforce it. (Linehan, 1993a, pp. 222–223; emphasis in original)

Two things are important to note here. First, validation means the acknowledgment of that which is valid. It does not mean "making" valid. Nor does it mean validating that which is invalid. The therapist observes, experiences, and affirms, but does not create validity. Second, "valid" and "scientific" are not synonyms. Science may be one way to determine what is valid, but the following are also bases for claiming validity: logic, sound principles, generally accepted authority or normative knowledge, and experience or apprehension of private events (at least when these are similar to the same experiences of others or are in accord with other, more observable events).

Validation can be considered at any one of six levels. Each level is correspondingly more complete than the preceding one, and each level depends on one or more of the previous levels. The first two levels of validation encompass activities usually defined as empathic, and the third and fourth levels are similar to empathic interpretations as those terms are used in the general psychotherapy literature. Although surely most therapists use and support Levels 5 and 6 of validation, they are much less often discussed in the literature. They are, however, definitional of DBT and are required in every interaction with the client. These levels are described most fully in Linehan (1997), and the following definitions are taken from her discussion.[1]

> [At Level 1], validation requires listening to and observing what the client is saying, feeling, and doing as well as a corresponding active effort to understand what is being said and observed. The essence of this step is that the therapist is *interested* in the client. The therapist pays attention to what the client says and does. The therapist notices the nuances of response in the interaction. Validation at [Level 1] communicates that the client *per se*, as well as the client's presence, words, and responses in the session have "such force as to compel serious attention and [usually] acceptance" [see definitions of "validation" above]. (pp. 360–361; emphasis in original)

> The second level of validation is the accurate reflection back to the client of the client's own feelings, thoughts, assumptions, and behaviors. The therapist conveys an understanding of the client, a hearing of what the client has said, and a seeing of what the client does, how he or she responds. Validation at [Level 2] sanctions, empowers, or authenticates that the individual is who he or she actually is. (p. 362)

> [At Level 3] of validation, the therapist communicates to the client understanding of aspects of the client's experience and response to events that have not been communicated directly by the client. At [this] level . . . the therapist "reads" the client's behavior and figures out how the client feels and what the client is wishing for, thinking, or doing just by knowing what has happened to the client. It is when one person can make the link between precipitating event and behavior without being given any information about the behavior itself. Emotions and meanings the client has not expressed are articulated by the therapist." (p. 364)

> [At Level 4], behavior is validated in terms of its causes. Validation here is based on the notion that all behavior is caused by events occurring in time and, thus, in principle is understandable. Behavior is justified by showing that it is caused. Even though information may not be available to know all the relevant causes, the client's feelings, thoughts, and actions make perfect sense in the context of the person's current experience, physiology, and life to date. At a minimum, what is can always be justified in terms of sufficient causes. That is, what is "should be" in that whatever was necessary for it to occur had to have happened. (p. 367)

---

[1] All quotations are from Linehan (1997). Copyright 1997 by the American Psychological Association. Reprinted by permission.

[At Level 5], the therapist communicates that behavior is justifiable, reasonable, well-grounded, meaningful, and/or efficacious in terms of current events, normative biological functioning, and/or the client's ultimate life goals. The therapist looks for and reflects the wisdom or validity of [the] client's response and communicates that the response is understandable. The therapist finds the relevant facts in the *current* environment that support the client's behavior. The therapist is not blinded by the dysfunctionality of some of the client's response patterns to those aspects of a response pattern that may be either reasonable or appropriate to the context. Thus, the therapist searches the client's responses for their inherent accuracy or appropriateness, or reasonableness (as well as commenting on the inherent dysfunctionality of much of the response if necessary). (pp. 370–371; emphasis in original)

[At Level 6], the task is to recognize the person as he or she is, seeing and responding to the strengths and capacities of the individual while keeping a firm empathic understanding of the client's actual difficulties and incapacities. The therapist believes in the individual and his or her capacity to change and move towards ultimate life goals. The client is responded to as a person of equal status, due equal respect. Validation at the highest level is the validation of the individual as "is." The therapist sees more than the role, more than a "client," or "disorder." [This level of] validation is the opposite of treating the client in a condescending manner or as overly fragile. It is responding to the individual as capable of effective and reasonable behavior rather than assuming that he or she is an invalid. Whereas [Levels 1–5] represent sequential steps in validation of a kind, [Level 6] represents both change in level as well as kind. (p. 377)

Cheerleading strategies are another form of validation, and are the principal strategies for combating clients' active passivity and tendencies to hopelessness. In cheerleading, therapists communicate the belief that clients are doing their best and validate their ability to eventually overcome their difficulties (a type of validation that, if not handled carefully, can simultaneously invalidate clients' perceptions of their helplessness). In addition, the therapists express a belief in the therapy relationship, offer reassurance, and highlight any evidence of improvement. Within DBT, cheerleading is used in every therapeutic interaction. Although active cheerleading by therapists should be reduced as clients learn to trust and validate themselves, cheerleading strategies always remain an essential ingredient of a strong therapeutic alliance.

Problem-Solving Strategies

We have previously discussed how therapies with a primary focus on client change are typically experienced as invalidating by highly emotionally dysregulated clients. However, therapies that focus exclusively on validation can prove equally problematic. Exhortation to accept one's current situation by itself offers little solace to an individual who experiences life as painfully unendurable. Within DBT, problem-solving strategies are the core change strategies, designed to foster an active problem-solving style. With emotionally dysregulated clients who have BPD or borderline features, however, the application of these strategies is fraught with difficulties. The therapist must keep in mind that the process will be more difficult than with many other client populations. In work with emotionally dysregulated clients, the need for sympathetic understanding and interventions aimed at enhancing current positive mood can be extremely important. The validation strategies just described, as well as the irreverent communication strategy to be described below, can be tremendously useful here.

Within DBT, problem solving is a two-stage process that concentrates first on understanding and accepting a selected problem, and second on generating and implementing alternative solutions. The first stage employs behavioral analysis, which also involves insight into recurrent behavioral context patterns, and the giving of didactic information about principles of behaviors, norms, and so on. The second stage specifically targets change by employing solution analysis, which also involves orienting the client to the specific therapeutic change procedures likely to bring about desired changes, and strategies designed to elicit and strengthen commitment to these procedures. The following discussion specifically addresses behavioral and solution analyses. (See also Chapter 8 for an illustration of how to conduct behavioral analysis and solution analysis with a client.)

Behavioral Analysis

Behavioral analysis is one of the most important strategies in DBT. It is also the most difficult. The purpose of a behavioral analysis is to select a problem and to determine empirically what is causing it, what is preventing its resolution, and what aids are available for solving it. Behavioral analysis addresses four primary issues:

1. Are ineffective behaviors being reinforced, are effective behaviors followed by aversive outcomes, or are rewarding outcomes delayed?
2. Does the client have the requisite behavioral skills to regulate emotions, respond skillfully to conflict, and manage his or her own behavior?
3. Are there patterns of avoidance, or are effective behaviors inhibited by unwarranted fears or guilt?
4. Is the client unaware of the contingencies operating in the environment, or are effective behaviors inhibited by faulty beliefs or assumptions?

Answers to these questions will guide the therapist in the selection of appropriate change procedures, such as contingency management, behavioral skill training, exposure, or cognitive modification. Thus the value of a behavioral analysis is in helping the therapist assess and understand a problem fully enough in order to guide effective therapeutic response.

The first step in conducting a behavioral analysis is to help the client identify the problem to be analyzed and describe it in behavioral terms. Problem definition usually evolves from a discussion of the previous week's events, often in the context of reviewing diary cards. The assumption of facts not in evidence is perhaps the most common mistake at this point. Defining the problem is followed by conducting a chain analysis—an exhaustive, blow-by-blow description of the chain of events leading up to and following the behavior (i.e., antecedents and consequences).

In a chain analysis, the therapist constructs a general road map of how the client arrives at dysfunctional responses, including where the road actually starts, notated with possible alternative adaptive pathways or junctions along the way. Additional goals are to identify events that automatically elicit maladaptive behavior, behavioral deficits that are instrumental in maintaining problematic responses, and environmental and behavioral events that may be interfering with more appropriate behaviors. The overall goal is to determine the function of the behavior, or, from another perspective, what problem the behavior was instrumental in solving.

Chain analysis always begins with a specific environmental event. Pinpointing such an event may be difficult, as clients are frequently unable to identify anything in the environment that set off a problematic response. Nevertheless, it is important to obtain a description of the events co-occurring with the onset of the problem. The therapist then attempts to identify both environmental and behavioral events for each subsequent link in the chain. Here the therapist must play the part of a very keen observer, thinking in terms of very small chunks of behavior. The therapist asks the client, "What happened next?" or "How did you get from there to there?" Although from the client's point of view such links may be self-evident, the therapist must be careful not to make assumptions. For example, a client who had frequently attempted suicide stated once that she tried to kill herself because her life was too painful to live any longer. From the client's point of view, this was an adequate explanation for her suicide attempts. For the therapist, however, taking one's life because life was too painful was only one possible solution. One could decide life was too painful, then decide to change one's life. Or one could believe that death might be even more painful and decide to tolerate life despite its pain. In this instance, careful questioning revealed that the client actually assumed she would be happier dead than alive. Challenging this assumption then became a key to ending her persistent suicide attempts.

It is equally important to pinpoint exactly what consequences are maintaining the problematic response. Similarly, the therapist should also search for consequences that serve to weaken the problem behavior. As with antecedent events, the therapist probes for both environmental and behavioral consequences, obtaining detailed descriptions of emotions, somatic sensations, actions, thoughts, and assumptions. A rudimentary knowledge of the rules of learning and principles of reinforcement is crucial.

The final step in behavioral analysis is to construct and test hypotheses about events that are relevant to generating and maintaining the problem behavior. The biosocial theory of BPD suggests several factors of primary importance. For example, DBT focuses most closely on intense or aversive emotional states; the amelioration of negative affect is always suspected as among the primary motivational variables in dysfunctional behavior. The theory also suggests typical behavioral patterns, such as deficits in dialectical thinking or behavioral skills, that are likely to be instrumental in producing and maintaining problematic responses.

Solution Analysis and Change Procedures

Once the problem has been identified and analyzed, problem solving proceeds with an active attempt at finding and identifying alternative solutions. Sometimes solutions will be suggested during the conduct of the behavioral analysis, and pointing to these alternative solutions may be all that is required. At other times a more complete solution analysis will be necessary. Here the first task is to "brainstorm" or generate as many alternative solutions as possible. Solutions should then be evaluated in terms of the various outcomes expected. The final step in solution analysis is choosing a solution that will somehow be effective. Throughout the evaluation, the therapist guides the client in choosing a particular behavioral solution. Here it is preferable for the therapist to pay particular attention to long-term gain rather than short-term gain, and for solutions to be chosen that render maximum benefit to the client rather than benefit to others.

DBT employs four sets of change procedures taken directly from the cognitive and behavioral treatment literature:

- Skills training: Teaching the client new skills.
- Contingency procedures: Providing a consequence that influences the probability of preceding client behaviors' occurring again.
- Exposure: Providing nonreinforced exposure to cues associated previously but not currently with a threat.
- Cognitive modification: Changing the client's dysfunctional assumptions or beliefs.

These four areas are viewed as primary vehicles of change, since they influence the direction that client changes take. Although they are discussed as distinct procedures by Linehan (1993a), it is not clear that they can in fact be differentiated in every case in clinical practice. The same therapeutic sequence may be effective because it teaches the client new skills (skills training), provides a consequence that influences the probability of preceding client behaviors' occurring again (contingency procedures), provides nonreinforced exposure to cues associated previously but not currently with threat (exposure), and/or changes the client's dysfunctional assumptions or schematic processing of events (cognitive modification). In contrast to many cognitive and behavioral treatment programs in the literature, these procedures (with some exceptions noted below) are employed in an unstructured manner, interwoven throughout all therapeutic interactions. Thus, although the therapist must be well aware of the principles governing the effectiveness of each procedure, the use of each is usually an immediate response to events unfolding in a particular session. The exceptions are in skills training, where skills training procedures predominate, and Stage 2, where exposure procedures predominate.

Skills Training

An emphasis on skill building is pervasive throughout DBT. In both individual and group therapy, the therapist insists at every opportunity that the client actively engage in the acquisition and practice of behavioral skills. The term "skill" is used synonymously with "ability," and includes in its broadest sense cognitive, emotional, and overt behavioral skills, as well as their integration (which is necessary for effective performance). Skill training is called for when a solution requires skills not currently in the individual's behavioral repertoire, or when the individual has the component behaviors but cannot integrate and use them effectively. As listed earlier, skills training in standard DBT includes training in mindfulness, interpersonal effectiveness, emotion regulation, and distress tolerance. The training process incorporates three types of procedures: (1) skill acquisition (modeling, instructing, advising); (2) skill strengthening (encouraging *in vivo* and within-session practice, role playing, feedback); and (3) skill generalization (phone calls to work on applying skills, taping therapy sessions to listen to between sessions, homework assignments). In working with adolescents, we find it useful to include family members in skills training as well, since they can provide coaching for the adolescent and often themselves have important skills deficits.

Contingency Procedures

Every response within an interpersonal interaction is a potential reinforcement, punishment, or withholding/removal of reinforcement. Contingency management requires therapists to organize their own behaviors so that client behaviors that represent progress are reinforced, while unskillful or maladaptive behaviors are extinguished or lead to aversive consequences. The most important contingencies with most clients are therapists' interpersonal behaviors with the clients. The ability of a therapist to influence a client's behavior is directly tied to the strength of the relationship between the two. Thus contingency procedures are less useful in the very beginning stages of treatment (except possibly in cases where the therapist is the "only game in town"). A first requirement for effective contingency management is that therapists attend to their clients' behaviors and reinforce those behaviors that represent progress toward the clients' treatment goals. Equally important is that therapists take care not to reinforce behaviors targeted for extinction. In theory this may seem obvious, but in practice it can be quite difficult. The problematic behaviors of emotionally dysregulated clients are often followed by positive increases in desired outcomes or cessation of painful events. Indeed, the very behaviors targeted for extinction have been intermittently reinforced by mental health professionals, family members, and friends. Note that contingencies operate no differently with family members involved in an adolescent's treatment, and that family sessions and skills training sessions can at times highlight these contingencies (e.g., a parent may be reinforcing a teen's maladaptive behaviors and ignoring adaptive behavior attempts). In fact, in the new Walking the Middle Path module of skills training, learning principles are taught explicitly to adolescents and family members, to help facilitate awareness of the contingencies operating in their interactions.

Contingency management will at times require the use of aversive consequences, similar to "setting limits" in other treatment modalities. Three guidelines are important here. First, punishment should "fit the crime," and the client should have some way of terminating its application. For example, in DBT a detailed behavioral analysis follows a self-injurious act, and this analysis is an aversive procedure for most clients. Once it has been completed, however, the client's ability to pursue other topics is restored. Second, it is crucial that therapists use punishment with great care, in low doses, and very briefly, and that a positive interpersonal atmosphere be restored following any client improvement. Third, punishment should be just strong enough to work. Although the ultimate punishment is termination of therapy, a preferable fall-back strategy is putting clients on "vacations from therapy." This approach is considered when all other contingencies have failed, or when a situation is so serious that a therapist's therapeutic or personal limits have been crossed. When utilizing this strategy, the therapist clearly identifies what behaviors must be changed, and clarifies that once the conditions have been met, the client can return. The therapist maintains intermittent contact by phone or letter, and provides a referral or backup while the client is on vacation. (In colloquial terms, the therapist kicks the client out and then pines for his or her return.)

Observing limits constitutes a special case of contingency management involving the application of problem-solving strategies to client behaviors that threaten or cross a therapist's personal limits. Such behaviors interfere with the therapist's ability or willingness to conduct the therapy, and thus constitute a special type of therapy-interfering behavior. Therapists must take responsibility for monitoring their own personal limits, and clearly communicate to their clients which behaviors are tolerable and which are not. Therapists who do not do this will eventually burn out, terminate therapy, or otherwise harm clients.

DBT favors natural over arbitrary limits. Thus limits will vary between therapists and within the same therapist over time and circumstances. Limits should also be presented as for the good of a therapist or treatment agency, not for the good of a client. The effect of this is that while clients may argue about what is in their own best interests, they do not have ultimate say over what is good for their therapists. Also, for adolescents this approach is often refreshing, compared to hearing parents' requests of them as being "for their own good."

Exposure

All of the change procedures in DBT can be reconceptualized as exposure strategies. Many of the principles of exposure as applied to DBT have been developed by researchers in exposure techniques (see Foa & Kozak, 1986; Foa, Steketee, & Grayson, 1985). These strategies work by reconditioning dysfunctional associations that develop between stimuli (e.g., an aversive stimulus, hospitalization, may become associated with a positive stimulus, nurturing in the hospital; the client may later work to be hospitalized) or between a response and a stimulus (e.g., an adaptive response, healthy expression of emotions, is met with aversive consequent stimuli, rejection by a loved one; the client may then try to suppress emotions). As noted earlier, the DBT therapist conducts a chain analysis of the eliciting cue, the problem behavior (including emotions), and the consequences of the behavior. Working within a behavior therapy framework, the therapist operates according to three guidelines for exposure in DBT: (1) Exposure to the cue that precedes the problem behavior must be nonreinforced (e.g., if a client is fearful that discussing suicidal behavior will lead to being rejected, the therapist must not reinforce the fear by ostracizing the client); (2) dysfunctional responses are blocked, in the order of the primary and secondary targets of treatment (e.g., self-injurious behavior related to shame is blocked by getting the client's cooperation to throw away hoarded medications); and (3) actions opposite to the dysfunctional behavior are reinforced (e.g., the therapist reinforces the client for talking about painful, shame-related self-injurious behavior).

Therapeutic exposure procedures are used informally throughout the whole of DBT and may be formally implemented when clients have suicidal behaviors under control and can cooperate in therapy. These procedures involve first orienting the client to the techniques and to the fact that exposure to cues is often experienced as painful or frightening. Generally, the therapist encourages the client to stay in contact with the cue—particularly when the cue is an image, an emotion, or a topic under discussion. The therapist does not remove the cue to emotional arousal, and at the same time helps the client block the action tendencies (including escape responses) associated with the problem emotion. In addition, the therapist works to assist the client in achieving enhanced control over the aversive event. A crucial step of exposure procedures is that the client be taught how to control the event. It is critical for the client to have some means of titrating or ending exposure when emotions become unendurable. The therapist and client should collaborate in developing positive, adaptive ways for the client to end exposure voluntarily. At a minimum, however, the client should be encouraged to continue exposure until some habituation occurs, marked by a noticeable reduction in the problem emotion (see Linehan, 1993a).

Cognitive Modification

The fundamental message given to clients in DBT is that cognitive distortions are just as likely to be caused by emotional arousal as to be the cause of the arousal in the first place. The overall message is that for the most part, the source of a client's distress is the extremely stressful events of his or her life, rather than a distortion of events that are actually benign. Although direct cognitive restructuring procedures, such as those advocated by Beck and by Ellis (Beck, Rush, Shaw, & Emery, 1979; Beck, Freeman, Davis, & Associates, 2003; Ellis, 1962, 1973) are used, they do not hold a dominant place in DBT. In contrast, contingency clarification strategies are used relentlessly, highlighting contingent relationships operating in the here and now. Emphasis is placed on highlighting both immediate and long-term effects of clients' behavior, both on themselves and on others; clarifying the effects of certain situations on the clients' own responses; and examining future contingencies the clients are likely to encounter. An example here is orienting clients to DBT as a whole and to treatment procedures as these are implemented.

Stylistic Strategies

Stylistic strategies have to do with the style and form of therapist communication—the "how" rather than the "what" of therapy. DBT balances two quite different styles of communication. The first, "reciprocal" communication, is similar to the communication style advocated in client-centered therapy. The second, "irreverent" communication, is quite similar to the style advocated by Whitaker (1975) in his writings on strategic therapy. Reciprocal communication strategies are designed to reduce a perceived power differential by making the therapist more vulnerable to the client. In addition, they serve as a model for appropriate but equal interactions within an important interpersonal relationship. Irreverent communication, in contrast, is designed to push the often rigid client off track so that new learning can take place. Irreverence by definition is an unexpected, somewhat "off-the-wall" response to a client. It can facilitate problem solving or produce a breakthrough after long periods when progress has seemed glacial. To be used effectively, irreverent communication must balance reciprocal communication, and the two must be woven into a single stylistic fabric. Without such balancing, neither strategy represents DBT.

Reciprocal Communication

Responsiveness, self-disclosure, and genuineness are the basic guidelines of reciprocal communication. Responsiveness requires taking the client's agenda and wishes seriously. It is a friendly, affectionate style reflecting warmth and engagement in the therapeutic interaction. Both self-involving and personal self-disclosure, used in the interest of the client, are encouraged. Disclosure of immediate, personal reactions to the client and his or her behavior is frequent. For example, a therapist whose client complained about his coolness said, "When you demand warmth from me, it pushes me away and makes it harder to be warm." Similarly, when a client repeatedly failed to fill out diary cards but nevertheless pleaded with her therapist to help her, the therapist responded, "You keep asking me for help, but you won't do the things I believe are necessary to help you. I feel frustrated, because I want to help you but feel you won't let me." Such statements serve both to validate and to challenge a client. They are also instances of contingency management (because therapist statements about the client are typically experienced as either reinforcing or punishing) and of contingency clarification (because the client's attention is directed to the consequences of his or her interpersonal behavior). Self-disclosure of professional or personal information is used to validate and model coping and normative responses.

Irreverent Communication

Irreverent communication is used to push the client "off balance," get the client's attention, present an alternative viewpoint, or shift affective response. It is a highly useful strategy when the client is immovable, or when therapist and client are "stuck." It has an "offbeat" flavor and uses logic to weave a web the client cannot get out of. Although it is responsive to the client, irreverent communication is almost never the response the client expects. The therapist highlights some unintended aspect of the client's communication, or "reframes" it in an unorthodox manner. For example, if the client says, "I am going to kill myself, the therapist might say, "I thought you agreed not to drop out of therapy." Irreverent communication has a matter-of-fact, almost deadpan style, which is in sharp contrast to the warm responsiveness of reciprocal communication. Humor, a certain naiveté, and guilelessness are also characteristic of the style. A confrontational tone is irreverent as well, communicating "bullshit" to responses other than the targeted adaptive response. For example, the therapist might say, "Are you out of your mind?" or "You weren't for a minute actually believing I would think that was a good idea, were you?" The irreverent therapist also calls the client's bluff. For the client who says, "I'm quitting therapy," the therapist might respond, "Would you like a referral?" The trick here is to time the bluff carefully, with the simultaneous provision of a safety net; it is important to leave the client a way out.

Although all clients can benefit from this approach, the irreverent communication style works particularly well with adolescents. It helps command their respect and strengthens the alliance, and often differs greatly from the responses they are accustomed to from parents, teachers, doctors, or other authority figures. It is essential, however, never to use it in a mean-spirited way; the therapist must be mindful of his or her intentions and attitudes while using irreverence.

Case Management Strategies

When there are problems in the client's environment that interfere with the client's functioning or progress, the therapist moves to the case management strategies. Although not new, case management strategies direct the application of core strategies around case management problems. There are three case management strategy groups: the consultation-to-the-patient[2] strategy, environmental intervention, and the consultation team meeting.

Consultation-to-the-Patient Strategy

The consultation-to-the-patient strategy is deceptively simple in theory and extremely difficult in practice. As its name indicates, the strategy requires the therapist to be a consultant to the client rather than to the client's network. The overriding implications of this are that in general, a DBT therapist does not intervene to adjust environments for the sake of the client, and does not consult with other professionals about how to treat the client unless the client is present. According to this philosophy, the client, not the therapist, is the intermediary between the therapist and other professionals. The therapist's job is to consult with the client on how to interact effectively with his or her environment, rather than to consult with the environment on how to interact effectively with the client. The consultation-to-the-patient strategy is the preferred case management strategy and perhaps the most innovative aspect of DBT.

This strategy was developed with three objectives in mind. First, clients must learn how to manage their own lives and care for themselves by interacting effectively with other individuals in the environment, including healthcare professionals. The consultant strategy expresses belief in clients' capacities and targets their ability to take care of themselves. By doing too much for an adolescent client in particular, a therapist inadvertently interferes in the teen's capacity to build mastery—a necessary ingredient in the treatment of depression. Second, the consultation-to-the-patient strategy was designed to decrease instances of so-called "splitting" between a DBT therapist and other individuals interacting with a client. Splitting occurs when different individuals in the person's network hold differing opinions on how to treat the client. By remaining in the role of a consultant to the client, the therapist stays out of such arguments. Table 3.3 lists key corollaries to the consultation-to-the-patient strategy. Finally, this strategy promotes respect for clients by imparting the message that they are credible and capable of performing interventions on their own behalf.

With an adolescent, a practitioner might be tempted to alter the balance of consultation to the client versus consultation to the client's network, believing that since the client is a minor, more consultation on his or her behalf is needed. Although this may be true at times, it is also beneficial to serve as consultant directly to the adolescent whenever possible. Adolescents can themselves benefit from enhancing their effective interactions with others, from re-

---

[2]Although we prefer to use the term "client," the strategy outlined in Linehan (1993a) is "consultation to the patient," and we will use that term here to avoid confusion.

TABLE 3.3. Corollaries to the Consultation-to-the-Patient Strategy

1. Give other professionals general information about the treatment program.
2. Outside of the treatment team, do not discuss the client or his or her treatment without the client present.
3. Within the treatment team, share information, but keep the spirit of the strategy (i.e., let go of attachment to what other team members do with the client).
4. Do not tell other professionals how to treat the client.
5. Teach the client to act as his or her own agent in obtaining appropriate help.
6. Do not intervene or solve problems for the client with other professionals before giving the client a chance to solve the problem.
7. Do not defend other professionals.

Note. For further details, see Linehan (1993a, pp. 412–416).

ductions in "splitting," and from the message that they are capable of advocating for themselves. For example, the therapist can consult with an adolescent regarding how to speak effectively with family members, other care providers, teachers, or bosses.

Traditionally, health care professionals routinely exchange information helpful to whichever professional is currently treating the client. Thus routine use of the consultation-to-the-patient strategy will ordinarily require attention to orienting professionals in one's own community to the strategy. Although consultation between professionals is actually encouraged, not discouraged, the requirement that the client be present (and, preferably, arrange the consultation) is almost always going to be different and require expenditure of some extra time. In our experience, however, once the community is oriented, the strategy works well and actually can save time in the long run. With adolescents, the idea of orienting professionals in the community to this strategy would apply when a therapist interacts regularly with school or healthcare professionals regarding teen clients. Orienting the community helps to ensure that the adolescents will be taken seriously rather than punished for direct communication and appropriate self-advocacy (e.g., when an adolescent assertively discusses troubling side effects of a medication with a treating physician).

Environmental Intervention

As outlined above, the bias in DBT is toward teaching the client how to interact effectively with his or her environment. The consultation-to-the-patient strategy is thus the dominant case management strategy and is used whenever possible. There are times, however, when intervention by the therapist is needed. In general, the environmental intervention strategy is used over the consultation-to-the-patient strategy when substantial harm may befall a client if a therapist does not intervene. The general rule for environmental intervention is that when clients lack abilities that they need to learn, are impossible to obtain, or are not reasonable or necessary, the therapist may intervene.

Consultation Team Meeting

Consultation with therapists is integral, rather than ancillary, to DBT. Consultation to the therapist, as a treatment strategy, balances the consultation-to-the-patient strategy discussed above. DBT, from this perspective, is defined as a treatment system in which (1) therapists apply DBT to the clients and (2) the consultation team applies DBT to the therapists. Thus the team actually "treats" the therapist, and in doing so it provides a dialectical balance for therapists in their interactions with clients.

There are three primary functions of consultation to the therapist in DBT. First, the consultation team helps to keep each individual therapist in the therapeutic relationship. The role here is to cheerlead and support the therapist. Second, the team balances the therapist in his or her interactions with the client. In providing balance, consultants may move close to the therapist, helping him or her maintain a strong position. Or consultants may move back from the therapist, requiring the therapist to move closer to the client to maintain balance. With adolescents and family members, the team will often help the therapist maintain balanced allegiances (e.g., helping with such struggles as seeing the parents as entirely to blame). Third, within programmatic applications of DBT, the team provides the context for the treatment. At its purest, DBT is a transactional relationship between and among a community of clients and a community of therapists.

CHAPTER 4

DBT Program Structure
Functions and Modes

In the first part of this chapter, we look at how the responsibility for meeting treatment functions and Stage 1 behavioral targets is spread among various treatment modes. As we will show, the hierarchy of Stage 1 targets shifts, depending on each mode's function. In the latter part of the chapter, we address issues involved in setting up a DBT program for adolescents, including factors to consider both within and across treatment modes.

HOW DBT PRIORITIZES TREATMENT TARGETS ACROSS FUNCTION AND MODE

As outlined in the preceding chapter, the primary targets of DBT Stage 1 are decreasing life-threatening behaviors, decreasing therapy-interfering behaviors, decreasing quality-of-life interfering behaviors, and increasing behavioral skills. These specific treatment targets can only be met if the therapy program as a whole serves the following five functions: to motivate clients by reducing emotions, beliefs, and reinforcers conducive to dysfunctional behaviors; to increase clients' capabilities and skills; to ensure that clients' new behaviors generalize to the natural environment; to structure the environment to support both clients and therapists; and to improve therapists' motivation and capability for conducting effective therapy. As we have noted in Chapter 3, it is not the mode itself that is critical, but its ability to address a particular function. An overview of each function, and examples of potential modes of treatment to address each function, are presented in Table 4.1. The arrangement of functions and modes in a DBT program determines who does what and when. In what follows, we discuss potential modes in adolescent DBT that address each function.

Function: Improving Motivation to Change
Primary Mode: Individual Therapy with Adolescents

Individual therapy sessions constitute the primary setting in which adolescents learn to apply skills taught in the skills training group to their own lives. Thus individual therapists address not only skill capabilities, but also motivational and environmental factors that inhibit effective coping styles or reinforce dysfunctional coping behaviors. The individual therapist is the primary therapist and is responsible for (1) assessing all problem behaviors and skill deficits, all relevant antecedents and consequences of targeted behaviors, and motivational problems; (2) problem solving for these problem behaviors; and (3) organizing other modes to address

TABLE 4.1. Functions of Comprehensive Treatment for Adolescents, and Examples of Potential Modes to Address Them

Function	Outpatient modes	Inpatient modes	Other possible modes
Improving motivation to change	Individual therapy Family therapy Pharmacotherapy	Individual therapy Milieu-based system of rewards and consequences	Adolescent egregious behavior protocol
Enhancing capabilities	Multifamily skills training group Individual therapy Pharmacotherapy	Adolescent-only skills training group Pharmacotherapy Group therapy	Individual skills training Single-family skills training Behavior analysis group Bibliotherapy
Ensuring skill generalization	Phone coaching Inclusion of family members in skills group As-needed family sessions	Milieu-based coaching and reinforcement	Parallel family-member-only groups Phone coaching for Parents Hotline for coaching with rotating staff Homework groups E-mail consultation
Structuring the environment to support clients and therapist	Consultation with family members, school personnel, other care providers	Training the milieu Family meetings Discharge planning	Consultation with other relevant individuals or institutions Admin. support Ongoing workshops for education of family members
Improving therapists' motivation and capabilities	Therapist consultation/ supervision team	Therapist consultation/ supervision team	Individual supervision Didactic training/ continuing education Adjusting caseload to facilitate work with difficult cases.

problems in each area. Individual outpatient therapy sessions are usually scheduled once weekly for 50–60 minutes each, although biweekly sessions may be held during crisis periods or at the beginning of therapy.

The priorities of specific targets within individual therapy are the same as the overall Stage 1 priorities of DBT discussed above. Therapeutic focus within individual therapy sessions is determined by the highest-priority treatment target relevant at the moment. This ordering does not change over the course of therapy; however, the relevance of a target does change. Relevance is determined either by a client's most recent day-to-day behavior (since the last session) or by current behavior during the therapy session; problems not currently in evidence are not considered relevant. If satisfactory progress on one target goal has been achieved, has never been a problem, or is currently not evident, the therapist shifts attention to the immediately following treatment target.

The consequence of this priority allocation is that when high-risk suicidal behaviors or NSIB, therapy-interfering behaviors, or serious quality-of-life-interfering behaviors are occurring, at least part of the session agenda must be devoted to these topics. If these behaviors are not occurring at the moment, then the topics to be discussed are set by the client. The therapeutic focus (within any topic area discussed) depends on the hierarchy of primary targets, the skills targeted for improvement, and any secondary targets. For example, if suicidal behavior has occurred during the previous week, attention to it would take precedence over attention to therapy-interfering behavior. In turn, focusing on therapy-interfering behaviors would take precedence over working on quality-of-life-interfering behaviors. Although it is ordinarily possible to work on more than one target (including those generated by the client) in a given session, higher-priority targets always take precedence.

Determining the relevance of targeted behaviors is assisted by the use of diary cards. These cards are filled out and brought to weekly sessions. Failure to complete or bring in a card is considered a therapy-interfering behavior. Diary cards record daily instances of suicidal acts or NSIB, suicidal ideation, urges to commit suicide or NSIB, "misery," use of substances (licit and illicit), and use of behavioral skills. Other targeted behaviors (e.g., bulimic episodes, daily productive activities, flashbacks, etc.) may also be recorded on the blank area of the card. The therapist doing DBT must develop the pattern of routinely reviewing the card at the beginning of each session. If the card indicates that a suicidal act or an NSIB has occurred, it is noted and discussed. If high suicidal ideation is recorded, it is assessed to determine whether the client is at risk for suicide. If a pattern of substance abuse or dependence appears, it is treated as a quality-of-life-interfering behavior.

Work on targeted behaviors involves a coordinated array of treatment strategies, as described in Chapter 3 (see also Figure 3.1). Essentially, each session is a balance between change and acceptance strategies. More specifically, following behavioral analysis, this is a balance between structured as well as unstructured problem solving (including simple interpretive activities by the therapist) and unstructured validation. The amount of therapist time allocated to each (problem solving or validating) depends on the urgency of the behaviors needing change or problems to be solved on the one hand, and the urgency of the client's needs for validation, understanding, and acceptance without any intimation that change is needed on the other.

Some settings with a high patient-to-staff ratio conduct individual behavioral analysis and problem solving in a group therapy mode. Other settings—ones that have limited resources or time, or that are just beginning a DBT program for the first time and wish to start gradually—might forgo this mode entirely and provide only skills training. However, research indicates that training in DBT skills with no DBT individual therapy may be no more effective than treatment as usual (Linehan, 1993a). So if individual DBT therapy is not possible, we recommend that some provision for coaching and generalization be made. For example, skills training would be enhanced by the availability of telephone coaching (outpatient settings) or reinforcement by the milieu (inpatient/residential settings).

Function: Enhancing Capabilities

Primary Mode: Skills Training with Adolescents

Increasing behavioral skills is a Stage 1 primary treatment target. However, skills acquisition within individual psychotherapy is very difficult because of the need for crisis intervention and attention to other issues. Thus a separate component of treatment directly targets the acquisition of behavioral skills. Skills training is typically addressed in a group format. If it is not feasible to get a group started in particular a setting, teaching skills individually might be considered; this can be done either by the primary therapist or by another therapist at another time. If the primary (individual) therapist teaches skills, we recommend actually scheduling a separate session each week to address only skills. If getting to the clinic is an issue for a client, then double sessions might be scheduled (in which the first half focuses on skills, a break occurs, and then the second half focuses on individual behavioral analysis and problem solving). We recommend a clear break between modes; trying to shore up capabilities while handling ongoing crises is like trying to build a shelter in the midst of a storm. One cannot address crises without skills; one cannot learn skills while responding to crises. Thus a clear break between the two modes allows for a separate and distinct focus on each important goal without interference.

As can be seen in Table 4.2, standard DBT teaches a comprehensive set of skills that are grouped within four skills modules: Mindfulness Skills, Emotion Regulation Skills, Interpersonal Effectiveness Skills, and Distress Tolerance Skills. A fifth module, Walking the Middle

TABLE 4.2. Overview of Specific DBT Skills by Module

Module: Core Mindfulness Skills

"Wise mind" (state of mind)
"What skills" (observe, describe, participate)
"How skills" (don't judge, focus on one thing mindfully, do what works)

Module: Emotion Regulation Skills

Observing and describing emotions
Reducing vulnerability to emotion mind: PLEASE MASTER (treat PhysicaL illness, balance Eating, avoid mood-Altering drugs, balance Sleep, get Exercise; build MASTERy)
Increasing positive emotions
Mindfulness of current emotion
Acting opposite to current emotion

Module: Interpersonal Effectiveness Skills

DEAR MAN (Describe, Express, Assert, Reinforce; stay Mindful, Appear confident, Negotiate)
GIVE (be Gentle, act Interested, Validate, use an Easy manner)
FAST (be Fair, no Apologies, Stick to values, be Truthful)

Module: Distress Tolerance Skills

Distracting with "Wise mind ACCEPTS" (Activities, Contributing, Comparisons, Emotions, Pushing away, Thoughts, Sensations)
Self-soothing the five senses (vision, hearing, smell, taste, touch)
Pros and cons
IMPROVE the moment (Imagery, Meaning, Prayer, Relaxation, One thing in the moment, Vacation, Encouragement)
Radical acceptance
Turning the mind
Willingness

Module: Walking the Middle Path Skills

Employing behavioral principles: Self and other
Validation: Self and other
Thinking dialectically
Acting dialectically

Path Skills, is adolescent-specific and can be taught as well. (We describe this module in more detail later in this chapter.) Because there is a great deal of material to cover, skills training in DBT follows a psychoeducational format. In contrast to individual therapy, where the agenda is determined primarily by the problem to be solved, in skills training the agenda is set by the skill to be taught. Thus the fundamental priorities here are skill acquisition and strengthening. Although stopping client behaviors that seriously threaten life (e.g., potential suicide or homicide) or continuation of therapy (e.g., not coming to skills training sessions, verbally attacking others in group sessions) is still a first priority, less severe therapy-interfering behaviors (e.g., refusing to talk in a group setting, restless pacing in the middle of sessions, attacking the therapist and/or the therapy) are not given the attention in skills training that they are given in the individual psychotherapy mode. If such behaviors were a primary focus, there would never be time for teaching behavioral skills. Generally, therapy-interfering behaviors are put on an extinction schedule while the client is "dragged" through skills training and simultaneously soothed. In DBT, all Stage 1 skills training clients are required to be in concurrent individual psychotherapy. Throughout, each client is urged to address other problematic behaviors with his or her primary therapist; if a serious risk of suicide develops, the skills training therapist (if different from the primary therapist) refers the problem to the primary therapist.

In some settings, therapists, while not doing DBT as the primary treatment approach, nevertheless reserve a portion of each session to cover DBT skills from the skills training manual (Linehan, 1993b). This is often because a client or therapist has learned of the treatment and wishes to incorporate aspects of it into the therapy. In such cases, we recommend that the therapist coach the client and consider ways to enhance generalization, since these factors are essential in the client's truly learning and applying the skills.

Finally, many DBT programs offer some type of maintenance or graduate group to clients who complete Stage 1 of treatment. Such groups are designed to continue addressing the treatment functions of improving capabilities, improving motivation, and promoting generalization of skills. Often such graduate groups are structured in a less intensive manner (in terms of both the adolescents' participation and the resources of the program). These groups are discussed later in this chapter and in Chapter 11.

Function: Ensuring Skill Generalization

Primary Modes: Telephone Consultation, Individual therapy, Family Therapy

Telephone calls between sessions are an integral part of outpatient DBT. When DBT is conducted in other settings, such as inpatient units, other extratherapeutic contact can be arranged. Phone calls have several important purposes: (1) to provide coaching in skills and promote skill generalization; (2) to provide emergency crisis intervention; (3) to break the link between suicidal behaviors and therapist attention by inviting contact for "good news"; and (4) to provide a context for repairing the therapeutic relationship without requiring the client to wait until the next session. When a phone call is made to seek help, the focus of the phone session varies, depending on the complexity and severity of the problem to be solved and the amount of time the therapist is willing to spend on the phone. In a situation where it is reasonably easy to determine what the client should do, the focus is on helping the client use behavioral skills (rather than dysfunctional behaviors) to address the problem. With a complex problem or with a problem too severe for the client to resolve soon, the focus is on ameliorating and tolerating distress and inhibiting dysfunctional problem-solving behaviors until the next therapy session. In the latter case, resolving the problem that set off the crisis is not the target of the phone session.

With the exception of taking necessary steps to protect a client's life when suicide is threatened, all calls for help are handled as much alike as possible. This is done to break the association between suicidal behaviors and increased phone contact. To do this, a therapist can do one of two things: refuse to accept any calls, including suicide crisis calls, or insist that a client who calls during such crises also call during other crises and problem situations. Because experts on suicidal behaviors uniformly say that therapist availability is necessary with suicidal clients (see Linehan, 1993a), DBT chooses the latter course; it encourages (and at times insists) on calls during nonsuicidal crisis periods, as well as calls to share good news. In DBT, calling the therapist too infrequently, as well as too frequently, would be considered therapy-interfering behavior.

The final priority for phone calls to individual therapists is relationship repair. Clients with BPD or borderline features often experience delayed emotional reactions to interactions that have occurred during therapy sessions. From a DBT perspective, it is not reasonable to require clients to wait up to a whole week before dealing with these emotions, and it is appropriate for clients to call for a brief "heart-to-heart." In these situations, the role of the therapist is to soothe and reassure. In-depth analyses should wait until the next session.

In milieu settings, the function of ensuring skill generalization will need to occur through other modes, such as coaching from nursing staff and other members of the milieu, homework groups, or other means. Chapter 8 provides additional discussion on the use of telephone consultation.

In addition to telephone calls, individual therapy helps with the generalization of skills, as the therapist works with the adolescent during behavioral analyses to understand where capability deficits led to problem behaviors and to apply specific skills to those situations. Homework assignments assigned by the individual (as well as group) therapist also promote generalization, by ensuring that the adolescent takes what is learned and applies it in real-life contexts. Individual sessions can also be audiotaped, and the adolescent can listen to the tapes between sessions to further promote generalization. Finally, family therapy sessions (as well as family participation in group) also contribute to skills generalization by providing the adolescent with skills coaches at home, as well as *in vivo* opportunities to practice in therapeutic contexts.

Function: Structuring the Environment to Support Clients and Therapists

Primary Modes: Various Interventions with Family Members and Contacts with Ancillary Treatment Providers

One of the essential components of DBT is attention to contingencies throughout the entire treatment program. The aim is to be sure that all programmatic rules and all program staff members reinforce skillful rather than maladaptive behaviors. This is especially important with respect to suicidal behaviors. The premise is that if clients can only get help that they want or need by getting more suicidal or engaging in other maladaptive behaviors, then it is doubtful that the treatment as a whole will be effective.

Unlike most adults, however, adolescents are usually still in the original invalidating environment in which they learned dysfunctional patterns. Therefore, to be effective, DBT with adolescents needs to address any invalidating behaviors between family members. It does so by intervening with family members in three different ways: including family members in skills training groups, offering telephone consultation for family members on implementing skills, and integrating family members as needed into individual therapy sessions.

In addition, structuring the environment can be achieved through contact with providers of ancillary treatments, such as psychiatrists or school counselors. Ideally, providers of these treatments will in some way be linked with the DBT treatment team or be familiar with principles of DBT. An example would be a psychiatrist who provides pharmacotherapy at the same clinic that houses the treatment, or, better yet, who is actually a member of the treatment team. In the program at Montefiore Medical Center, we regularly include psychiatrists as part of the consultation team. Thus clients in our DBT program who require medication see one of the team psychiatrists. When it is not possible to include an ancillary treatment provider as part of the DBT team, maintaining contact between the team and the provider, while offering some education and orientation to DBT strategies, is the preferable strategy. For example, we coach the client on how to present DBT to the ancillary provider, including reviewing the skills notebook, assumptions, and rules. For teenagers, ancillary treatment modes often include treatments administered through the school. In residential and day treatment facilities, schooling might be integrated into the treatment; in this case, there should be close contact and cooperation between the treatment and the educational staff. In outpatient settings, therapists deciding to engage school personnel must put in additional effort to arrange meetings, orient these personnel to DBT, and develop treatment plans. This is easier to do when the treatment staff has a continuing relationship with school professionals through a history of referrals and working together.

Function: Enhancing Capabilities and Motivation of Therapists

Primary Mode: Consultation Team

DBT assumes that effective treatment of BPD must pay as much attention to a therapist's behavior and experience in therapy as it does to a client's. Treating clients with suicidal behaviors and/or borderline characteristics is enormously stressful, and staying within the DBT frame can be tremendously difficult. Thus an integral part of the therapy is the treatment of the therapist. All therapists are required to be in a DBT consultation team. DBT team meetings are held weekly and are attended by therapists currently utilizing DBT with clients. Note that this meeting is distinct from staff meetings, morning rounds, or similar meetings that address issues such as clients' medication status, discharge planning, unit procedures, and the like. When settings or time constraints require incorporating administrative/client management functions into DBT team meetings, it is helpful to set an agenda and limit the time devoted to the former issues, or cover them only after therapist consultation issues have been addressed. This preserves the goal of the consultation meetings: to allow therapists to discuss their difficulties providing treatment in a nonjudgmental and supportive environment that also helps improve their motivation and capabilities. The role of consultation is to hold each therapist within the therapeutic frame and address problems that arise in the course of treatment delivery. Thus the fundamental target is increasing adherence to DBT principles for each member of the consultation team. The DBT team is viewed as an integral component of DBT; it is considered group therapy for the therapists. Each member is simultaneously a client and a therapist in the group.

Team Meeting Format

The DBT consultation team is an essential and ongoing part of the DBT program. That is, the team does not end after any individual's completion of treatment. Rather, it continues as clients come and go, serving as a sort of backbone of the entire treatment program. Depending on the setting, of course, team members may come and go as the staff turns over. However, almost any setting will ask a practitioner to commit to the team for at least the duration of his or her involvement with DBT. In training settings (e.g., graduate department clinics, teaching hospitals), student team members (i.e., psychology graduate students, residents, social work interns) often remain team members throughout the duration of their placement.

In our programs, we start each team meeting with a brief mindfulness exercise (e.g., observing thoughts, focusing all of one's attention on one's breathing, etc.), led by different therapists on a rotating basis, to forge a break with the previous activities of the day and cue a DBT mindset. These exercises also serve to enhance therapists' skills in leading mindfulness exercises and coaching mindfulness skills. We then read one of the team agreements (to be described below), review the team notes from the previous week, and set an agenda for the meeting. The agenda is set by the team, and the order in which items are discussed is based on the DBT hierarchy of targets: (1) therapist needs for consultation around suicidal crises or other life-threatening behaviors; (2) therapy-interfering behaviors (including client absences and dropouts, as well as therapist therapy-interfering behaviors); (3) therapist team-interfering behaviors and burnout; (4) severe or escalating quality-of-life-interfering behaviors; (5) good news and therapists' effective behaviors; (6) summary of the previous week's skills group and graduate group sessions by group leaders; and (7) administrative issues (e.g., requests to miss the next team meeting or be out of town; new client contacts; changes in skills trainers or group time, format of consultation group, etc.). This agenda spans the first hour of the team meeting. Although the agenda may look impossibly long, ordinarily the time is managed by therapists' being explicit about where they need help and consultation from the team. At the University of Washington, all therapists are asked to come to each team meeting prepared to state what help they need and the importance of their need for time on a scale from 1 to 3. The other half to full hour of the meeting is devoted to maintaining DBT training, including a review of skills corresponding to those being taught in group that week, skills practice, videotapes, or other new teaching materials/exercises. At some sites the training hour is set at a different time of the week, with therapists from all DBT teams attending.

The in-depth discussions of clients and of therapists' difficulties in delivering competent DBT center around enhancing the therapists' ability to deliver treatment effectively. This involves validating the therapists' reactions while still eliciting effective treatment behaviors. Often the team helps a depleted therapist to regain a nonjudgmental, empathic stance toward a client's behaviors by pointing out perspectives the therapist may no longer be able to generate. Furthermore, the team can help the therapist get unstuck by coaching issues such as handling difficult communications or planning effective contingency management strategies. Teams also address such issues as burnout and personal difficulties or limits that interfere with treatment. In addition, the consultation meeting is focused on therapist behaviors that interfere with team functioning, such as failure to keep agreements made in team, coming late or leaving early, taking responsibility for one's own clients but not for other clients, talking too much or too little, annoying habits evident in team, and the differences of opinion or conflicts that inevitably arise between members of the treatment team.

Team Agreements

DBT promotes a set of agreements for consultation team members that help facilitate interactions between colleagues within the meetings. The agreements are intended to facilitate maintaining a DBT frame. They help to create a supportive environment for managing client–therapist and therapist–therapist difficulties. These agreements apply equally to consultation groups working with adolescent clients. In addition, we have noticed that most of the agreements contain principles that facilitate work with family members as well, as explicated below.

Dialectical Agreement

The group agrees to accept a dialectical philosophy. Essentially, this involves adhering to the notion that there is no absolute truth, and thus searching for a synthesis of polarities when extreme viewpoints arise.

We find that extreme viewpoints often arise when therapists are working with adolescent clients. A polarity that arises is "blaming" a teen versus "blaming" a parent. When strong differences of opinion emerge among the team members, this situation is normalized according to the dialectical world view; that is, truth is neither absolute nor relative, and reality exists in opposing forces. Team members are urged to search for the grain of truth in the opposing perspective and work toward a synthesis. It can be helpful to consider whether one is aligning with one of the extreme behavior patterns described in Chapter 5, such as invalidating the client or pathologizing normal behavior.

Consultation-to-the-Patient Agreement

The second agreement involves consulting to clients on how to interact effectively with others in their environment, rather than consulting with the environment on interacting effectively with clients. This provides clients with opportunities to practice skillful interactions and avoids the trap of reinforcing clients' tendencies to elicit help from others while themselves remaining passive (see the discussion of "active passivity" in Chapter 5). The agreement implies that if a client tells the individual therapist that he or she is angry with the skills trainer for saying something upsetting in group, the individual therapist consults to the client on how to interact effectively with the skills trainer, instead of telling the skills trainer how to interact with the client.

With adolescents, in contrast to adults, there is typically a need to do more consulting with the environment. For example, minors cannot be expected to initiate contact with ancillary treatment providers (e.g., consultation with a psychiatrist), be fully responsible for getting themselves to sessions when they rely on transportation from parents, or arrange meetings with school personnel. On the other hand, within these constraints, adolescents can nevertheless be coached on how to communicate effectively and play an appropriate and active role in such situations (such as accurately describing medication side effects to a psychiatrist, asserting to parents the importance of making it to therapy and behaving in a way that facilitates this, or speaking with school staff members in a way that helps them to be taken seriously).

Consistency Agreement

Consistency of therapists is not necessarily expected. Treatment team members not only "agree to disagree" with one another; they are also not necessarily expected to be consistent from client to client or over time with the same client. Clashes or mix-ups are regarded as inevitable and as presenting opportunities for clients and treatment staff alike to practice DBT skills. In work with parents of adolescents, it is useful to extend this principle to parents. Therapists and adolescents alike must understand that it is not realistic to expect parents to be perfectly consistent, due to factors such as mood, stress level, or a teen's presentation. Thus this agreement helps team members accept variations within other members and within the family members of teens attending treatment.

Observing-Limits Agreement

Therapists agree to observe their own personal limits without judging others. They also agree not to make inferences about team members' limits that seem narrow (e.g., seeing a therapist as withholding, rigid, or self-centered) or broad (e.g., seeing a therapist as needing to rescue a client or as having boundary problems).

This agreement stems from the observation that therapists working with suicidal, emotionally dysregulated clients tend to attribute violations of their own personal limits to *clients'* problems with "boundaries." This makes little sense, as specific therapists' limits are idiosyncratic. For example, one therapist may be able to tolerate working with a hostile, argumentative adolescent, but not one who calls several times over each weekend. Another may openly receive weekend phone calls, but may quickly burn out with a belligerent teen. Thus notions of clients' violating boundaries often pathologize the clients, when in fact "crossed boundaries" often say more about therapists' sensitivities and standards than about clients' judgment. Furthermore, part of negotiating an interpersonal relationship involves accepting feedback about the other person's limits, and, just as importantly, developing some ability to "read" the other's limits. Thus setting universal rules in treatment (e.g., no more than four phone calls per week) would not only be arbitrary and fail to appease every therapist, but would also hinder this potentially therapeutic aspect of the therapist's self-disclosure. Thus DBT therapists carefully identify their own personal limits and then clarify these limits to clients, while explicitly taking responsibility for them rather than giving the clients responsibility for them. For example, a therapist might tell a client the following: "When you mimic me, insult me, and frequently compare me (unfavorably) to your last therapist, it makes it hard for me to want to keep working with you. A different therapist might not have a big problem with this, but it just crosses my personal limits."

The team might step in, however, if it becomes apparent that a therapist has drawn limits that interfere with effective therapy. For example, if an overwhelmed therapist begins to stop accepting phone calls outside of ordinary working hours and an adolescent thus loses an opportunity for skills generalization, the team would seek to understand and validate the therapist's experience, but would also problem-solve to help the therapist become more available to the client (e.g., delay assignment of additional cases or find some way to reduce the therapist's workload; coach the therapist in keeping phone calls brief and focused or in otherwise handling them in a way that feels more manageable). On the other hand, the team must truly work toward being nonjudgmental about a therapist's limits and simply accept them when they are not harmful to the therapist's clients (even if they are narrower than the limits of other team members). For example, one therapist who was threatened with a knife by a college-age client wanted to cease working with the client altogether. Despite the client's desire to continue working with this therapist, the team supported the therapist in ceasing contact after ensuring that appropriate care was offered to the client (switching to another therapist plus taking additional steps to protect the new therapist's safety and ease in working with the client).

In working with parents, it is also helpful to keep in mind the principle of observing limits. Parents can often be so anxious about their child's welfare that they make unreasonable demands on the therapist. Parents who are overwhelmed with other obligations may want the therapist to be unreasonably available to their child or may make unnecessarily frequent calls for advice or reassurance. Parents who are used to having control in their lives may try to control the process of therapy or make insistent demands that confidentiality be broken. In each case, it is the task of the team to assist the therapist in clarifying and managing his or her own limits with the parents.

Phenomenological Empathy Agreement

All therapists agree to search for nonpejorative, phenomenologically empathic interpretations of a client's behavior. The agreement is based on the DBT assumptions that patients are doing the best they can and want to improve. For example, when a therapist attends a consultation meeting and reports that his or her client is "a manipulative, insensitive, crazy adolescent who makes me want to quit therapy today," the other team members try to (1) help the therapist generate nonjudgmental, phenomenologically empathic descriptors of the client's behavior; and (2) validate the therapist's sense of feeling overwhelmed, angry, and frustrated. To do so might require a colleague to refer to the biosocial theory of BPD. For example, the client's childhood history of abuse and chronic invalidation may be helpful in explaining the client's current emotion dysregulation and interpersonal deficits, which quickly alienate those close to him or her. In DBT, a client's behavior is not considered manipulative without an assessment of the client's actual motivation. The fact that the therapist feels manipulated does not mean that manipulation was the client's intent. Nonpejorative descriptions include reminding therapists that clients are doing the best they can, given their limited skills repertoires; indeed, the limitations of their skills repertoires have gotten them into treatment. Moreover, it is difficult for clients to give up their current coping strategies because they are often reinforced, at least in the short term. This dialectical, empathic, nonpejorative thinking reduces the all-or-none thinking often pervasive among clients with BPD or borderline characteristics, and even among the staff members who treat them.

This stance toward empathy for the client's experience extends to family members as well. This is often difficult; we have seen numerous therapists on our teams become angry or frustrated with parents for their invalidation, noncompliance, or outright therapy-destroying behavior. However, the best chance of forming an alliance with such parents involves maintaining a phenomenologically empathic view of their experience. Keeping in mind the transactional development of BPD, one can consider the difficulty (often spanning the adolescent's life) of raising an adolescent who seems overly emotional, demanding, and difficult. This is only exacerbated by the pain, fear, and guilt parents often experience as a result of the teen's suicidal and otherwise self-destructive behavior. Such behaviors place a great strain on parents, who often feel lost or "at their wits' end." When the team takes the time to bolster a therapist's empathic understanding of such a parent's experience, progress can often be made.

Fallibility Agreement

The group members agree that all therapists are fallible. DBT follows the assumption that therapists will make mistakes, and will even violate the present consultation group agreements. The job of the treatment team will be to balance problem solving aimed toward directing a therapist back into a DBT framework with validation of the wisdom present in the therapist's actions or position.

Again, it is helpful to apply this principle to clients' family members as well. Parents will inevitably make mistakes. The team can help a therapist accept this inevitability while problem-solving about how to repair the damage from a mistake or otherwise get a parent back on track toward working effectively with a teen.

DBT is the treatment of a community of clients by a community of therapists. Thus therapists agree that they are in fact the therapeutic community for all clients being seen by team members. That is, each person takes responsibility for working to ensure that each client receives the best treatment possible. Therapists agree to speak out actively, both to recognize effective therapy behaviors and to modify or eliminate ineffective therapy behaviors of team members. The suicide of one therapist's client is the suicide of a client of all therapists.

Team Members' Roles

There are various ways of dividing up responsibilities for conducting DBT teams. We have found that a team does much better when there is an active team leader who is given primary responsibility for knowing, remembering, and articulating the DBT principles when necessary, and for overseeing the fidelity of the treatment provided. This job should be given to the person on the team with the best training in DBT, or, among equally trained (or untrained) therapists, the person with the best leadership qualities. Most teams rotate responsibility for developing and managing the agenda and for writing the team notes among members on either a weekly or monthly basis. Because the team is an integral part of the therapy itself, it is of course important that team notes be taken and kept in the therapy records. At many clinics, the "observer" task of helping team members stay on track with their agreements also rotates among members. At the University of Washington, the observer has a small "mindfulness bell" and rings it whenever team members make judgmental comments (in content or tone) about themselves, each other, or a client; stay polarized without seeking synthesis; fall out of mindfulness by doing two things at once; or jump in to solve a problem before assessing the problem. An entire meeting rarely goes by without the bell's ringing at least once. (DBT is not for the faint of heart.) We have found that over time team members almost jump over the observer to ring the bell, often catching themselves with judgmental words or thoughts. The secret, of course, is to ring the bell nonjudgmentally.

ADAPTING DBT FOR ADOLESCENTS: SETTING UP PROGRAMS

Anyone who considers starting a DBT program for adolescents needs to answer questions such as the following: How will the adolescent client population be defined? Who will constitute the treatment team? In what modes will clients be treated? Should any adaptations to standard DBT be made? We next discuss these and other issues to consider in setting up a DBT treatment program for adolescents and their families. For much of the discussion that follows, we draw on our personal experiences in DBT programs with adolescents at Montefiore Medical Center (Miller); Long Island University, C. W. Post Campus (Rathus); and the University of Washington Behavioral Research and Therapy Clinic (Linehan). We have also surveyed numerous adolescent DBT programs around the world to help inform this discussion.

How Will the Adolescent Client Population Be Defined?

Adolescent DBT programs employ varying inclusion criteria, depending on the treatment setting. For example, some DBT programs for adolescent inpatients use suicidal behavior as an inclusion criterion (Katz et al., 2004). Several residential programs employ some degree of injury directed toward self or others as the primary inclusion criterion (Miller, Rathus, et al., in press). One forensic DBT program included those teens with criminal offenses who also engaged in violence toward self or others (Trupin, Stewart, Beach, & Boesky, 2002). One high school selected "at-risk" teens for a lunchtime 22-week DBT skills training group; these youth were defined as truant, violent, self-injurious, and/or substance-abusing (Sally, Jackson, Carney, Kevelson, & Miller, 2002). Most adolescent outpatient DBT programs include teens with histories of suicidal behavior, NSIB, and current suicidal ideation *plus* BPD features, since these criteria most closely resemble the inclusion criteria used in Linehan's original outcome studies with suicidal adults (see Miller, Rathus, et al., in press) Among the adolescent DBT programs we surveyed, the youngest clients were 12 and the oldest were 19 years of age, with a median age of 16 (Miller, Rathus, et al., in press).

Most adolescent DBT programs, regardless of setting, exclude teens who present with psychotic disorders, severe cognitive impairment (i.e., IQ lower than 70), or severe receptive or expressive language problems. For example, actively psychotic or actively manic adolescents are excluded from the Montefiore program's multifamily skills training group and instead are taught skills individually or with their family members, since their psychotic or manic behaviors may become too disruptive to a group. The differential diagnosis between BPD and a bipolar disorder is sometimes difficult to make in adolescents. Also, for reasons discussed in Chapter 1, many clinicians will make Axis I diagnoses but not Axis II diagnoses in adolescents. In the Montefiore program, all clients referred receive a thorough diagnostic evaluation even if they have recently had one somewhere else. We are particularly careful to reassess clients referred with bipolar disorders to clarify the differential diagnosis, since treatments may vary accordingly.

Teens with moderate to severe learning disabilities and those with borderline IQ scores are often included in DBT treatment programs. Accommodations typically include teaching fewer skills at a slower pace, simplifying the terms used to teach, simplifying the diary card, and possibly having clients repeat the skills training curriculum. The following sections take a closer look at other factors (age, gender, diagnosis, and cultural factors) that need to be considered in setting a program's inclusion and exclusion criteria.

Age

Although adolescents as a group are generally defined as ranging in age from 12 to 19 (Berk, 2004) and some suggest even older, this is not a homogeneous group. Early adolescence (roughly age 11 or 12 to age 14) is characterized by recent entry into puberty; often by first-time experimenting with things such as dating and substance use; and by attending middle school or junior high school. Those in middle to late adolescence (roughly ages 14 to 18) are typically attending high school and are sandwiched in between the childhood years and adulthood, often facing increased demands, pressures, and responsibility. For example, they may be working, learning to drive, and entering more serious romantic relationships. The oldest adolescents might be considered to range from roughly age 18 to age 20, 21, or even 25. For example, Arnett (1999) has defined a period from ages 18 to 25 called "emerging adulthood" or "transitional adulthood." According to Arnett, this stage is primarily a middle- and upper-class phenomenon that occurs prior to early adulthood and reflects a sort of extended adolescence. Emerging adulthood is marked by continued financial dependence (and sometimes continued residence in the parents' home), continued identity development, continued exploration rather than commitment in terms of relationships and vocation, and possible continued engagement in risky or impulsive behaviors.

Given this diversity among age subgroups, how does one define the population of adolescents in terms of age, and should a program mix these various ages or limit treatment to early, middle, or late adolescence or some combination thereof? Moreover, should practitioners base inclusion decisions solely on age, or also on level of functioning? For example, an 18-year-old living at home, attending high school, and dependent on his or her family of origin seems more adolescent-like than an 18-year-old who is working full-time and living independently with a stable partner. Advantages to limiting treatment to particular age groups within adolescence include increased homogeneity in terms of life issues (which may lead to a greater connection to peers in group settings) and the potential for development of greater specialization in a particular stage of adolescence among staff members (e.g., a setting could have its "early adolescence expert" who runs these groups or takes on many of the individual cases). However, a setting must have either enough of a referral base that it can afford to turn away adolescents outside a specific age range, or enough referrals *and* staff members to fill and run various groups, each limited to specific ages. Some settings might have several groups running simultaneously and might thus choose to have them divided into two (e.g., 12–15, 16–19) or three (e.g., 11–14, 14–17, 17–20) age groupings. Some settings, such as hospitals, may have institution-wide criteria for ages, in which clients ages 17 and younger are treated in a child/adolescent program and clients ages 18 and above automatically receive services in the adult outpatient, day treatment, or inpatient department. Still other settings without a large enough teen referral base may include adolescents ages 16 and older within adult programs.

Because of staff or referral limitations or other reasons, providers may prefer to run mixed-age programs for adolescents. Advantages include the ability to accept a greater range of clients to fill groups, less need to differentiate between age and level of functioning, and the potential for older participants to serve as mentors and models for younger ones. In our Montefiore program, clients are adolescents ranging in age from 12 to 19 years, mixed together in skills groups. We have found that older clients will often play a sort of "big sibling" role to younger clients, coaching them and imparting advice and wisdom. This is inspirational for younger attendees and a source of pride and motivation for older attendees. One risk is accepting an "outlier" in age for a particular group who then ends up feeling alienated—for example, a 19-year-old in a group of mostly 14- and 15-year-olds. To prevent this, the skills trainer may encourage the older teen to play a special role in the group in order to capitalize on the age discrepancy. Other alternatives are referring an outlier adolescent to another group or conducting skills training individually.

Gender

Gender is another factor to consider. Will a program include both girls and boys, and if so, will it place them together in groups? Some residential treatment settings are limited to treating one gender, or else separate the genders into different residences. But most other settings admit both boys and girls. Some advantages of limiting a skills group to a single gender are similar to those of limiting a group to a narrow age range: Doing so allows for greater homogeneity of issues brought into the group and perhaps greater comfort with self-disclosure. Furthermore, it may minimize the degree of disruption or distraction due to sexual interest, flirting, or increased social anxiety due to the presence of the opposite sex. (The issue of sexual interest would obviously remain for homosexual adolescents, regardless of group type.)

In our Montefiore and Long Island University programs, however, we combine males and females for several reasons. First, this practice allows us to treat boys in settings that get a low percentage of male referrals, There might not otherwise be enough male participants to fill a group. In our Montefiore settings, only 15–20% of our DBT referrals are male, resulting in about one male adolescent per group of five to six clients and their families. This is typical, given the much higher rates of BPD diagnoses, suicide attempts, and NSIB in females. Second, the presence of both genders allows for developing skillful opposite-sex friendships, role-playing boyfriend–girlfriend conversations with opposite-sex participants, and gaining insight on issues from the other gender's perspective. This promotes generalization of skills. In a mixed gender group, it is very important to make it clear to members that both boys and girls will be in the group, even if at some points there are no male members. In our University of Washington program, this communication broke down at one point recently. And when a male was accepted into the group, there were extreme emotional reactions and near-panic on the part of two members who had been previously raped. Although we did not rescind our decision, several extra individual sessions and much coaching were needed to smooth out the transition. The mixed-gender group is now doing very well, and the lone male is "radically accepted," in the DBT sense (see Linehan, 1993b).

Diagnosis

What will a program's diagnostic entry criteria be? Will clients be suicidal, and if so, how will "suicidality" be defined? Will clients need to meet full criteria for BPD, exhibit subthreshold BPD features, or simply manifest emotional or behavioral dysregulation? How will these criteria be measured? Will clients with comorbid disorders be included, or will certain comorbid disorders be cause for exclusion? Will clients be combined into mixed diagnostic groups, or will they be assigned to relatively homogeneous groups?

Groups with high diagnostic homogeneity would be hard to come by in this field, since suicidal individuals with borderline features tend to be characterized by multiple problems and multiple comorbidities. However, minimal entry criteria (e.g., meeting full criteria for BPD and displaying evidence of recent suicidal behaviors and NSIB) can result in a relatively homogeneous group with the advantage of close similarity to the original group with whom DBT was validated (Linehan et al., 1991; Linehan, 1993a). This may also allow for similar problems raised in group sessions, and thus possibly a greater feeling of connection to the group. Diagnostically mixed groups, however, may also be beneficial; more evidence is emerging that DBT can be successfully adapted for a range of populations and target behaviors (see Miller & Rathus, 2000). Casting a wider net also has the potential to benefit more people, but certain cautions are warranted in combining diagnostic groups or having varied inclusion criteria. First, individuals with certain diagnoses, though appropriate for DBT, might be better served in a DBT or other program specifically tailored for those diagnoses (e.g., primary diagnoses of eating disorders or substance abuse/dependence). Second, certain diagnostic groups may not be best served in group settings. For example, recent evidence finds that youth with conduct disorder or antisocial features fare *worse* when treated in group formats, because of the modeling, training, and peer validation of antisocial behaviors that occurs (Dishion, McCord, & Poulin, 1999). Third, if entry criteria become too loose, individuals' severity levels and treatment targets may differ so drastically from one another that group skills training may lose its focus: What is being treated may become unclear, the biosocial theory underlying the treatment may no longer apply, and the group may disintegrate. We thus recommend at least having an identifiable unifying theme that brings group members together.

Our Montefiore program's entry criteria are that adolescents must both be suicidal (suicide attempt within past 16 weeks or current suicidal ideation) and exhibit borderline personality features (a full BPD diagnosis, or at least three diagnostic criteria). Exclusion criteria consist of active psychosis, severe learning disabilities, or severe cognitive impairment. In addition to BPD, the primary comorbid diagnoses have included mood, anxiety, eating, substance-related, and disruptive behavior disorders.

Cultural Factors

Will a program be homogeneous or heterogeneous in terms of SES and ethnicity? In general, we have found that the answer to this question tends to be determined by setting. For example, our Montefiore inner-city population consists of mostly lower-SES adolescents who represent ethnic minority groups (predominantly various Hispanic groups, African American youth, and youth of African descent from the Caribbean). Our suburban population consists of mostly middle- to upper-SES American teens. Thus we have no decision to make about whom to assign to groups. However, one might consider whether cultural factors are disparate enough within a given setting that there would be reason to consider assigning clients to groups on this basis. For example, one consideration might be the primary language spoken by the family; some settings have implemented skills groups taught in Spanish to allow family members' participation when little or no English is spoken. On the other hand, definitions of culture vary widely (see the discussion of culture in Rathus & Feindler, 2004), and culturally diverse groups have the potential to enhance members' experience.

Who Will Constitute the Treatment Team?

The treatment team consists of everyone involved with the DBT program across modes—that is, skills trainers, individual therapists, and providers of additional modes within a particular setting (such as nurses in a milieu setting). At a bare minimum, it should consist of at least two mental health professionals trained in DBT and, ideally, experienced in working with adolescents. Having at least one other colleague with whom to discuss one's own difficulties in providing DBT serves the essential DBT function of enhancing therapist capabilities and motivation, as described earlier in this chapter. And having at least a third DBT therapist can help the team achieve a synthesis when the other two are stuck highlighting opposite poles of a particular dialectic.

The ideal treatment team will depend on the nature of the particular setting, but there are some common elements. First, the more previous DBT training that team members have, the easier DBT is to implement. At a minimum, the team leader should be intensively trained in DBT. Second, experience in working with adolescents is helpful for team members because of the many developmental issues that make adolescents a unique population to work with. Third, family therapy experience is helpful. Many teen programs will include family members. Practitioners must be comfortable working with multiple family members at once. Even when family members are not included in the skills training, they will probably be involved in some way with treatment and have contact with the treatment providers, since their teens are minors. Team members experienced in group work can also make helpful contributions as group skills leaders themselves or as consultants to the skills trainers. In essence, the more experience the team members have in the related aspects of treatment, the better, since the treatment is complex and the populations treated are challenging.

If providers in a setting are inexperienced in DBT, we recommend a structured reading group for self-teaching, plus attendance at available trainings, workshops, and conferences. In-house training can be conducted by team members with expertise in the treatment, and therapist consultation meetings include didactic portions. We have held team meetings in which didactics are taught on a rotating basis; each team member does readings on a skill, strategy, or principle on his or her week to teach, and then runs the didactic portion of that week's team meeting, teaching peers. We also recommend ongoing individual supervision by a well-trained and experienced therapist or even by outside consultants, in addition to therapist consultation team meetings, for novice DBT therapists. The bottom line is that all participating therapists agree to provide DBT and adhere to the DBT team agreements.

Depending on the setting, the disciplines of team members will vary. Some teams may be multidisciplinary, and others may be limited to one or two disciplines. In our inner-city Montefiore Medical Center setting, our treatment teams have included psychologists, psychologists in training, psychiatrists, and social workers. Representatives of other disciplines can participate as well, such as nurses, caseworkers, or mental health aides. Members of multiple disciplines can be trained to deliver this treatment, and multidisciplinary teams offer various areas of expertise in consulting on each case. For example, when possible, it is helpful to have a nurse practitioner or physician on the team to handle medication issues, rather than having a client's pharmacotherapy handled by an outside party who is unfamiliar with DBT. In inpatient DBT settings, it is common to have direct care staff members as part of the treatment team—serving as primary therapists or skills coaches, or playing other roles. In our suburban Long Island University psychology training clinic setting, the team initially consisted of one intensively trained psychologist (Rathus) and several graduate students in clinical psychology. Such single-discipline teams are possible and allow for training of new therapists. However, such a team composition (one leader and many trainees) poses a risk of burning out the team leader. The leader in such a situation is advised either to seek outside peer consultation or to require a minimal 2-year commitment from students. That way, once trainees acquire a certain level of experience, they are more skilled and can play more of a senior role on the team (see also Chapter 12).

In What Modes Will Clients Be Treated?

Whenever possible, we recommend delivering the "gold standard" comprehensive treatment as outlined in Chapter 3 and as originally developed and researched with documented efficacy (Linehan et al., 1991; Linehan, 1993a). We define "comprehensive treatment" as achieving all five of the functions discussed earlier in this chapter (i.e., increasing motivation, enhancing capabilities, generalizing skills, structuring the environment, and enhancing therapists' capabilities). In a traditional DBT outpatient program, motivational issues are addressed in individual therapy; capabilities are primarily enhanced via a skills training group; skills generalization is achieved by having the client call his or her primary therapist for coaching when the client is in distress; structuring the environment is often achieved through family sessions and/or contacts with the school or other agencies; therapists' capabilities are enhanced by participation in the therapist consultation meetings and continuing education. (See Table 4.1 on the functions of comprehensive treatment for adolescents.)

As described earlier (and also outlined in Table 4.1), different modalities can be effectively used to achieve these functions, depending on the treatment setting. For example, inpatient and residential units often utilize milieu therapists instead of primary therapists to achieve skills generalization, since the clients can receive *in vivo* coaching on the unit as soon as they become distressed. Sometimes a setting is unable to identify enough clients who meet criteria to form a skills training group, so they choose to provide individual (or family) skills training in order to address the function of enhancing the client's capabilities. These adjustments are typically indicated for various settings, and these programs still maintain the five functions and thus the overall comprehensiveness of the DBT model.

What does it mean if an adolescent DBT program does not want to, or is unable to, deliver all five functions? First, providers have to admit to themselves and to clients and families that they are not delivering DBT as it was originally developed and studied. Second, it may be perfectly acceptable to start out on a smaller scale! Furthermore, it remains an empirical question as to which functions are required to achieve treatment efficacy, so we recommend testing the effectiveness of particular interventions in particular settings. We have encountered several situations in which programs, for various reasons, do not deliver the comprehensive treatment. We describe a few examples below.

One common obstacle among new programs is having a limited number of therapists (as few as two) on a team. Although it is entirely possible to conduct the comprehensive treatment with only two therapists, some providers like to start out more slowly. For example, some providers have begun their program with a weekly therapist consultation meeting and a weekly skills group that is led jointly by the two therapists. The goal in this situation would be to identify ways of achieving the other functions over time. Another common difficulty is that some outpatient providers are unable or unwilling to provide telephone coaching between sessions. If a provider is unwilling to provide telephone coaching, then he or she should not be providing DBT if a client does not have someone to serve as a coach to increase skills generalization. Some private practitioners have developed a two-person team model: Each therapist sees his or her own clients for individual therapy, is available by pager for telephone coaching, and conducts collateral family sessions on an as-needed basis; each therapist also conducts weekly family skills training sessions for the other therapist's individual clients and their families. The two therapists have a weekly consultation meeting to discuss their difficulties in providing treatment. Even though it may be less than ideal, many practitioners, especially those in rural settings, opt to have weekly consultation meetings over the telephone.

It is not yet known whether these less-than-comprehensive approaches can achieve the same degree of effectiveness as the well-researched comprehensive treatment. Is applying certain elements of DBT more helpful than applying none at all? One study (Linehan, 1993a) found that clients who received comprehensive DBT did better than clients who received a DBT skills group and a non-DBT individual therapy. No one has studied this with adolescents. Anecdotally, we find that the more comprehensive the treatment, the better the outcomes. Hence we suggest that programs or outpatient therapists offer and then provide comprehensive treatment whenever possible. If they start out smaller, they should set a goal to build up the comprehensive treatment model within a reasonable amount of time. One of the biggest obstacles for clinicians starting a comprehensive DBT program is fear that they (1) do not know enough to make it work and (2) will not be able to achieve all of the functions, usually because of the resources available to them. Our opinion is that with proper supervision and consultation, even two motivated therapists can conceivably start a comprehensive program. We certainly encourage teams of two to assertively invite other potentially interested parties to join their team.

Should Standard DBT Be Adapted for Adolescents?

DBT as originally described and evaluated (Linehan et al., 1991; Linehan, 1993a) included older adolescents and young adults in the sample, so using the original standard treatment with adolescents is certainly an option. However, when the entire client population consists of adolescents, we and other practitioners have found that several modifications to the treatment are helpful, based on developmental and contextual considerations (Miller, Rathus, et al., in press). In making any changes, we and others have tried to maintain the essence of DBT. In a survey of DBT service providers for adolescents, Miller, Rathus, et al. (in press) found that the most common adaptation is inclusion of families in skills training. Other common adaptations included abbreviating treatment length, simplifying the skills handouts, including skills handout examples that are more relevant to teen females and males, changing the "homework" label, simplifying diary cards, including family therapy sessions, adding new skills relevant to parents or other family members, and conducting an orientation for adolescents' support networks. Details on these and other adaptations are woven throughout the rest of this book. It is important to note, however, that some adolescent programs follow the standard model and use the standard handouts and diary cards. The central modification, regardless of setting, is to relate all topics and behavioral skills to the issues faced by adolescents while delivering the treatment. Generally we have found that the main factor in determining what adaptations to make is a therapist's own comfort and experience with materials used.

As an example of one potential outpatient modification, we describe our Montefiore program for adolescents here. The central modifications for adolescents in this program consist of (1) the inclusion of family members with adolescents in a multifamily skills group; (2) the inclusion of family therapy sessions; (3) provision for family members to receive telephone coaching and consultation between skills group sessions; (4) the development of adolescent–family dialectical dilemmas and secondary treatment targets that are addressed in the skills group, as well as in individual and family therapy (described later in Chapter 5 and Appendix B); (5), a reduction in treatment length from standard DBT's 1 year to 16 weeks, with an optional 16–32 additional weeks of a graduate group; (6) a slightly reduced number of standard skills to fit within the 16-week format; (7) the addition of a fifth skills module, Walking the Middle Path, developed specifically for adolescents and families, and (8) modified handouts, written to present fewer ideas per page in simplified language, and designed to be more "adolescent-friendly." An overview of the Montefiore program is given in Table 4.3. Below we briefly discuss each of these adaptations and how they work within this program.

Inclusion of Family Members in Skills Training Groups

To enhance generalization and help structure each adolescent's environment, we have found it helpful to include family members in skills training sessions. When skills training is conducted as a separate individual session each week, parents may attend this session regularly,

---

TABLE 4.3. Overview of Montefiore Program for Suicidal Adolescents

Orientation to mental health clinic and intake evaluation (1–2 visits)

Diagnostic interviewing, history taking, formal behavioral analysis of targeted behaviors

Pretreatment orientation and commitment stage

Teen, teen's family, and therapist reach mutually informed decision to work together; negotiate a
   common set of expectancies to guide initial steps of therapy
Adolescents and their families attend orientation group

First phase of treatment—16 weeks

Individual therapy for adolescent
Multifamily skills group for adolescent and family
Phone consultation (individual therapist with adolescent)
Phone consultation (family members with skills group leaders)
Family sessions as needed (usually 4–6 over the 16 weeks)
Therapist consultation meetings (weekly, for treatment team)

Second phase of treatment: Graduate group—16-week modules[a]

Graduate group for adolescent (weekly)
Phone consultation (graduate group coleader with adolescent)
Family sessions as needed (typically with group coleader)
Therapist consultation meetings
Individual therapy (in some cases that require ongoing individual work)
Ancillary treatment modes

Note. All aspects of the Montefiore program address the Stage 1 aims of achieving stability and safety, and reducing suicidal behaviors and other forms of severe behavioral dyscontrol.

[a]Clients can contract for additional 16-week modules during the continuation phase, as long as they can identify behavioral goals.

for single-family skills training. Depending on the setting, family members can also attend skills training *groups* or participate in skills training in other ways. In our Montefiore program, we include a weekly multifamily skills training group. Family members were included to increase generalization of skills by training parents and thus allowing them to serve as models as well as potential coaches. Our further hope was to target the invalidating environment directly and enhance family members' capacity to provide validation, support, and effective parenting. We find that this works well for several reasons—including teaching the family members the same skills at the same time as their children for coaching and reinforcement value; providing *in vivo* opportunity to role-play skills with the family members; improving ineffective and invalidating interactions from family members; providing interfamily support (both parent to adolescent and parent to parent); reducing the adolescents' disruptive behaviors in group by having other adults in attendance; and (ideally) enhancing treatment compliance by having parents accompanying their teens into the group.

However, some programs conduct separate groups for parents. These might take the form of parallel skills groups in which parents are seen separately but are taught the same curriculum. Alternatively, some programs run separate parent groups with overlapping but not identical content; for example, some parent training, stress management, psychoeducation, supportive, or other material might be brought in. Some of these groups bring parents and adolescents together once every third or fourth week, perhaps for 2 weeks in a row, for conjoint topic presentations. Others keep the groups completely separate and conduct them at different times and on different days. The main reasons for separating parent and adolescent groups include belief in the importance in covering some different material; belief that the inclusion of parents might inhibit adolescents' self-disclosure (or parents' ability to speak freely); or, in the case of severely dysfunctional families, belief that family members' presence might increase emotional and behavioral dysregulation within the group. In one case, we conducted individual skills training for a teen's parents, paralleling the multifamily skills group, because the parents' interactions with their teen were so volatile that they would have been strongly disruptive to the group. Chapter 10 details the workings of a skills training group.

Finally, some programs do not include family members in skills training—particularly in settings that make such participation impractical, such as inpatient, residential, or forensic settings. In such cases, practitioners might hold family meetings to orient family members to skills.

Family Therapy Sessions in DBT for Adolescents

Since much of the turmoil in the lives of suicidal adolescents involves their primary support systems (i.e., their immediate families in many cases), we have found it helpful to include family members during some of the time scheduled for individual sessions. This occurs on an as-needed basis when (1) a family member provides a central source of conflict, and the adolescent needs more intensive coaching or support in attempting to resolve this conflict; (2) a crisis erupts within the family and needs immediate attention; (3) the therapist determines that the treatment would be enhanced by orienting/educating a particular family member to a set of skills (if the family member is not attending a skills group), treatment targets, or other aspects of treatment; or (4) the contingencies at home are too powerful for the client to ignore or avoid and continue to reinforce dysfunctional behavior. Typically, a selected family member will attend 3–4 sessions out of the adolescent's 16 weeks of individual therapy, although on occasion we have had family members attend as many as 12–14 sessions. In addition, depending on the treatment program, some individual therapists will divide their individual sessions in half in order to accommodate the family therapy portion in the latter half. Other therapists may invite the families in for a separate third session during the week (i.e., family therapy in addition to individual therapy and a skills training group). Chapter 9 and Table 9.1 summarize conditions under which it is appropriate to schedule a family session.

When family members will participate in groups, we recommend limiting the number of clients in each group, since parental involvement makes groups about two to three times as large. In Montefiore's inner-city program, where many teens live in single-parent households, typically 5–6 adolescents per group are ideal, for a total of 10–12 members when family members are included. In our suburban graduate school clinic program at the C.W. Post Campus of Long Island University, and in our suburban private practices in which both parents often attend, we restrict the number of adolescents to 4–5, since this typically results in 10–15 participants in the group. Our rule of thumb is to make sure the skills trainers have at least 4–5 minutes per member to review homework. With a larger size, the leaders risk not having enough time to review the take-home practice exercises. In addition, the leaders are likely to have more difficulty keeping all members engaged in a larger group. A limitation to a smaller group is the periodic absence from the regular rotation of "senior members" who can help to orient new members. Ideally, those who have been there for 8 and 12 weeks tell the new members why they should participate and how the program has been helpful to them. The senior adolescents learn their role from those who precede them. When referrals slow down or clients drop out precipitously, the group develops gaps where there are no new members at a given entry point or a "senior class" is no longer present. This is far from catastrophic, but it is something to keep in mind when providers are forming a group and considering client flow and rates of dropout. In understanding the utility of working with parents or other family members, therapists should note that the inclusion of family members in treatment can actually address all five functions of treatment. By serving as models and coaches of effective behavior, parents can help increase their children's capabilities, as well as helping with generalization of skills outside the session. When family sessions can address parents' reinforcement of ineffective behavior and punishment of skillful behavior, clients' motivation can improve, and gains can be maintained. And working cooperatively with helpful parents can increase the capabilities and motivation of therapists, as well as help to structure the environment to reinforce the clients' progress.

Of course, adolescents do not always welcome the participation of family members in their treatment. Commonly, there is a background of invalidation and conflict with parents; adolescents may fear that therapy will offer yet another setting in which to be criticized, or yet another personal space that will be intruded upon. They might also wonder where a therapist's loyalties will ultimately lie if their parents become involved. Adolescents may thus appear sullen and uncommunicative in the initial sessions that include parents. It is thus critical to privately assess the adolescents' thoughts and concerns about including family members, orient the teens to the role parents will play in treatment, validate any accurate concerns, clarify misunderstandings about the process, clarify issues of confidentiality, and point out the benefits of including parents.

In some cases, family members will not be available to attend an individual session for a variety of reasons. These include conflicting work schedules, transportation difficulties, language barriers, or refusal for other reasons. In such cases, a therapist has several options. One is to determine whether the therapist can help parents solve practical problems in attending by problem-solving with them over the phone. Another is to try again at a later date, rather than giving up completely. Parents' views on attending or abilities to attend may change. Another option is to solicit the participation of another family member or someone in a caregiver or close interpersonal role, if this is relevant to ongoing work in individual therapy. For example, we have occasionally brought in grandmothers, godmothers, older siblings, and even boyfriends, when we felt it would be beneficial to do so. Finally, a therapist can decide to work with a teen without parental involvement, helping the adolescent to accept this lack of involvement in treatment while at times coaching him or her on effective interactions with the parent(s). See Chapter 9 for an in-depth discussion of the inclusion of family members in individual therapy.

Telephone Consultation to Family Members

In running numerous multifamily skills groups, we began to observe that family members attending these groups could benefit as much as their adolescents from telephone consultation. This posed a dilemma, since parents in skills training do not have an individual therapist to call. We had no model for this, since standard DBT does not include family members as regular participants in therapy. We decided to offer parents the opportunity to call the skills group leaders, but to limit this to as-needed phone consultations for skills generalization (as opposed to other purposes, such as asking for help appropriately, repairing the relationship, or sharing good news). In cases where one of the skills group leaders is the primary therapist for their child, the parents may only call the other group leader, to avoid placing the child's primary therapist in a potentially compromised position. In settings in which the primary therapist is also the skills trainer, allowing the parents to call the adolescent's therapist risks hindering the client's trust. Thus, in such situations, it may be best to have a policy of setting clear guidelines on what is to be discussed in a therapist–parent skills coaching call that the parent and adolescent agree to, and to follow each phone call with a disclosure of it in the next session. Alternatively, skills coaching for parents may need to be restricted to the context of skills training or family sessions. Even if a parent's phone coach is someone other than the adolescent's primary therapist, we encourage parents to tell their adolescent when such a phone contact has been made, so the adolescent remains confident that nothing about his or her treatment is occurring in a deceptive manner.

Reducing Length of Treatment for Adolescents; Adding a Graduate Group

Abbreviated length of treatment is a common adaptation in work with adolescents. Our Montefiore-based adolescent program reduced treatment length for the following reasons. First, we wanted to offer a treatment that would appear easier to sell to an adolescent population, given results from other studies showing that many suicidal adolescent clients tend to complete only a limited number of therapy sessions, coupled with their world view that anything more than a couple of months feels daunting. Second, we wished to offer a brief treatment in light of the fact that we were including many clients with first-time NSIB or suicide attempts, many of whom did not meet full criteria for BPD; thus we felt we could treat many with a short-term format and offer optional additional therapy (i.e., either a graduate group or, if needed, a repeat of the first phase of treatment) for those who needed it (i.e., those who remained at a severe level of disorder with extreme behavioral dyscontrol). Third, we wanted to offer a meaningful treatment for clients who could not afford longer-term treatment. Finally, we wished to provide a treatment that was more in keeping with the current health care climate (e.g., acceptable to insurance companies), provided that we could demonstrate its effectiveness at this length. The concept of shorter-term treatment is consistent with data from two recent randomized controlled studies of suicidal adolescents that achieved reductions in deliberate self-harm and suicide attempts in treatments lasting typically between 3 and 6 months (Huey et al., 2004; Wood et al., 2001). After some experimentation, we chose to increase the length of our initial phase of treatment from 12 to 16 weeks, in order to add the 4-

week Walking the Middle Path Skills module (see below) to the skills training curriculum and to leave additional time to address family issues. Even if longer-term treatment appears indicated, therapists who "sell" longer-term treatment do themselves and their clients a disservice. Adolescents appear to respond well to time-limited, measurable treatment segments. Thus a 16-week treatment, even if repeated, sounds more feasible to some teens than a 32-week treatment.

Since documented rates of relapse and recurrence among depressed adolescents are high, clinical researchers have recommended either booster or continuation treatment to address this problem (Birmaher et al., 2000). Thus we have implemented a second phase of treatment—a graduate group, with other treatment modes as needed—because of the clinical sense it makes to have a continuation phase (at least 4 months) in treating multiproblem suicidal adolescents, most of whom have mood disorders (e.g., Rathus, Wagner, & Miller, 2005).

In our Montefiore program, the two phases together comprise 32 weeks of treatment (see Table 4.3). Both phases address the DBT Stage 1 overarching targets of achieving stability and safety, and reducing suicidal behaviors and other forms of severe behavioral dyscontrol. The DBT later-stage targets (e.g., decreasing PTSD) are not formally addressed in our DBT program for adolescents. However, programs wishing to address later-stage targets could offer continuation of treatment for their adolescent clients. Some clients continue in individual therapy to address Stage 2 targets, while also participating in a graduate group.

Many DBT programs for adolescents offer some type of maintenance or graduate group to clients who complete the initial phase of treatment. Such groups are designed to continue to address the functions of improving capabilities, improving motivation, and promoting generalization of skills, but in a way that requires less intensive adolescent participation and fewer program resources. Continuing treatment in a separate, second phase with reduced intensity has the following advantages: It (1) allows adolescents to feel a sense of mastery earlier (by completing the first phase, similar to graduating from eighth grade and entering ninth); (2) addresses teens' common apprehension about committing to a longer-term treatment by offering a "foot-in-the-door" approach to an extended treatment (the first commitment is to only a shorter time period; only later are they asked to contract for more time); (3) allows additional opportunity to address treatment goals once the initial, highest-priority targets are reduced; and (4) reallocates staff resources, such that openings for more intensive treatment are provided to those adolescents beginning DBT, with life-threatening and severe quality-of-life-interfering behaviors. (Note that the therapist consultation/supervision team continues through this second phase, addressing the function of treating the therapist; the function of structuring the environment occurs as needed.)

There are many options for conducting this second phase, in terms of length, format, and modes offered. In our 16-week program, adolescent participants graduating from the DBT program have the option of continuing in a weekly client consultation group for at least an additional 16 weeks. Again, adolescents are asked to make a 16-week commitment to the graduate group, with an explicit understanding that they may recontract for another 16 weeks, and then another (and so on), if they are so inclined and able to identify specific goals on which to work. Some teens stay in a graduate group for 2 years before leaving for college.

Adolescents are "graduated" if they complete the first 16 weeks of treatment in terms of attendance requirements and demonstrate a significant control of life-threatening behaviors, as well as commitment to continue working on treatment goals. At the end of the initial 16 weeks, individual therapy, the multifamily skills group, and telephone consultation with the individual therapist end. There are some teens, however, who retain their primary therapist and phone coaching with that therapist. For those who terminate treatment with their primary therapist, however, telephone consultation responsibilities are turned over to one of the two leaders of the graduate group. Each coleader is considered a primary leader for half of the group members; clients contact their primary group coleader for phone consultations. These graduate group coleaders make use of the therapist consultation/supervision meeting just as the therapists do who are treating clients in the comprehensive 16-week program. The graduate group is described in detail in Chapter 11.

Depending on the needs of the setting, one could offer graduate groups with continued individual therapy, phone contact, family sessions, or other modes. The essence is to find the synthesis between acknowledging progress and reduction in highest-priority target behaviors on the one hand, and the common need for additional treatment to work on the multitude of targets with which a teen might present on the other.

Reduced Overall Number of Skills to Fit Shortened Treatment

When shortening the length of treatment, we had to decide whether to prioritize breadth or depth for coverage of skills. That is, we could cover more skills in a shorter amount of time or devote more time to fewer skills. Teaching fewer skills in more depth helps increase clients' expertise in those skills. Teaching many skills in a short time exposes clients to the skills but leaves little time for mastery or practice. We have tried to balance breadth and depth. We have slightly reduced the number of skills taught within each module (see Table 10.4, which lists the skills taught in adolescent DBT), but have also added a new module that seemed essential for working with adolescents and family members (see below). Although there still are many handouts to cover in our shortened treatment, we opted to maintain a large number of the original DBT skills because (1) we had no basis for determining which, if any, were nonessential; (2) clients are idiosyncratic with regard to which skills they "latch onto," so we felt that exposure to more would be helpful; (3) although we do not expect clients to master the skills in group, they have opportunities for mastery during take-home practice exercises, practice exercise review, application in problem solving during individual therapy, and phone coaching; and (4) clients relearn (and have the opportunity to teach) the skills in the graduate group.

A New Skills Module: Walking the Middle Path

After several years of conducting DBT with adolescents and families in several contexts, it became apparent to us that three issues required regular additional attention and were not sufficiently addressed in Linehan's original skills package developed for adults. These issues were validation of self and other (which will be included in the second edition of Linehan's [1993b] skills training manual); the use of behavioral principles with self and other; and the identification of three common and specific adolescent–family dialectical dilemmas.

In standard DBT, validation and invalidation are discussed during the monthly orientation when we describe the biosocial theory and during the interpersonal skill lecture entitled GIVE (in which V stands for validation). However, our adolescents and families required more time for learning and practicing their validation skills. Thus we developed one lecture devoted exclusively to validation skills, addressing validation of both self and others.

Another skills deficit identified in this population was the inability to apply behavioral principles effectively. Although the emphasis began with teaching parents how to reinforce, extinguish, punish, and shape their adolescents' behaviors effectively, we quickly realized the value of teaching adolescents how to apply the same principles with people in their lives, including themselves. For example, adolescents benefited greatly from learning how to reinforce their younger siblings for playing more quietly while they were trying to study. In addition, many adolescents were pleasantly surprised to learn the concept of self-reinforcement (e.g., watching a movie only after they had completed their homework assignments).

A third issue, adolescent–family dialectical dilemmas, presented itself consistently in our work with this population. As explicated in Chapter 5, a suicidal adolescent and/or family member, and sometimes even a therapist, learn over time to alternate between one behavioral pattern that underregulates emotion and another that overregulates emotion. These patterns are introduced in the multifamily skills training group, and they are specifically targeted in the DBT family therapy. We thus teach the following three common patterns to teens and families: excessive leniency versus authoritarian control, normalizing pathological behaviors versus pathologizing normative behaviors, and forcing autonomy versus fostering dependence. We describe this new skills module in more detail in Chapter 10. Lecture and discussion points for the module can be found in Appendix B, and handouts for it are provided in Appendix C.

Modified Handouts for Adolescents

Depending on the age range and functioning level of a particular adolescent population, providers may decide to modify the original DBT (Linehan, 1993b) skills training handouts. Whether they are modified or not, it is crucial that therapists adapt examples of each skill to fit the adolescents in their treatment program. At Montefiore, we modified the skills handouts in a number of ways to help the adolescents grasp the concepts more readily. First, we simplied some of the terminology. For example, the term "doing what works" is used instead of "effectively" as one of the mindfulness skills, and the term "can't decide" is used in lieu of "indecision" as one of the factors reducing interpersonal effectiveness. Second, the language on the handouts was streamlined, with fewer words on each page. Many of our teens, especially those with reading problems, reported difficulty comprehending the handouts that contained more elaborate descriptions of concepts. Therefore, we simplified the visual layouts of the handouts as much as possible, to decrease the chances of visual overstimulation by reducing the amount of variability in font size, bold print, underlining, and italicizing. We modified homework sheets as well, with the same aims in mind. Finally, we included some graphics to make the handouts appear more "adolescent-friendly." The handouts included in the DBT skills manual (Linehan, 1993b) can be copied for distribution to clients. Across many specialized settings, treatment teams have taken modified the terminology and layout of the published handouts to fit their own clinical situations.

CHAPTER 5

Dialectical Dilemmas for Adolescents
Addressing Secondary Treatment Targets

As discussed in Chapters 2 and 3, DBT considers suicidal and other behaviors associated with BPD as products of emotion dysregulation. The behavioral patterns resulting from this dysregulation are characterized by vacillations between polarized positions. Each pattern represents transactions between an emotionally vulnerable individual and his or her invalidating environment. Over time, the individual with BPD learns to alternate between behavioral extremes that either underregulate or overregulate emotion; in this sense, such behavior patterns can be understood as dialectical failures (Linehan, 1993a). DBT views these patterns of shifting between behavioral extremes as "dialectical dilemmas" for the client, in that the client alternately tries, but is unable to make work, each extreme approach to emotion regulation. The first three primary treatment targets discussed in Chapter 3 (life-threatening behaviors, therapy-interfering behaviors, and quality-of-life-interfering behaviors) are themselves expressions of these dialectical dilemmas. Because these behaviors endanger the client's life or the therapy itself, or impair the quality of the client's life, they must be immediately addressed and so take precedence. But the overall patterns help sustain the dysfunctional behaviors, and so the patterns themselves need to be targeted by treatment if there is to be long-term change. Therefore, DBT has a set of secondary treatment targets. These treatment targets involve finding syntheses of the client's extreme behavioral styles. The therapist attends to these secondary targets throughout treatment, weaving them into behavioral analysis, insight strategies, and discussion of other issues as relevant.

The standard DBT dialectical dilemmas are as follows:

Emotional vulnerability versus self-invalidation
Active passivity versus apparent competence
Unrelenting crises versus inhibited grieving

The three additional adolescent-specific dialectical dilemmas we have developed (Rathus & Miller, 2000) are these:

Excessive leniency versus authoritarian control
Normalizing pathological behaviors versus pathologizing normative behaviors
Forcing autonomy versus fostering dependence

At each polar extreme, there are two secondary treatment targets: one aimed at decreasing the maladaptive behavior, the other aimed at increasing a more adaptive response. Table

5.1 lists the dialectical dilemmas and corresponding secondary treatment targets in standard DBT, and Table 5.2 lists those developed for an adolescent population. Note that while these behavior patterns are helpful in conceptualizing clients' behavior, they are not universal; thus, for a given case, they should be assessed rather than assumed (Linehan, 1993a). In the following sections, we discuss each dialectical dilemma as it tends to present in adolescent clients, and then also discuss its corresponding treatment targets.

STANDARD DIALECTICAL DILEMMAS IN ADOLESCENTS, AND THEIR TREATMENT TARGETS

Emotional Vulnerability versus Self-Invalidation

DBT regards "emotional vulnerability" as a core feature of BPD; the term as used here refers to the experience of intense emotional suffering. At this pole, emotional vulnerability is the experiential side of emotion dysregulation (see Chapter 3 on biosocial theory). Individuals with emotional vulnerability are often highly emotionally aroused, which creates not only behavioral instability but also dyscontrol over cognitions, physiological arousal, facial expressions, body language, and communications. Moreover, emotional vulnerability is accompanied by the phenomenological experience of being out of control, which stems from a lack of influence over emotionally evocative stimuli, combined with the inability to modulate reactions to these stimuli.

Four characteristics accompany the frequent, intense, and tenacious emotional arousal of clients with BPD (Linehan, 1993a). The first is that emotions are not unidimensional physiological events, but rather full-system responses involving also cognitive, experiential, and expressive/behavioral responses. Thus such clients must attempt to regulate this entire system of responses associated with emotional states (e.g., internal arousal, facial expression, action patterns)—a formidable task. Second, this intense emotional arousal disrupts even behaviors that are usually planned, regulated, and functional, causing the client to become demoralized and making negative emotions even worse. Third, the inability to regulate the high emotional arousal gives the client a frightening sense of the uncontrollability and unpredictability of emotional reactions. Fourth, this lack of control leads to fears of both situations over which the

TABLE 5.1. Standard DBT Dialectical Dilemmas, with Corresponding Secondary Treatment Targets

Dilemma	Targets
Emotional vulnerability versus self-invalidation	Increasing emotion modulation; decreasing emotional reactivity
	Increasing self-validation; decreasing self-invalidation
Active passivity versus apparent competence	Increasing active problem solving; decreasing active passivity
	Increasing accurate communication of emotions and competence; decreasing mood dependency of behavior
Unrelenting crises versus inhibited grieving	Increasing realistic decision making and judgment; decreasing crisis-generating behaviors
	Increasing emotional experiencing; decreasing inhibited grieving

TABLE 5.2. Adolescent Dialectical Dilemmas, with Corresponding Secondary Treatment Targets

Dilemma	Targets
Excessive leniency versus authoritarian control	Increasing authoritative discipline; decreasing excessive leniency
	Increasing adolescent self-determination; decreasing authoritarian control
Normalizing pathological behaviors versus pathologizing normative behaviors	Increasing recognition of normative behaviors; decreasing pathologizing of normative behaviors
	Increasing identification of pathological behaviors; decreasing normalization of pathological behaviors
Forcing autonomy versus fostering dependence	Increasing individuation; decreasing excessive dependence
	Increasing effective reliance on others; decreasing excessive autonomy

client has little control and expectations of valued others. Thus new situations, challenging situations, and even praise from a therapist (which can be accompanied implicitly by expectations of maintaining or furthering progress) can be terrifyingly daunting, further maintaining the vulnerability.

The suffering that accompanies the inability to regulate emotion can create despair that one is doomed to a life of unending misery. In fact, one can make the analogy that clients with BPD or borderline features are the "psychological equivalent of third-degree burn patients. They simply have, so to speak, no emotional skin. Even the slightest touch or movement can create immense suffering" (Linehan, 1993a, p. 69). At one extreme, these clients can sink into such despair that suicide appears the only way out. At the other, the clients can become so angry that suicide to punish others appears reasonable, because others either do not understand their pain or cannot help them. Thus extreme statements such as "I've suffered through all this—it's amazing I haven't killed myself yet," or "I'll die and I'll show you!" may appear dramatic, and yet may reflect clients' attempts to convey their actual overwhelmed, hopeless experience.

Emotional vulnerability may be harder to discern in adolescent clients than in others. Compared to younger children or adults, adolescents report more negative moods, greater extremes of mood, and more mood lability (Buchanan, Eccles, & Becker, 1992; Csikszentmihalyi & Larson, 1984; Larson & Richards, 1994). This increase in moodiness has been attributed primarily to cognitive and environmental factors (Larson & Richards, 1994), rather than to the biological changes of puberty. For example, adolescents not only experience an increase in negative life events and personal transitions; they also have the abstract reasoning capacity to consider the far-reaching implications of these events (Arnett, 1999; Larson & Ham, 1993; Larson & Richards, 1994). In fact, changes in emotional development include the increase in frequency of a range of psychological conditions, including mood disorders, conduct disorders, eating disorders, and suicide attempts (Brooks-Gunn & Petersen, 1991; Garner, 1993; Rutter, 1986; U.S. Department of Justice, 1994; U.S. Department of Health and Human Services, 1994). Conflicts with parents increase, and tensions commonly arise (Galambos & Almeida, 1992). Furthermore, adolescents' increased sense of the uniqueness of their experiences, and increased self-consciousness due to a feeling of being "on stage" (Berk, 2004; Lapsley, 1991), often result in their being perceived as "melodramatic." Moreover, adolescents today face unique sets of stressors, including increased drug and alcohol use (Substance Abuse and Mental Health Services Administration, 1996), violent crimes (as either victims or perpetrators; CDC, 1992), and gang membership.

Despite these characteristics of adolescence, Arnett (1999) has suggested a modified "storm and stress" view of this period. He asserts that although there is indeed an increase in moodiness, argumentativeness, and stressors in adolescence compared with other stages of the life span, emotional instability is not inevitable, and many teens in fact adjust well. Thus, while many youth encountering such stressors will suffer a deteriorating course, many will grow up to be successful adults. A key task of therapists, then, involves distinguishing true signs of emotional vulnerability from the expected vicissitudes of adolescence. Signs that emotional variability is going beyond normative adolescent moodiness and dramatic presentation include *intransient* states of depressed or otherwise negative moods; *continuous* extreme sensitivity and emotional arousal, with marked difficulty returning to baseline mood; identification of diagnosable conditions (e.g., major depression, substance abuse, conduct disorder); and evidence of severely maladaptive coping with moodiness or stressors (e.g., self-harm behavior, drug use, school problems, association with a delinquent peer group, or social withdrawal).

"Self-invalidation" refers to taking on characteristics of the emotionally invalidating environment (see Linehan, 1993a). These include invalidating one's own emotional experiences, and thus trying to suppress the experience or expression of emotions; distrusting one's own perceptions, thus undermining identity and looking to others to define one's reality; responding to one's own emotional states with negative secondary emotions such as shame, disgust, or anger; and oversimplifying the ease of problem solving, expressed by denying one's problems or blaming oneself for them (e.g., "I'm overreacting," "I should be able to do more," etc.). At this end of the polarity, clients may want to commit suicide to punish themselves, believing that they deserve to die. Alternatively, suicide can be an outcome of unrealized perfectionism associated with invalidation of one's true difficulties in achieving goals.

This behavior may be especially difficult to identify and change in adolescents at the beginning of treatment. It is typical for children not to trust themselves, and to engage in "social referencing"—that is, looking to parents and other authority figures for cues as to how to react, interpret situations, and feel (Berk, 2004). In this sense, self-invalidation is rather normative, particularly in younger adolescents. Yet adolescence is a time when increasing separation from parents occurs, and a greater sense of trusting oneself develops. Certainly by later adolescence (i.e., ages 16–18), greater trust in oneself and stronger self-validation should be apparent.

In regard to targeting self-invalidation in treatment, adolescent clients present several challenges. First, adolescent clients are typically residing within their original invalidating environment, which serves as a powerful model for self-invalidation. Second, adolescents are increasingly susceptible to influence by peers. When peers are invalidating (e.g., "That's ridiculous!", "You are such a loser!"), adolescents are likely to internalize such messages. Third, adolescence is the primary period for identity development. According to Erikson (1968), the major psychological conflict of adolescence is identity versus identity diffusion. Those with trouble formulating an identity (identity diffusion) have a poor sense of themselves, their values, and their goals. Related to identity formation is the notion of self-concept. In adolescence, the self-concept evolves to include an expanded definition of self, including insight into one's psychological qualities (Barenboim, 1977), personal values and aspirations, and the need to be liked by others (Berk, 2004). Thus weakly established identities and self-concepts may make teens more likely to question their perceptions and look to others to define themselves—hallmarks of self-invalidation.

For minority youth or recent immigrant youth, the development of an identity comes with even more challenges than for youth from the mainstream culture. Teens from ethnic minority backgrounds face the task of reconciling the values of their own ethnic culture with those of the dominant culture (Phinney & Rosenthal, 1992). Too strong an identity with their own minority group may limit their opportunities in the dominant culture, while allying too strongly with the dominant culture may lead to being ostracized by their own group (Phinney & Rosenthal, 1992). Discrimination, lack of successful role models, and reduced SES are further conditions faced by many minority adolescents as they struggle to form an identity (O'Conner, 1989; Spencer, Dornbusch, & Mont-Reynaud, 1990) and may further intensify self-invalidation.

On a more hopeful note, the development of formal operational thinking provides adolescents with the capacity to make choices about their world views, their personal values, and their future occupations. Adolescents become able to imagine various options and roles without having actually experienced them (Kahlbaugh & Haviland, 1991). Self-concept during adolescence becomes based on an expanded range of areas, including romantic relationships, peer acceptance, and academic and job success (Harter, 1990). Thus there is the potential to integrate new information and change the pattern of self-invalidation.

To summarize this first dialectical dilemma, it involves vacillating between self-blame (e.g., "I was so stupid to react that way!", "I'm the cause of all my troubles") and blaming or attacking others ("How could he do that to me and make me this upset?", "I'm a helpless victim"), and between oversimplifying life's problems and feeling so overwhelmed by life that suicide seems the only option. The extremes of self-invalidation mean that teens consider themselves inadequate, shameful, responsible for their difficulties, and even deserving to die. On the other hand, teens' accentuation of emotional vulnerability means blaming their troubles on everyone or everything other than themselves. Self-blame is consistent with the adolescent tendency toward egocentrism (Lapsley, 1991). At the same time, externalizing blame is common to adolescents as they increase their argumentativeness and criticism (Elkind, 1984).

In dealing with this pattern, the therapist must also be dialectical. He or she has to avoid colluding with the self-invalidation that can occur with badly timed or too strong an emphasis on change and problem solving. On the other hand, the therapist has to avoid colluding with emotional vulnerability by badly timed or too strong a stance of acceptance and validation. The therapist's task is to find a balance between acceptance and change. As the therapist's stance shifts, so too do the secondary behavioral treatment targets aimed at increasing and decreasing specific behavior. See Table 5.3 for an overview of this dialectical dilemma, its corresponding treatment targets, and related strategies and techniques.

Treatment Targets: Increasing Emotion Modulation; Decreasing Emotional Reactivity

The treatment targets of increasing emotion modulation and decreasing emotional reactivity are both aimed at the emotional vulnerability pole of the dialectical dilemma. Together they involve "turning down the volume" on the intense, dysregulated emotional states characteristic of emotional vulnerability. The goal is not completely inhibiting emotions, but helping teens to moderate the extremity of their emotional responses. A therapist teaches a client emotion regulation skills to modulate emotional responses, such as observing and describing emotions (mindfulness skills are required here as well), reducing emotional vulnerability through self-care and building a sense of mastery, and acting opposite to the current emotion.

TABLE 5.3. Targeting Emotional Vulnerability versus Self-Invalidation

Dialectical pattern	Secondary treatment targets	Specific techniques/strategies
Emotional vulnerability (unstable anger, depression, anxiety)	Increasing emotion modulation; decreasing emotional reactivity	Emotion regulation skills: observing/ describing emotions; encouraging self-care; building sense of mastery; acting opposite to current emotion
		Mindfulness skills
Self-invalidation (distrust, dismissal of own perceptions, emotions, and problem-solving approaches)	Increasing self-validation; decreasing self-invalidation	Attending to client's emotional cues and rational thoughts, to promote self-trust
		Nonjudgmental observation and description of emotion
		Lessening inhibition of emotion
		Exposure for unrealistic primary emotions causing negative secondary emotions
		Acting opposite to self-invalidation by stopping it and replacing with self-validation
		Promoting teen's use of behavioral shaping (small positive reinforcements for small steps in the desired direction)

Treatment Targets: Increasing Self-Validation; Decreasing Self-Invalidation

In targeting self-invalidation, the therapist works to overcome the influence of the invalidating environment. The teen needs to learn to validate his or her emotions, perceptions, and approach to problem solving, in place of extreme emotional displays to elicit such validation from one's environment. The therapist employs strategies to (1) enhance the adolescent's self-trust through attending to emotional cues and rational thoughts; (2) encourage nonjudgmental observation and labeling of emotional states, rather than inhibition of them; (3) expose the teen to primary emotions that are unrealistic for the situation and that cause negative secondary emotions; (4) invoke the emotion regulation skill of opposite action to activate self-validating behaviors (i.e., the therapist stops a self-invalidating statement and has the client replace it with a self-validating statement); and (5) promote the teen's use of shaping (i.e., rewarding him- or herself for small increments of progress toward goals.

Active Passivity versus Apparent Competence

"Active passivity" describes a coping style characterized by approaching difficulties with passivity and helplessness, while actively eliciting the help of *others* in solving problems. This coping style stems in large part from the inability of individuals with BPD or borderline/suicidal features to prevent the experience of extreme aversive emotions, coupled with a sense of helplessness in resolving their own problems. At this point, they become especially vulnerable to the threat of loss of relationships and may frantically attempt to prevent abandonment. Because of a helpless yet demanding style, individuals manifesting active passivity are likely to alienate caregivers and ultimately experience rejection or invalidation.

Active passivity in an adolescent is in some ways strikingly different from expected behavior. This is because most teens strive for increased individuation from parents, spend more time with peers, and experiment with their new decision-making and planning capacities (Elkind, 1984; La Greca & Prinstein, 1999; Larson & Richards, 1991). Teens typically want to drive a car or use public transportation themselves, begin to earn their own money, and handle personal problems with less intrusion from parents (e.g., Lapsley, 1991).

On the other hand, other aspects of adolescent development may exacerbate a state of active passivity. First, teens may realistically be more dependent upon others to solve their problems, if they are indeed dependents living at home. That is, they may need others for things like money or transportation. Second, in the areas in which they can help themselves, they may be overwhelmed by their growing cognitive capacities and have trouble with systematic decision making (Elkind, 1984). Third, they may have been punished by parents for independent decision making when this led to problematic behaviors in the past.

"Apparent competence" refers to the tendency of others to misperceive clients with BPD or borderline/suicidal characteristics as more competent, effective, and in control, and less in need of help, than they actually are. Generally such misperceptions are due to one of two problems: (1) The verbal expressions of difficulty and vulnerability are not synchronous with the nonverbal expressions of control and calmness, and an observer assumes that the nonverbal messages are more accurate than the verbal ones; and (2) competence in one set of situations or when certain people are nearby does not generalize to other situations. Apparent competence contrasts, of course, with the opposite pole of active passivity. That is, it contrasts with the alternate presentation within the same individual of having few areas of competence and strongly requesting help. This contrasting presentation often earns such clients the label of "manipulative." Apparent competence stems largely from the fact that emotionally vulnerable individuals are more competent within some affect states than others. Since their moods shift substantially and unpredictably, the competence of such individuals likewise shifts rapidly and with little warning. Teenagers' increased moodiness, combined with an emerging but as yet unstable identity, means that shifting affective and behavioral patterns are to be expected. In addition, clients with BPD or borderline features have often not learned how to communicate effectively about a need for help, and also tend to fare better in emotion regulation within the context of a supportive, secure relationship. Since the therapy relationship often provides such a setting, a therapist may not have access to the full range of affective dysregulation within a client's repertoire.

To summarize this second dialectical dilemma, it involves shifts between the extremes of helplessness on the one hand, and exaggerated or inaccurately assessed competence on the other. In dealing with this pattern, the therapist needs to be able to recognize and reinforce the client's actual areas of competence, and not the client's extreme helplessness. At the other extreme, the therapist needs to avoid developing unrealistic expectations about the client's competence level and thus disregarding minor indications of distress. Table 5.4 summarizes this dialectical dilemma, together with its treatment targets and useful techniques and strategies.

Treatment Targets: Increasing Active Problem Solving; Decreasing Active Passivity

One of the central goals of DBT is to increase clients' active problem-solving ability and expand their repertoire of effective coping strategies. At the same time, clients need to be more motivated to use these new strategies and to communicate more accurately when they do and don't need help. DBT addresses this goal through increased reliance on clients' behavioral skills. For example, mindfulness skills such as accessing "wise mind" (see Chapter 10) help clients to identify needs and determine what they need to do to achieve their objectives. Interpersonal effectiveness skills help clients assert their needs more effectively. Contingency management procedures increase clients' motivation to rely on their own abilities, and behavior analysis and solution analysis strategies increase their problem-solving capacity.

TABLE 5.4. Targeting Active Passivity versus Apparent Competence

Dialectical pattern	Secondary treatment targets	Specific techniques/strategies
Active passivity (helplessness while actively eliciting others' help)	Increasing active problem solving; decreasing active passivity	Interpersonal effectiveness skills Behavior and solution analyses to increase problem solving Mindfulness skills to identify needs Contingency management
Apparent competence (displaying emotional, behavioral, and interpersonal competence, often in conjunction with suddenly shifting mood states or in interpersonal relationship contexts perceived as safe)	Increasing accurate communication of emotions and competence; decreasing mood dependency of behavior	Recognizing vulnerabilities and asking for help appropriately Mindfulness skills to disengage mood from behavior Emotion regulation skills Distress tolerance skills

Treatment Targets: Increasing Accurate Communication of Emotions and Competence; Decreasing Mood Dependency of Behavior

In the next pair of treatment targets, the first one involves teaching clients to become more adept at communicating emotional states, recognizing and anticipating vulnerabilities, and asking for help appropriately. The second one involves teaching clients how to disengage mood from behavior—a central goal of DBT skills. This ability requires practice in mindfulness, emotion regulation, and distress tolerance skills.

Unrelenting Crises versus Inhibited Grieving

Among adolescents, the dialectical dilemma of unrelenting crises versus inhibited grieving involves the contrasting behavior patterns of either immediate, impulsive escape from emotional pain or pervasive avoidance of emotional pain. The term "unrelenting crises" (i.e., "crisis-of-the-week syndrome") describes a pattern of responses in which an initial precipitant evokes intense emotional pain, which the client then escapes through impulsive actions because of an inability either to tolerate or to diminish this pain. The combined consequences of impulsive behaviors, emotional vulnerability, and faulty interpersonal relations create conditions for encountering additional aversive events. The unrelenting nature of these aversive events hinders the ability to recover fully from any one stressful event, trapping the client in a vicious cycle in which he or she becomes more vulnerable to further emotion dysregulation. Even normal adolescents may appear to present a pattern of unrelenting crises, as adolescents' thinking is characterized by egocentrism, including the subjective sense that they are continually "on stage" and remain the focus of others' attention. The belief in this self-directed attention, referred to as the "imaginary audience," contributes to adolescents' self-consciousness, self-focusing, and nearly obsessive concern with appearance and behavior (Lapsley, 1991). It is also thought to contribute to adolescents' strong desire for privacy and low threshold for regarding parents' solicitations as intrusive. Another aspect of adolescents' egocentric thinking involves the "personal fable," or the belief that no one can understand their experiences or their emotional life, such as being in love. As such, everyday events may be related with a sense of high drama. Along with believing that their experiences are unique comes a sense of feeling special and invulnerable, which may relate to such adolescent risk-taking behaviors as experimentation with substances, sexual promiscuity, risky automobile driving, or criminal behavior (Lapsley, 1991). In general, impulsiveness increases at this time (CDC, 1995). Yet these behaviors, along with increased conflict with parents, moodiness, and impulsiveness, may set the stage for actual crisis situations, and a therapist must assess them (rather than assuming that they are just examples of an adolescent acting like an adolescent).

Note also that some adolescents are simply unlucky, and have chains of crises occur through factors not of their own making. For example, being born into poverty and not having supportive adults in one's life are circumstances that will in themselves generate crises. Yet much of the approach to targeting unrelenting crises (see below) will apply, regardless of whether an adolescent generates crises through his or her own actions.

In contrast with this tendency to move rapidly from crisis to crisis, individuals with BPD or borderline features also tend to *avoid* the full emotional processing of intensely painful losses or traumas. "Inhibited grieving" refers to involuntary, automatic avoidance of cues that evoke past losses and trauma, in which individuals shut down the natural progression of normal stages of grieving, and thus never become habituated to the sadness associated with loss and grief, as well as to anger, shame, and other painful emotions. Since everyday life provides frequent cues of loss, these clients enter a vicious cycle in which they become exposed to loss cues, begin mourning, interrupt this process by automatically avoiding the cues, become exposed to additional loss cues, and so on. For teens, avoidance of emotional processing may be facilitated by distractions such as peer group involvement, substance use, or experimenting with a variety of high-risk behaviors (CDC, 1995; U.S. Department of Health and Human Services, 1994; Zuckerman, 1979).

To summarize this third dialectical dilemma, it involves vulnerability to the unrelenting crises occurring in a client's life at one extreme, and at the other, overly inhibiting the affect related to these crises. Thus the client often fails to elicit needed social support and often handles the crises through impulsive behaviors designed to blunt painful emotions. The therapist's dialectical dilemma entails providing balanced responses to the fluctuating displays of intense affect or completely inhibited affect. Table 5.5 summarizes this dialectical dilemma, its associated treatment targets, and specific techniques and strategies.

Treatment Targets: Increasing Realistic Decision Making and Judgment; Decreasing Crisis-Generating Behaviors

The first two DBT targets for this dialectical dilemma are to decrease crisis-generating behaviors and to increase realistic decision making and judgment. These targets are based on the assumption that individuals with BPD or borderline characteristics participate in generating the crises they experience, through engaging in mood-dependent behaviors and having difficulty predicting realistic outcomes of those behaviors. Approaches to these behaviors include increasing consequential thinking (e.g., "If I curse out the teacher and storm out of the classroom, I'll probably get suspended, which would lead to lots of other problems"); mindfulness skills to practice observing emotional states and action urges rather than acting on them; emotion regulation skills to change extreme emotional reactions; and distress tolerance skills to avoid impulsive responding to emotional distress. In addition, DBT insight strategies address these behavioral targets by highlighting dysfunctional patterns involving faulty judgment and decision making. Teens possess the ability to benefit from these interventions because of their increases in hypothetical reasoning, ability to view situations from more than one angle, and capacity for self-regulation (Elkind, 1984; Overton, 1991; Romaine, 1984). Along with the capacity for abstract reasoning comes further development of moral principles: Teens are beginning to move from reward- and punishment-based moral choices to a more principled and ab-

TABLE 5.5. Targeting Unrelenting Crises versus Inhibited Grieving

Dialectical pattern	Secondary treatment targets	Specific techniques/strategies
Unrelenting crises (immediate, impulsive escape from emotional pain)	Increasing realistic decision making and judgment; decreasing crisis-generating behaviors	Increasing consequential thinking Mindfulness practice in observing emotions and urges, rather than acting on them Emotion regulation skills to change extreme emotional reactions Distress tolerance skills to avoid impulsive responding to emotional distress Increasing insight into dysfunctional patterns
Inhibited grieving (pervasive avoidance of emotional pain)	Increasing emotional experiencing; decreasing inhibited grieving	Exposure to rather than inhibition of/escape from negative emotions Mindfulness to current emotional states without changing them Distress tolerance skills of self-soothing, distracting, or radically accepting the emotion

stract morality, informed by increased perspective-taking ability (Kohlberg, 1984). (However, it should be noted that few individuals actually reach the highest stages of moral development proposed by Kohlberg.)

Treatment Targets: Increasing Emotional Experiencing; Decreasing Inhibited Grieving

The second part of targets involves increasing clients' ability to experience sadness and other negative emotions as they occur, rather than inhibiting them. This ability is a critical aspect of reducing both the intensity of these emotions and the impulsive behaviors that are likely to result from pervasive yet ineffective attempts at blocking them. The central approaches to addressing the targets involve exposure procedures, such as practicing mindfulness to current emotional states without changing them. Or clients can employ distress tolerance skills, including self-soothing, distracting, or radical acceptance of the emotion, to help them modulate and thereby tolerate the distress without acting impulsively to escape from it.

DIALECTICAL DILEMMAS SPECIFIC TO WORKING WITH ADOLESCENTS AND FAMILIES

Linehan's (1993a) original set of dialectical dilemmas and secondary targets remain applicable to the treatment of adolescents—as do other behavioral extremes she identified, such as skill enhancement versus self-acceptance, transparency versus privacy, trust versus suspicion, emotion control versus emotion tolerance, and self-focusing versus other-focusing.

However, we subsequently found that in work with suicidal adolescents and their parents, additional dialectical dilemmas specific to this family constellation become apparent. The parents of suicidal adolescents, the adolescents themselves, and even the treating therapists commonly vacillate and become polarized along three dimensions:[1]

---

[1]We would like to express our appreciation to Laura B. Silver McGuire, who helped us formulate the adolescent dialectical dilemmas.

Excessive leniency versus authoritarian control
Pathologizing normative behaviors versus normalizing pathological behaviors
Fostering dependence versus forcing autonomy

Excessive Leniency versus Authoritarian Control

Parents, the therapist, and the adolescent can all vacillate between being excessively lenient and being authoritarian. "Excessive leniency" refers to making too few behavioral demands of adolescents (or to adolescents' making too few demands on themselves). One way that parents display excessive leniency involves capitulation to an adolescent's demands. In this style of excessive leniency, parents of a suicidal adolescent relinquish many of the rules or standards that they would ideally apply, or that they actually do apply to their other children. Thus they defy their own values, or they apply different rules to different children. Many parents report feeling coercively controlled (e.g., Patterson, 1976) by their children's suicidality and emotion dysregulation, making statements such as "I know the stakes are too high if I say no and get her angry, so I just let her stay home from school," or "She says the smoking calms her down and there's always the threat of suicide, so I buy her cigarettes," or "I feel like I'm always walking on eggshells, so I let him go out with his friends until all hours, because it's better than the consequences of telling him he can't go." Although they may indulge their adolescents, these parents report often feeling conflicted, restrained, guilty, and resentful, unsure of themselves and their parenting decisions. Adolescents' increased tendency to argue and criticize endlessly (Elkind, 1984) only intensifies these feeling of defeat.

Excessive leniency may also be demonstrated through a laissez-faire style of parenting. This excessive permissiveness typically occurs in the context of parents' raising several children with little help, which often results in a rather chaotic household. In such cases, parents may acquiesce to adolescents demands because it requires the least effort in the moment. Or adolescents may do whatever they wish in the absence of parental supervision. Both the capitulation and the laissez-faire expression of excessive leniency may be in part a result of adolescents' reinforcing ineffective parenting and punishing effective parenting.

Adolescents themselves face similar conflicts with excessive leniency, often pushing their environments to let them live according to their own standards, but then later facing negative consequences due to this lack of controls on their behavior. Although initially gaining what they want, they may face increased emotion dysregulation as a result (e.g., through consequences of their actions, such as disrupting their sleep schedules or missing classes and then failing a test). Those whose parents exhibit a laissez-faire parenting style may frequently behave in a reckless manner without any model for negotiating the difficult situations in which they consequently find themselves. In addition, these adolescents may experience some degree of anxiety or disappointment in response to this lack of parental supervision. Following a period of few or no externally imposed or self-imposed controls (and the resulting negative consequences), an adolescent, parents, and/or other involved authority figures will commonly flip to the other extreme of overly tight controls on the adolescent's behavior. This represents a move to the authoritarian control pole of the dilemma.

"Authoritarian control" refers to holding tight reins on behavior, by coercive methods of limiting freedom, autonomy, and independent decision making. This pattern might include enforcing overly strict or even unrealistic rules about curfew, contact with boyfriends or girlfriends, schoolwork, or even TV watching. Parents of adolescents often attempt to hold tighter reins as their children mature physically and cognitively, demand more autonomy, and experiment with new behaviors to fit their more adult-like bodies and minds. Yet these controls can become extreme in parents who are desperate to suppress the behavioral dysregulation in their suicidal adolescents with BPD or borderline features. Parents may apply hasty punishments or novel rules that are excessive and unlikely to be carried out (e.g., "You are grounded until the end of the school year"). Or adolescents, especially within the suburban population, will similarly apply such unrealistic punishments to themselves (e.g., "I won't watch any TV after school until after the next marking period, so I can get my grades up"). When these extreme methods of exerting control fail, are violated, or are given up on, parents and adolescents alike seem to become demoralized and commonly revert to an excessively lenient approach.

The behavioral extremes described here closely parallel Baumrind's (1991a) child-rearing dimension of "permissiveness–restrictiveness" in her research on parenting styles. Perhaps because of the strikingly labile nature of mood and behavior in suicidal adolescents with borderline features, we have observed a tendency for parents of such adolescents to vacillate between these two extremes, rather than to adhere consistently to one style. Even if parents stably exhibit tendencies toward one end of the pole or the other, they frequently switch to the opposite pole when a crisis arises or when they are feeling ineffective and demoralized. Moreover, overly permissive or overly restrictive (i.e., authoritarian) parenting styles have been linked with more negative child outcomes (e.g., Baumrind, 1991b; DeKovic & Janssens, 1992), and may comprise part of DBT's theorized environmental contribution to the etiology of BPD or borderline features. This may especially apply in situations in which such styles prove a particularly poor fit with children's temperaments or needs. In other words, somewhat extreme parenting styles along this dimension may contribute to negative child outcomes, while problematic child outcomes may contribute to rendering parents' styles more extreme.

To summarize this dialectical dilemma, for parents it involves vacillating between the extremes of being overly permissive with their adolescents (and feeling ineffectual, coerced, and partly responsible for the adolescents' continued difficulties) on the one hand, and setting unreasonable, overly restrictive limits on the other (often to compensate for a period of perceived overpermissiveness). The parents face the quandary of not reinforcing maladaptive behavior while not stifling normal development. For example, parents may wonder whether they should permit marijuana use by a 17-year-old because it serves as an effective soothing mechanism in lieu of self-cutting, or whether they should give in when other demands are linked with suicide threats.

This dialectical dilemma for the adolescent involves the question "When do I let myself off the hook, and when do I buckle down?" For the therapist, the dilemma involves balancing supporting the parents in enforcing effective limits while exhorting them to reinforce small improvements and to allow a reasonable level of freedom. For example, a parent must recognize a C+ as improvement when past grades were failing, instead of grounding an adolescent for not making the honor roll. The therapist also needs to support the adolescent in adhering to limits, as well as in rewarding him- or herself for small accomplishments. Table 5.6 summarizes this dialectical dilemma and its associated treatment targets and strategies/techniques.

Treatment Targets: Increasing Authoritative Discipline; Decreasing Excessive Leniency

The first pair of targets for this dilemma involves establishing a reasonable degree of parental authority (or self-discipline) while reducing excessive leniency. In fact, what Baumrind (1991a, 1991b) has labeled the "authoritative" parenting style offers a useful model for an effective middle ground for parents in this domain. The authoritative style of parenting consists of high restrictiveness and high demands for mature behavior, balanced with demonstrations of reasoning, support, love, and respect for the child's viewpoint. Children raised

TABLE 5.6. Targeting Excessive Leniency versus Authoritarian Control

Dialectical pattern	Secondary treatment targets	Specific techniques/strategies
Excessive leniency (placing too few behavioral demands or limits on the adolescent's behavior)	Increasing authoritative discipline; decreasing excessive leniency	Balancing restrictiveness and demands with reasoning, love, and respect Providing clear rules; rewarding desired behavior, along with establishing consequences for not following them (contingency management strategies) Following "wise mind" values in placing limits; using interpersonal effectiveness skills to communicate with teens
Authoritarian control (placing overly tight controls on the adolescent's behavior)	Increasing adolescent self-determination; decreasing authoritarian control	Rewarding effective behaviors while minimizing excessive rule setting, punishments, and coercive control strategies Using interpersonal effectiveness skills in discussions with teens, rather than unilateral, inflexible rules

in this fashion tend to show good outcomes in peer socialization, school performance, self-reliance, and self-esteem (Baumrind, 1991b; Dumas & La Freniere, 1993).[2] And parents who learn authoritative parenting methods can still be satisfied that they can exert some control over their children (as opposed to feeling they must surrender authority to appease the volatile adolescents).

Ways of increasing the characteristics of an authoritative parenting style include an emphasis on rewarding (and thus shaping and maintaining) desired behavior; providing clear rules and expectations, along with consequences for not following them; and enforcing the rules and consequences consistently. Therapists can work with parents on these issues primarily during as-needed family sessions, although some of these points can also be worked into discussions within multifamily skills training groups. Consequences should not be excessive to the point of being unlikely to be carried out. Yet teaching parents the behavioral principle of "correction–overcorrection" can be useful for applying consequences to adolescents. In correction–overcorrection, a parent applies a consequence that either withholds something that an adolescent wants or adds an aversive condition. Next the parent has the adolescent engage in a behavior that not only corrects effects of the maladaptive behavior, but goes beyond this to overcorrect its effects (Linehan, 1993a). As soon as the correction and overcorrection are completed, the initial consequence is removed. The consequence should relate to the problem behavior and ideally teach the adolescent client something as well. For example, if a newly licensed adolescent "borrows" the parents' car without permission and gets into a fender bender, the parents might withhold driving privileges, then ask the adolescent to pay for the damage (correction), and then apply new rules involving much closer monitoring of the adolescent (e.g., earlier curfews, frequent phone calls, etc.) for 1 month (overcorrection).

---

[2]This research was correlational, suggesting that we cannot conclude that this parenting style *caused* the observed child outcomes. Child behavior may elicit certain parenting responses, or a third factor may cause both parenting styles and child outcomes. Or, consistent with the biosocial theory of DBT, parent and child responses may co-create each other over time.

These consequences would hold the adolescent responsible for the damage to the car (teaching responsibility) and also require a temporary increase in communication and decrease in autonomy. Upon the adolescent's taking care of the damage and abiding by the agreements of 1 month's increased supervision, access to the car would be reinstated. An important factor to consider in applying consequences is what was lost or damaged by the egregious behavior. Ideally, whatever was lost in the infringement needs to be repaired. In this example, both the car and the parents' trust have been damaged; the consequences are thus intended to repair both.

In addition to enhancing parents' authoritative parenting, therapists can also teach parents to follow their "wise mind" values in determining which behaviors to restrict or permit; teach them the principle of observing their own limits (since if they do not, parents, much like therapists, are likely to feel resentful, overwhelmed, burned out, and ineffective); and emphasize the use of interpersonal effectiveness skills in communicating with adolescents in a way that helps parents attain their objectives while maintaining the relationship and keeping their self-respect. Other interpersonal effectiveness skills lend additional support, such as identifying thoughts that interfere with effectiveness (e.g., "This will never work") and identifying factors to consider when considering interpersonal objectives with an adolescent child (e.g., "Is this a good time?", "Does she have the capability to give me what I am asking for?").

For adolescents, these targets involve applying similar contingency management strategies in self-discipline, including favoring reward over punishment as a method of influencing their own behavior. They also need to set realistic goals for and apply realistic consequences to their behavior. For example, rather than canceling all social plans for an entire marking period (a strategy bound to be abandoned), the adolescent might try building in small, frequent rewards for movement toward goals (e.g., completing 2 hours of homework before turning the TV on). We should note that many teens in our inner-city population have trouble with this model of self-reinforcement. Because of exposure to violence and other traumas, many such adolescents have a sense of a foreshortened future and other pessimistic views. The concept of delayed gratification may prove hard to sell. But therapists can also work with adolescents individually, teaching enhanced judgment, planning, and decision-making skills (e.g., using distress tolerance skills to reduce impulsive responding, and then considering likely consequences of various behavioral choices). Furthermore, adolescents can benefit from the practice of accepting and tolerating parental inconsistency.

One of our cases concerned a 17-year-old boy who would come home drunk and past curfew. At some times when he did this, his parents would not outwardly respond, to avoid creating a scene. They nevertheless remained concerned and angry about it. At other times, for similar transgressions, they would unpredictably lose their tempers and punish him excessively, due in part to feeling impotent and exploited. They would think, "We are tolerant and let him get away with murder, and instead of appreciating it and behaving according to the rules, he takes advantage of us." The goals in this case were to encourage parental communication of rules and expectations, as well as consistent and appropriate discipline (e.g., "The punishment should fit the crime"). Importantly, the parents also needed to become familiar with principles of shaping, and to reward their son for progress in adhering to rules. Therapists have sometimes found themselves in the precarious position of nearly invalidating parents and oversimplifying dilemmas while trying to help them to find a middle path in this area. For example, a parent may say, "How could I have insisted she go to school that day? I had to get to work myself, and I just could not have dealt with an explosion at that point!" On the other hand, "How can I *not* insist she attend school? There are only 2 months left in the school year, and she's in danger of not graduating!"

Treatment Targets: Increasing Adolescent Self-Determination;
Decreasing Authoritarian Control

The next pair of targets involves establishing a reasonable degree of parental permissiveness without having parents abdicate all parental authority or neglect the adolescent's needs for external controls. As with the targets of increasing authoritative discipline and decreasing excessive leniency, an effective middle ground for parents consists of working toward more of an authoritative style of parenting. In particular, ways for parents to increase an adolescent's self-determination and reduce authoritarian control include rewarding instances of the adolescent's effective behaviors while minimizing excessive rule setting, application of punishments, and coercive control strategies (such as nagging, yelling, hitting, or inducing guilt). In place of unilateral rules, the therapist can work with parents to increase their use of interpersonal effectiveness skills with the adolescent to communicate behavior preferences with explanations of positive or negative consequences ("I'd like it if you did this, because . . . "). This approach not only grants adolescents more jurisdiction over their own behaviors, but also allows parents to model important aspects of effective functioning, such as skillful communication and consideration of consequences. For adolescents, increasing self-determination and decreasing an authoritarian style of self-control primarily involve self-applied contingency management strategies—a significant challenge for many of our teens.

Pathologizing Normative Behaviors versus Normalizing Pathological Behaviors

We define "pathological behaviors" as extreme manifestations of developmentally normative behavior that are also likely to harm an adolescent's quality of life or physical well-being in the long run. For example, rather than experimenting with marijuana at a party, an adolescent becomes involved in selling it at school; rather than experimenting with sexuality, an adolescent engages in unprotected sex that results in an unwanted pregnancy or in contracting HIV, or becomes subject to a gang rape after drinking excessively in a dangerous situation; rather than yelling at her parents and storming out of the room, an adolescent fights with her parents and ingests a bottle of pills.

Distinguishing between normative and pathological behaviors may become especially confusing for parents, since several behaviors typical of adolescents are also characteristic of BPD. These include unstable identity, a variety of high-risk behaviors, relationship instability, and emotional lability. Thus it may be difficult to distinguish behavioral patterns indicative of pathology from those falling within developmental norms for adolescents. Developmentally normative adolescent behaviors include those that are commonly observed and reported within the teenage years (e.g., experimentation with drugs, alcohol, and sexuality; changing goals or self-image; frequent breakups of romantic relationships; interpersonal conflicts, particularly with parents; moodiness), but that *do not* result in self-harm, hospitalization, school dropout, or other life-threatening or severe quality-of-life-impairing consequences.

To summarize this dialectical dilemma, for the parents it involves recognizing and allowing normative adolescent behaviors, while at the same time identifying and addressing those behaviors that are linked to severe dysfunction or negative consequences. This may pose a formidable challenge, as parents' judgments of what behaviors are "dangerous" or "abnormal" have become steadfastly colored by the shadow of past suicide attempts or hospitalizations. On the one hand, it may be easy for parents to fear and restrict developmentally normative behaviors, since they may view them as linked with high-risk situations or severe consequences in their children. For example, one father granted that it is typical for adolescents to experiment with alcohol with friends, but remembered that when his son recently drank, he also drove, got into a car accident, and got arrested. Another parent realized that kids miss school on occasion because of illness, but feared that her daughter's asking to stay home one day because of a migraine signaled a depression relapse; the previous depressive episode had begun with her daughter's finding reasons to stay home (and had ultimately led to a suicide attempt and hospitalization). A third parent could not determine whether her daughter's skipping classes in late spring reflected normal "senior-itis" (her daughter asserted that everyone was doing it) or the return of impulsive behaviors and ineffective judgment. Adolescents who have greatly improved after an initial suicidal crisis have at times complained that their parents have unrealistic expectations, and, rather than acknowledging their progress, require them to behave as "perfect teenagers."

On the other hand, parents of suicidal adolescents with BPD or borderline features may (1) become so desensitized to at-risk behaviors that they overlook signs of danger or dysfunction, or (2) knowingly ignore harmful behaviors because of relief that they are *less* harmful than other behaviors the adolescents have exhibited previously (e.g., accepting school truancy because an adolescent is no longer slashing her arms with a razor).

For the adolescent, this dialectical dilemma similarly involves recognizing normative versus pathological behaviors. Suicidal adolescents in treatment often fluctuate between second-guessing seemingly normative behavior patterns (e.g., "I failed my first road test—do you think this means I'm all screwed up?") and rationalizing clearly problematic and dysfunctional behavioral patterns (e.g., "I had to fight her 'cause she gave me a dirty look"). For the therapist, the dialectical dilemma involves maintaining as objective a view as possible of what constitutes normative versus non-normative adolescent behavior in general. It further involves noting which questionable behaviors have not been functionally related to other dysfunctional behaviors for a particular client and which behaviors have proven maladaptive for this client. For example, spending the night at a friend's house might be anything from beneficial to dangerous, depending on the nature and history of the relationship with the friend. Even therapists are susceptible to targeting developmentally normative behaviors on the basis of links that indicated dysfunction in the past but may have changed (e.g., arguing with a parent may no longer be an antecedent to self-injurious behavior or urges). Therapists may also become desensitized to maladaptive behaviors that are lower in magnitude than past behaviors (e.g., conflict with a parent may still be severe and adversely affecting quality of life, but goes unnoticed by the therapist as a target because it no longer escalates into violence toward the parent). Moreover, a therapist must take care not to impose personal values while determining session targets from the diary card, but instead must *assess for behaviors that are functionally related to treatment targets*. Issues that particularly tend to challenge a therapist's objectivity include teenage sexuality (e.g., abstinence, birth control, parenthood, abortion), substance use, nicotine use, gang membership, education, body piercing and tattoos, and use of physical force in self-defense. Table 5.7 summarizes this dialectical dilemma and its treatment targets.

Treatment Targets: Increasing Recognition of Normative Behaviors; Decreasing Pathologizing of Normative Behaviors

Increasing parents' or adolescents' recognition of developmentally normative behaviors while decreasing the pathologizing of these behaviors involves a combination of techniques. Psychoeducation on normative adolescent behaviors is used, and the therapist also encourages "wise mind" judgments about whether the behavior in question seems like what adolescents typically do. Handout C.5 in Appendix C provides examples of normative adolescent behaviors and of behaviors that are cause for concern. The therapist must also consider whether the

TABLE 5.7. Targeting Pathologizing Normative Behaviors versus Normalizing Pathological Behaviors

Dialectical pattern	Secondary treatment targets	Specific techniques/strategies
Pathologizing normative behaviors (viewing developmentally normal adolescent behaviors as deviant)	Increasing recognition of normative behaviors; decreasing pathologizing of normative behaviors	Psychoeducation about normative teen behaviors
		Considering whether behavior in question is functionally linked with target-relevant maladaptive behaviors
		For teens, accepting parents' fears/reactions and repairing or overcorrecting behaviors
Normalizing pathological behaviors (failing to address or perceive deviant adolescent behaviors as such)	Increasing identification of pathological behaviors; decreasing normalization of pathological behaviors	Psychoeducation
		"Wise mind" judgments of normative nature of behaviors
		Evaluation of risk level, as well as links with dysfunctional behaviors

behavior in question was carried out impulsively or dangerously, and assess whether the behavior is functionally linked with a target-relevant maladaptive behavior.

Adolescents may also be taught to work toward accepting their parents' tendency to make too much of what seems like "normal teenage behavior" to them. Therapists can explain to their adolescent clients that when a teen's behavior has reached an extreme (e.g., suicide attempt, school suspension, or unwanted pregnancy), it is typical for adults to hold this individual to stricter standards than others, even after the teen has shown improvement. Thus adolescents may have to (1) practice distress tolerance skills while their parents are applying overly demanding or perfectionistic standards; (2) use interpersonal effectiveness skills to ask for what they want and negotiate a way both to attain their goals and to address/allay their parents' concerns; and (3) overcorrect their own behavior to earn back their parents' trust and acceptance.

Treatment Targets: Increasing Identification of Pathological Behaviors; Decreasing Normalization of Pathological Behaviors

Increasing parents' or adolescents' identification of pathological (i.e., harmful) behaviors involves psychoeducation (e.g., educating an adolescent girl about risks of unprotected sex when she is normalizing it, saying that her boyfriend prefers it that way). Decreasing the normalization of harmful behaviors also involves "wise mind" judgments about the normative nature and comfort level of particular behaviors (e.g., encouraging the just-mentioned adolescent to follow her "wise mind" evaluation about performing a sexual act that feels coerced, despite her boyfriend's protestations that it is "no big deal"). "Wise mind" also encourages evaluations about the impulsiveness or risk level of a behavior. The therapist can point out that a client's decision occurred rashly and without consideration of consequences—for example, when a client challenges, "So what's the harm in quitting my after-school job? People quit jobs every day!" The therapist should consistently assess the behavior's functional links with target-relevant maladaptive behaviors (e.g., a link between a client's spending "normal" time with a boyfriend after school and consistently coming late to therapy appointments). The therapist's application of in-session behavioral analyses affords ample opportunities to address this target. Helping the client to recognize maladaptive behavior patterns and unwanted consequences can help in reducing the normalization of non-normative behavior.

Fostering Dependence versus Forcing Autonomy

"Fostering dependence" refers to acting in ways that serve to stifle an adolescent's natural movement toward autonomy. This may include parents' overt attempts to block a teen's independent functioning and growth, or more subtle actions that result in reduced autonomy. Parents may naturally attempt to monitor and maintain communication with their adolescents as the teens assert independence and engage in more risky behaviors. Yet the tendency to foster dependence is often extreme in parents of adolescents who have been suicidal, out of fear that loosening their grip will reduce their ability to protect their children and result in more harm to them. In addition, some parents report having developed an intense, special bond with an adolescent child as a result of seeing the teen through suicidal crises and then joining him or her in treatment (i.e., the multifamily skills training group), although this usually entails the exclusion of other siblings who do not share in this experience. For the adolescent, fostering dependence may include clinging to parents by behaving in an overly needy manner. Such clinginess may occur because of the suicidal adolescent's deep sense of self-doubt and lack of self-confidence.

One way that fostering dependence may manifest itself is through excessive caretaking by parents, to the extent that an adolescent does not learn to negotiate the world on his or her own. For example, one adolescent was experiencing increasing conflict with a teacher, had gotten to the point of yelling and cursing at her, and was expressing misery about these events to her mother. Her mother stepped in and, after a series of meetings with school personnel, arranged for her daughter to drop the class and receive individualized tutoring in the subject in its place. The mother reported her conflict about having intervened in this manner. On the one hand, she realized she had not let her daughter face the natural consequences of her actions; nor had she allowed the daughter to negotiate the situation on her own and possibly repair the relationship with the teacher, thus building mastery. On the other hand, she had been afraid of the potential consequences of continued problematic interactions with the teacher; moreover, she had been afraid of her daughter's increasing emotion dysregulation as school was becoming more stressful. Rather than risk a recurrence of suicidal behavior and hospitalization, this mother understandably took the immoderate step of terminating interaction with the teacher as rapidly as possible.

"Forcing autonomy," on the other hand, involves parents' severing (or at least strongly loosening) the ties with their adolescents, in such a way that the adolescents are thrust toward separation, greater self-sufficiency, and a more adult level of functioning. It might include kicking the adolescents out, or demanding that they earn the money required to support themselves. Although it is expected that adolescents will gradually increase their autonomy and reduce reliance on parents, this can occur to an extreme degree within the population of suicidal adolescents with borderline features. Parents of such teens will at times essentially push the adolescents toward independence or reject them, as a result of either giving up, feeling exasperated and burned out, or believing that such a push is needed to get the teens to "grow up" and "start taking some responsibility." Examples of this tendency are reflected in statements such as "Well, then, find a way to pay for therapy yourself!", "Fine, then don't come home at all!", and "You call up the principal and explain this!" At times forced autonomy can take the form of excessive responsibility thrust upon an adolescent (e.g., responsibility for feeding, washing, and dressing four younger siblings each morning before school; such parental directives are not uncommon in some of our families, where single parents are raising several children).

At the same time, adolescents may force their own autonomy by letting go too fast or too extremely. This may be the result of an impulsive reaction to conflict, a desire to prove themselves, a result of life circumstances their actions have created (e.g., becoming pregnant and moving in with a boyfriend), or trouble in regulating emotional distance with a parent. As an example of this last pattern, one of our adolescents, who was rather withdrawn and lacking in self-confidence, would go for a period of time depending on her mother for social companionship—accompanying her to movies, shopping, ball games, and so on, confiding in her all the while. After a while, she would get disgusted and fed up with her mother (they often argued), as well as humiliated that at age 17 she needed to rely on her mother as a friend. She would then flip to the other extreme—pushing her mother away, shutting her out of her life, and experiencing her as intrusive if she even asked how her day was. After a period like this, she would inevitably feel both guilty and alone, and would again revert to the dependent extreme of this behavioral dimension.

To summarize this dialectical dilemma, it necessitates the parents' finding the middle way between clinging or caretaking to the point of stifling the adolescent's individuation process, and pushing away or letting go precipitously. For the adolescent, it entails achieving a balance between an effective and comfortable degree of relatedness and dependence on the one hand, and an effective and comfortable degree of separation, individuation, and identity formation on the other. For the therapist, the dialectical dilemma concerns not only guiding the adolescent in finding a balanced level of dependence on and autonomy from parents, but in monitoring his or her own tendency to foster extreme dependence versus extreme self-reliance in the adolescent vis-à-vis the therapeutic relationship. Table 5.8 summarizes this dialectical dilemma and associated treatment targets and strategies.

Treatment Targets: Increasing Individuation; Decreasing Excessive Dependence

The targets of increasing individuation and decreasing excessive dependence involve teaching parents to balance consultation to their children in how to negotiate their environments with direct environmental interventions. This notion derives from the DBT concept of consultation to the patient (see Chapters 3 and 4). Thus, rather than stepping in and taking over a situation to spare an adolescent environmental consequences or emotion dysregulation, parents can work toward instructing or coaching the adolescent in negotiating and mastering difficult situations, while still intervening when essential.

Similarly, the therapist can encourage adolescents themselves to consult with appropriate adults (e.g., parents, teachers, guidance counselors, relatives, the therapist) about handling difficult situations, rather than behaving in a helpless manner and imploring others simply to handle the situations for them (i.e., acting in an actively passive manner—the opposite of acting to build mastery, a necessary component of emotion regulation). Although an adolescent might become overwhelmed and thus emotionally dysregulated in the face of a challenging situation, the therapist might coach the adolescent to get into "wise mind," evaluate the situation, and plan an effective course of action, even if this includes soliciting the help of others. Critical problem-solving skills (e.g., generating alternatives to impulsive behaviors, thinking through consequences, and enhancing general behavioral skills) all apply to these targets. The therapist can point out to the adolescent the long-term advantages of working toward competent self-reliance, such as being taken seriously when the adolescent wants to be, earning more privileges, and reducing emotional vulnerability while increasing a sense of mastery and building a life worth living.

TABLE 5.8. Targeting Fostering Dependence versus Forcing Autonomy

Dialectical pattern	Secondary treatment targets	Specific techniques/strategies
Fostering dependence (stifling the adolescent's natural movement toward autonomy)	Increasing individuation; decreasing excessive dependence	Balancing consultation to teens on how to act with direct environmental intervention
		Encouraging teen to consult with adults and make "wise mind" evaluations of how to handle situations
		Increasing teens' problem-solving skills
		Building parents' social support networks
Forcing autonomy (thrusting the adolescent toward separation and autonomy prematurely)	Increasing effective reliance on others; decreasing excessive autonomy	Regulating distance between parent and adolescent, rather than going to either extreme (by using distress tolerance, emotion regulation, and interpersonal effectiveness skills)
		Pointing out to teen the notion of effective reliance on others (rather than the concept of dependence)

Parents' dependence on their adolescents may be heightened because of the social stigma and isolation they often feel as parents of children who have made suicide attempts or who have features (or a full diagnosis) of BPD. Some of these parents have reported that no one in their lives understands what they experience on a day-to-day basis; to make matters worse, they feel they cannot confide in friends or family members, because these others will conclude that they are horrible parents. Thus the therapist may encourage parents to enhance social support through support groups, friends they can trust, or even other parents in the multifamily skills training group. To some degree, this happens naturally; in fact, in one of our suburban populations, a group of mothers started meeting each other for dinner monthly.

Treatment Targets: Increasing Effective Reliance on Others; Decreasing Excessive Autonomy

The targets of increasing effective reliance on others and decreasing excessive autonomy involve the parents' and adolescent's remaining connected enough to enhance effective outcomes for the adolescent. Although adolescents have entered a developmental stage that involves a natural quest for separation and individuation from parents, they lack the experience and judgment to negotiate situations entirely on their own. The therapist can make the assumption that adolescents with suicidal behaviors or borderline features lack critical behavioral capacities as well. Specific interventions here include working toward regulating the amount of distance between parents and adolescents (i.e., thwarting the tendency to exhibit one behavioral extreme as a reaction to another; this may require distress tolerance and emotion regulation skills) and enhancing interpersonal effectiveness skills between parent and child (so that parents can offer and adolescents can ask for guidance; also, forced autonomy often occurs following a severe conflict between an adolescent and a parent). The therapist might point out to the adolescent the ultimate advantages of increasing effective reliance on others (gaining needed help while preventing further emotional vulnerability), as well as the maturity it takes to recognize when one needs help and to ask for it.

POLARIZATION BETWEEN PARENTS OF TEENS IN TREATMENT

Because adolescents typically reside with their parents and the parents participate in therapy, the adolescent dialectical dilemmas and corresponding treatment targets apply to parents as well as to therapists and clients. Interestingly, an additional tendency we have observed with this population is polarization *between* parents along the dialectical dimensions (especially in our suburban Long Island University population, where both parents are often involved in treatment). That is, parents are at times polarized along the dimensions of excessive leniency versus authoritarian control, pathologizing normative behaviors versus normalizing pathological behaviors, or fostering dependence versus forcing autonomy. This polarization has presented itself in a number of forms: Parents may participate in a teen's treatment together but adhere to divergent extremes; divorced parents may appear at different times for as-needed family sessions and present with positions in dramatic opposition to each other; or a teen may report that an absent parent's behaviors are opposed to those of the participating parent (typically either embracing the teen's position wholeheartedly or firmly rejecting it). Parental relationship discord is associated with youth behavior problems as either a cause, correlate, or consequence (e.g., Cummings & Davies, 1994). In addition, researchers have identified polarization as a process occurring within the interactions of discordant couples in general (e.g., Jacobson & Christensen, 1996). The parents of suicidal multiproblem teens in particular seem to struggle against each other commonly with regard to issues of firm or lenient discipline, interpretation of a teen's behavior as pathological or normative, and encouraging versus discouraging dependence. When such polarizations have an adverse impact on an adolescent, the therapist may find him- or herself siding with one parent, feeling pulled into doing couples therapy, or spending time coaching the adolescent to manage the parents' differences. Psychoeducational approaches can be helpful in leading parents to a middle path, such as teaching parents effective discipline strategies, educating them about developmental norms, and helping them to consider consequences of choices regarding the teen's level of autonomy. Furthermore, looking for the grain of truth in each parent's viewpoint and validating this is essential; working on a limited basis with parents to discuss these issues skillfully (e.g., nonjudgmentally listening to and validating each other's viewpoints) can also help reduce extreme positions. Ultimately, the therapist's goal might be to work with the adolescent to accept the parents' polarities and identify the behaviors that are most effective for the teen him- or herself.

SUMMARY: RESOLVING DIALECTICAL DILEMMAS

In essence, secondary targets in DBT share the overall goal with the primary targets of resolving dialectical dilemmas—that is, helping suicidal, emotionally dysregulated adolescents (and their parents) change their extreme behavioral patterns into a more balanced lifestyle. Regardless of the stage of therapy, the emphasis is on increasing the ability of adolescents and family members to "walk the middle path" and balance the many dialectical tensions inherent in their emotions, thoughts, and actions.

CHAPTER 6

Assessing Adolescents
Suicide Risk, Diagnosis, and Treatment Feasibility

This chapter reviews a variety of strategies for assessing adolescents in three primary domains: suicide risk, diagnosis, and DBT treatment feasibility. Information from these assessments informs the decision as to whether a given adolescent (and family) is clinically and lo-
gistically appropriate for a given DBT program. Moreover, initial treatment-planning data are
derived from these assessments. An assessment procedure that we find helpful with this high-
risk population in an outpatient setting includes evaluating suicide and NSIB risk, mental disorders, and eligibility for inclusion into the DBT program (Step 1); clarifying DBT Stage 1 target behaviors (Step 2); clarifying the feasibility of DBT for the specific adolescent client and
family (Step 3); and developing an initial treatment plan, together with establishing some initial commitment to treatment (Step 4). Other assessment methodologies should be considered
for other settings.

It is important for every new evaluation to include a suicide risk assessment. This assessment ideally includes an in-depth intake evaluation consisting of clinical interview, semistructured interview, and standardized questionnaires. Not all programs have the time and/or
resources to carry out this type of extensive assessment, which can take several hours and may
even be divided into two separate visits. Regardless of setting and resources, however, it is
critical to conduct an evaluation to gather history; determine behavioral problem areas, diagnoses, and suicide risk; ensure appropriateness for DBT; and identify major treatment targets
before treatment is officially started.

The assessment process typically begins when a referral is made from an emergency
room, an inpatient unit, a school, or a pediatrician's office. At this point we employ a brief (1-
page) telephone screening instrument that takes approximately 10 minutes to administer. Its
purpose is to assess quickly whether a prospective client meets the defined criteria for the
program. Our Montefiore-based outpatient Adolescent Depression and Suicide Program requires that prospective clients be between 12 and 18 years old, while also presenting with depression and/or suicidal or NSIB urges and actions (but not such acute ones that they need to
be rushed to an emergency room immediately). Our program's specific inclusion criteria are
as follows: at least one suicidal act and/or NSIB in the past 16 weeks or current suicidal ideation, *plus* a diagnosis of BPD or three features of BPD as measured by the SCID-II (see below). Other programs may choose to use less stringent criteria, inviting clients who exhibit
emotional or behavioral dysregulation without any apparent suicidal behaviors or NSIB.

If adolescents meet the preliminary inclusion criteria, they and their parents are invited
within 5 business days to an initial intake session. From this point on, the assessment process
can be distilled into the series of four general steps listed above and described in detail below.

STEP 1: ASSESSING SUICIDAL IDEATION, SUICIDAL BEHAVIORS, NSIB, AND MENTAL DISORDERS

It is the exception rather than the rule that clients actually present for treatment with us in a suicidal crisis. This is because referral to our program frequently *follows* an episode of acute suicidality, in which there has already been an inpatient hospitalization or at least an emergency room visit. Thus the suicidal crisis phase has passed, but the family or referring professional is looking for maintenance, stability, and prevention of future occurrences. Alternatively, an adolescent is referred because a school guidance counselor or a parent notices increasing depression or suicidal ideation, but it has not reached a crisis point. However, we certainly do see the exceptions—clients who are referred precisely because they are acutely suicidal, or for whom our initial assessment makes suicidality clear. We have occasionally walked a client to the emergency room following an initial evaluation if, after extensive efforts at crisis intervention, the adolescent refuses to stay alive even for 24 hours.

Although the protocol for handling a suicidal crisis is basically the same, regardless of whether the crisis occurs at the outset of treatment or sometime during the course of treatment (see Chapter 8), there are some important differences: At the initial evaluation, there is not yet a therapeutic alliance to use in handling the situation; the therapist does not know the client, including the client's biggest vulnerability factors or strengths; and the client has not yet learned skills to apply to the situation. Although these differences may seem to suggest higher risk and a necessarily poorer outcome, the converse may actually be true: Some evidence indicates that youth and their parents may be more likely to follow through with treatment when they present in a more acute state of distress (e.g., Kendall & Sugarman, 1997).

Strategies for Assessing Suicide and NSIB Risk

In work with high-risk adolescents, it is important to establish a sense of collaboration *before* assessing risk behavior. Researchers have found that the best predictor of a suicide attempt is a previous suicide attempt (Leon, Friedman, Sweeney, Brown, & Mann, 1990; Gould et al., 2003). However, since only 10–40% of those adolescents who commit suicide have made a previous attempt, it is necessary to assess for other risk factors, such as suicidal ideation and mental disorders (Brent et al., 1988; Marttunen et al., 1992). The assessment of suicide risk in adolescents is particularly difficult, because teenagers may provide evaluators with discrepant information and may be reluctant to disclose personal information to adult authority figures (Brent et al., 1988; Velting et al., 1998). Some research suggests that suicidal clients are more likely to disclose current suicidal ideation on a self-report measure than in a clinical interview (Kaplan et al., 1994; Velting et al., 1998). It is equally important not to rely exclusively on self-report measures. It is recommended that suicide risk assessments also include face-to-face interviews, since a clinical interview yields important information that cannot be obtained through questionnaires, such as the adolescent's quality of affect and compliance with the interviewer (Holinger, Offer, Barter, & Bell, 1994; Velting et al., 1998). Table 6.1 lists the instruments we use in our adolescent programs to assess suicide/NSIB risk and mental disorders and the frequency with which we administer them.

Examples of commonly used self-report inventories of suicidal ideation and attempts include the Suicidal Ideation Questionnaire (SIQ; Reynolds, 1987), the Scale for Suicide Ideation (Beck, Steer, & Ranieri, 1988), and the Harkavy–Asnis Suicide Survey (Harkavy–Friedman & Asnis, 1989). Our Montefiore program currently uses the SIQ, which is a brief (15-item) self-report inventory designed to assess thoughts about suicide in adolescents. Items

TABLE 6.1. Assessment Instruments Used with Adolescent Outpatients

When used	Instruments and areas assessed
Baseline/intake[a]	*Suicide/NSIB risk* Suicidal Ideation Questionnaire (SIQ; Reynolds, 1987) Lifetime Parasuicide Count (LPC; Linehan & Comtois, 1995) Suicide Attempt Self-Injury Interview (SASII; Linehan et al., 2006a) Reasons for Living Inventory for Adolescencts (RFL-A; Osman et al., 1998) DBT diary card *BPD features associated problems* Structured Clinical Interview for DSM-IV Axis II Personality Disorders, BPD module (SCID-II; First et al., 1997) Life Problems Inventory (LPI; Rathus et al., 2005) *General psychopathology and family functioning* Schedule for Affective Disorders and Schizophrenia for School-Age Children—Present and Lifetime Version (K-SADS-PL; Kaufman et al., 1997) Beck Depression Inventory—II (BDI-II; Beck et al., 1996) Symptom Checklist-90—Revised (SCL-90-R; Derogatis, 1994) Conners Rating Scale—Revised for parents and teachers (Conners et al., 1998) McMaster Family Assessment Device (FAD; Epstein et al., 1983) Children's Global Assessment Scale (CGAS; Shaffer et al., 1983)

Follow-up assessments:

Weeks 4, 8, 12, 16, 32, 48	SIQ, BDI-II, SCL-90-R, CGAS, LPI, SASII, diary card
Weeks 8, 16, 32, 48	LPC, RFL-A, FAD, Conners (P, T)
Week 16	DBT Skills Rating Scale for Adolescents (Parent and Teen forms; Rathus & Miller, 1995b)

[a]Typically, teens and parents complete self-report forms before participating in the diagnostic evaluation

are scored from 6 to 0. This instrument has demonstrated good content and construct validity, as well as internal consistency and test–retest reliability (Reynolds, 1987).

One problem with current self-report measures of suicidality is that they yield a high number of false positives, indicating that these measures alone are not sufficient to distinguish those adolescents who are truly at risk for suicidal behavior (e.g., Lewinsohn et al., 1996; Shaffer et al., 1996). To this end, reliable measures of intentionality are needed to help effectively distinguish those teens with intent to die from those without intent to die. The Suicidal Intent Scale (Beck, Herman, & Schuyler, 1974), the Lifetime Parasuicide Count (LPC; Linehan & Comtois, 1996), and the Columbia Suicide History Form (Malone, Szanto, Corbitt, & Mann, 1995), are measures of intentionality but have not been normed on adolescents. The Suicide Attempt Self-Injury Interview (SASII; Linehan, Comtois, Brown, Heard, & Wagner, 2006a) is a structured interview that obtains comprehensive information about any self-injury. The interview provides the information necessary to determine whether the self-injury was a suicide attempt or NSIB, and it gives information about events surrounding the episode. The

SASII is used on the most recent and most serious self-injury. It gives the clinician a good start on conducting a behavioral assessment of suicidal behaviors.

We use the LPC, since it assesses both suicide attempts and NSIB, determines intent to die, and establishes whether the self-harm required medical attention. The LPC is relatively short, is easy to administer, and has been employed in studies with our outpatient ethnic minority adolescent population (Velting & Miller, 1999). Regarding concurrent validity among similar minority outpatient adolescents, those youth diagnosed with three or more Axis I mental disorders were found to have more suicidal behaviors on the LPC than youth without these disorders (Velting & Miller, 1999).

One may consider administering another self-report measure that approaches suicide from a different vantage point. The Reasons for Living Inventory for Adolescents (RFL-A; Osman et al., 1998) is a modified version of the adult RFL, which taps expectancies about the consequences of living versus killing oneself and assesses the importance of reasons for living. The measure has six subscales; it is negatively and uniquely related to suicidal behavior, independent of its relationship to depression and hopelessness. It is not related to general psychopathology. The internal consistency of the global measure has been found to be .96 (Osman et al., 1998). This instrument functions to identify protective factors against suicide. Since many teens appear depressed and suicidal, this instrument helps to distinguish those at higher risk (i.e., teens who cannot identify any reasons to live) from those who can identify one or more reasons. After an adolescent completes the RFL-A and is unable to identify any reasons to live, the clinician may ask the adolescent directly, "So how would your mom feel if you killed yourself? Your dad? Your little sister?" Sometimes reassessing this question in a clinical interview format, instead of via self-report, elicits different information. From a risk assessment and family relations standpoint, the response to this question generates significant information.

Some adolescents engage in risk-taking behaviors without overt intent to self-injure or die. Although we cannot define such behaviors as suicidal, we do consider them extremely dangerous and potentially life-threatening. Some of these behaviors include "subway surfing" (standing on top of a moving subway car); riding a motorcycle without a helmet; driving while intoxicated; having unprotected sex with unknown partners; and using unclean needles or sharing needles to inject heroin. To date, there are no assessment measures to evaluate the broad range of these risk behaviors. However, it is important for clinicians to assess these types of activities while they conduct their initial assessments and throughout treatment. Some clients disclose these and other behaviors only after they have established a trusting alliance with their therapists.

During the course of the evaluation, it is helpful to take careful note of other suicide and NSIB risk factors highlighted in Chapter 1. Some of these risk factors (e.g., mental disorders, family discord, academic problems, stressful life events) become apparent during assessment for quality-of-life-interfering behaviors. Other risk factors are not always so apparent without further inquiry. For example, clinicians should inquire about an adolescent's sexual orientation, as well as physical or sexual abuse and neglect. Although the assessment of maltreatment is beyond the scope of this book (see Feindler, Rathus, & Silver, 2003; Wekerle, Miller, Wolfe, & Spindel, 2006), clinicians are advised to keep a number of things in mind when maltreatment seems probable. It is important to collect information from a number of different sources (including the adolescent, his or her nonoffending parent or caretaker, teachers, and any legal professionals), and to use a number of different formats as discussed below.

In addition to the usual components of a clinical evaluation (e.g., presenting problem; history of presenting problem; mental disorder; developmental, educational, family, and social histories; mental status; etc.), evaluations in case of potential maltreatment call for a few extra components. A description of the maltreatment, including identification of the perpetrator, duration, and type, should be elicited from as many sources as possible. Symptoms of PTSD and other problems associated with maltreatment (e.g., depression, disruptive behavior) should also be inquired about, including date of onset; however, the absence of PTSD symptoms does not indicate that maltreatment did not occur (Wonderlich et al., 2000). Finally, the evaluator should assess the adolescent's perceptions of the maltreatment, including his or her thoughts regarding what might have caused and maintained it, since this information will inform aspects of the psychotherapy. A comprehensive evaluation such as this will help the clinician develop a thorough case conceptualization, which in turn will guide treatment.

According to the National Clearinghouse on Abuse and Neglect Information (2004), the use of standardized assessments in combination with clinical judgment is the best approach to assessment. Standardized assessments include semistructured interviews and self-report measures. Semistructured interviews often assist in determining the presence of mental disorders. Self-report measures are useful supplements to structured or semistructured interviews, and can be completed by young victims and/or their nonoffending caregivers. Some measures, such as the Child PTSD Symptom Scale (Foa, Johnson, Feeny, & Treadwell, 2001), have been developed specifically to assess for abuse-related symptoms. Other instruments are available to assess for more general psychological impairment or adjustment distress (see Feindler et al., 2003, and "Assessing General Psychopathology and Family Functioning," below).

Strategies for Diagnostic Evaluation

To treat multiproblem suicidal teens effectively, it is critically important to conduct a thorough diagnostic evaluation. Some combination of mood disorders, anxiety disorders, substance-related disorders, disruptive behavior disorders, and eating disorders is common. In addition, certain mental disorders are clear risk factors for suicidal behavior in adolescents (as discussed at length in Chapter 1). Thus establishing a clear diagnostic picture early in the treatment helps to (1) assess risk, (2) inform the treatment planning, and (3) ensure that proper treatments are delivered. When it is possible, we recommend a comprehensive assessment battery that includes semistructured diagnostic interviews in addition to parent, teacher, and adolescent self-reports, as listed in Table 6.1. It should be noted, however, that some teens are reluctant to engage actively in the evaluation process. At times a clinician needs to check in with a client, potentially validate the client's feelings that this is a long and detailed process, and then either take a little break or establish a commitment that the client will reapply him- or herself to complete the evaluation.

Assessing BPD Features and Associated Problems

Although it would be ideal to assess for all Axis II disorders, Montefiore's program assesses only for BPD, due to our concern about burdening the clients with too many assessment measures and interviews. For example, some clients and family members have become burned out during the assessments, rendering the battery invalid by mindlessly writing 0 for each item on a questionnaire. As a reminder, according to the DSM-IV-TR (APA, 2000), it is permissible to diagnose BPD in adolescents (anyone under the age of 18) when maladaptive traits are pervasive, persistent (lasting at least 1 year), and unlikely to be limited to a developmental stage or an episode of an Axis I disorder.

Despite the increasing awareness of the presence of personality disorders among adolescents, no one has developed a semistructured interview to assess Axis II disorders among this age group. The Structured Clinical Interview for DSM-IV Axis II Personality Disorders (SCID-II; First et al., 1997) is a widely used semistructured interview to measure personality disorders among adults, and we use its BPD module to assess our adolescent population. Individuals must meet at least three of nine diagnostic criteria in the BPD module to be eligible to receive DBT in Montefiore's outpatient program. We chose three BPD criteria (coupled with current suicidal ideation or recent suicide attempt and/or NSIB) in order to cast a wider net and be overinclusive rather than underinclusive. Adolescents who present to our outpatient program with "only" three BPD criteria and some suicidal behaviors or NSIB typically have significant functional impairment and require intensive intervention. Clinically, these teens appear as appropriate for our outpatient DBT program as those who meet five or more BPD criteria. And teens with subthreshold BPD scores on the SCID-II (i.e., three or four criterion behaviors) were found to be more similar to clients formally diagnosed with BPD than to clients without BPD (i.e., those with two or fewer criterion behaviors) on features of emotional and behavioral dysregulation (Rathus et al., 2005).

We also administer a self-report measure we have developed to assess the major problem areas associated with BPD. The Life Problems Inventory (LPI; Rathus & Miller, 1995a; Rathus et al., 2005) is a 60-item self-report scale developed for adolescents as a baseline assessment and outcome measure, with four 15-item subscales assessing core aspects of BPD addressed in DBT: Confusion about Self, Interpersonal Difficulties, Emotion Dysregulation, and Impulsivity. Preliminary studies found the LPI to have good psychometric properties (Miller, Wyman, Glassman, Huppert, & Rathus, 2000). More recently, we conducted a larger study of this instrument's psychometric properties, using four groups: (1) outpatient adolescent mental health clients diagnosed with BPD features, (2) outpatient adolescent mental health clients without such features, (3) outpatient adolescent medicine clients, and (4) nondisordered college students. We found the LPI subscale scores to be internally consistent in both groups of psychiatric clients and the college control group. Moreover, the scores were stable over a 2-week period among the college students. Convergent validity was also demonstrated, since LPI scores were correlated with the SCID-II BPD module, depression, suicidal ideation, suicide attempts, and global psychopathology. Regarding criterion validity, the LPI scores discriminated among the outpatient adolescents with borderline features, the outpatient adolescents without borderline features, and the adolescent medicine outpatients (Rathus et al., 2005).

Assessing General Psychopathology and Family Functioning

One of the most commonly used semistructured diagnostic interviews to assess Axis I disorders in children and adolescents is the Schedule for Affective Disorders and Schizophrenia for School-Age Children—Present and Lifetime Version (K-SADS-PL; Kaufman et al., 1997). According to a review by Ambrosini (2000), the K-SADS-PL has demonstrated good reliability and criterion and predictive validity. The Demographic Data Questionnaire from the K-SADS screener obtains a wide range of demographic data, including age and ethnicity, as well as social, medical, and family history. The K-SADS screening module allows the interviewer to assess whether a client is symptomatic enough in a certain domain (e.g., mood disorder symptoms) to require the administration of the K-SADS-PL mood disorders module. Appropriate modules are provided for mood disorders, anxiety disorders, disruptive behavior disorders, substance-related disorders, eating disorders, and psychotic disorders. The adolescent and the parent/guardian are interviewed separately to obtain diagnostic information. The interview is scored categorically for the presence or absence of each diagnostic category.

Several self-report measures may also be useful to employ for assessing Axis I psychopathology with this multiproblem population. The Beck Depression Inventory–II (BDI-II; Beck, Stear, & Brown, 1996) is a 21-item self-report inventory of depression with established psychometric properties, including test–retest reliability with teens. The Symptom Checklist-90—Revised (SCL-90-R; Derogatis, 1994) is a 90-item self-report scale of symptoms experienced during the past week, spanning nine symptom areas: Somatization, Obsessive–Compulsive, Interpersonal Sensitivity, Depression, Anxiety, Hostility, Phobic Anxiety, Paranoid Ideation, and Psychoticism. The scale has acceptable internal consistency and test–retest reliability, and both concurrent validity and discriminant validity have been demonstrated. In addition, the adolescent DBT diary card (see Chapter 7 and Figure 7.3) is a self-report measure that is administered and collected each week. Adolescents are instructed to self-monitor their maladaptive behaviors (e.g., self-injury, drug use), the intensity of their emotions (e.g., anger = 5), and their use of new behavioral skills each day. This instrument thus collects a significant amount of information that is used clinically as well as for research purposes.

Observer ratings, including those by parents and teachers, are important to obtain as well to help round out the assessment of the suicidal multiproblem adolescent. Parents complete the Conners Rating Scale and the McMaster Family Assessment Device (FAD). The Conners Rating Scale—Revised (versions are available for parents and teachers; see Conners, Sitarenios, Parker, & Epstein, 1998a, 1998b) is a popular research and clinical tool for obtaining significant adults' reports of childhood behavior problems. Exploratory and confirmatory factor-analytic results revealed a seven-factor model: Cognitive Problems, Oppositional, Hyperactivity–Impulsivity, Anxious–Shy, Perfectionism, Social Problems, and Psychosomatic. The psychometric properties of the revised scale appear adequate, as demonstrated by good internal reliability coefficients, high test–retest reliability, and effective discriminatory power.

The McMaster FAD (Epstein, Baldwin, & Bishop, 1983) is a 53-item self-report questionnaire designed to measure family functioning. It is made up of seven scales: Problem Solving, Communication, Roles, Affective Responsiveness, Affective Involvement, Behavior Control, and General Functioning. Some items describe healthy functioning, while others describe unhealthy functioning. The FAD has adequate test–retest and internal consistency reliability, low correlations with social desirability, and cutoffs for the seven scales that have adequate levels of specificity and sensitivity (Miller, Epstein, Bishop, & Keitner, 1985). The parents and adolescent complete their own assessments of their perceived family functioning.

It is helpful during some part of the initial assessment with the parents to obtain a thorough family history (including history of mental disorders) and a clear picture of the current living situation, as well as the parents' and adolescent's reports of the current family stressors.

Therapists can rate clients' functioning on the Children's Global Assessment Scale (CGAS; Shaffer et al., 1983). The CGAS is an interviewer-generated measure of functional impairment used both as a continuous measure and as a marker of clinical impairment (i.e., CGAS score 60).

Employing assessments at regular intervals (see Table 6.1) allows clients, parents, and therapists to report changes in behaviors and symptoms. This not only enables clients to monitor their own target behaviors, but also guides ongoing treatment. In addition, data gathered at specific assessment points can be used for treatment outcome research.

Finally, we developed the DBT Skills Rating Scale for Adolescents (Rathus & Miller, 1995b), which is administered at the end of treatment to adolescents and family members who have participated in a skills training group. This instrument is a self-report of the helpfulness and overall effectiveness of the skills, as well as satisfaction with the overall DBT program. In one study, adolescents rated three mindfulness skills and one distress tolerance skill as the four most helpful skills taught (Miller et al., 2000). Interestingly, all four of these skills involve tolerating uncomfortable thoughts and feelings without actively attempting to change them. Given that many adolescents (especially those with borderline spectrum pathology) attempt to escape and avoid aversive emotions and those situations that create negative emotions, it is impressive and surprising that they experience tolerance and acceptance skills as most helpful (in contrast to the change-oriented skills, such as emotion regulation and interpersonal effectiveness skills).

In sum, administering this suggested assessment battery is aimed to help clinicians determine whether an adolescent meets the inclusion or exclusion criteria for a DBT program, as well as to provide additional data that will help inform the treatment planning. If clinicians do not have the time or financial resources to administer this aforementioned assessment battery, we recommend conducting at least a thorough clinical interview (with special attention to past and current suicidal ideation and attempts), and perhaps administering one relatively comprehensive self-report measure, such as the LPI (Rathus et al., 2005).

STEP 2: ASSESSING OF DBT STAGE 1 TARGET BEHAVIORS

The assessment of DBT Stage 1 targets can be woven into the Step 1 strategies for assessing suicide/NSIB risk and mental disorders. In order of descending priority, the Stage 1 targets are (1) reducing life-threatening behaviors, (2) reducing therapy-interfering behaviors, (3) reducing quality-of-life-interfering behaviors, and (4) increasing behavioral skills. Obtaining a detailed assessment of *all* Stage 1 target behaviors is extremely important in strengthening commitment to treatment and determining the treatment plan. Therapists who have more details about clients' problem areas typically have greater leverage in trying to obtain and strengthen commitment with clients. In addition, specific information about Stage 1 targets informs the development of a treatment plan (described in Chapter 7). To the extent possible, a clinician should prioritize these detailed assessments by using the DBT treatment target hierarchy.

Clinicians should assess the functions of their clients' life-threatening (suicidal, self-injurious, or homicidal) behaviors during the first session. Although this information can be obtained through clinical interview, it is often helpful to use an instrument such as the LPC (Linehan & Comtois, 1995) to obtain such information. This instrument includes questions about the most severe and the most recent examples of self-injurious behavior. Using these identified examples of life-threatening behaviors, the therapist can then question the client in order to identify specific antecedents and consequences that may help explain the function of these behaviors. Typically, these functional analyses begin to reveal important "warning signs" that can be used immediately in the treatment, such as feeling rejected by a romantic partner, feeling ashamed in front of peers, receiving a failing grade at school, or experiencing increasing amounts of love and affection after reporting suicidal ideation to the family. For example, if the therapist recognizes in a behavioral analysis that the client is being positively reinforced by family members after reporting suicidal ideation, the therapist would immediately address this by educating the client about this problem and teaching the family more effective contingency management in a family session as soon as possible.

If time permits, it is helpful to conduct a second detailed behavioral chain analysis of the most recent suicidal behavior and/or NSIB. As we will see in Chapter 8, DBT employs a behavioral analysis of any life-threatening behaviors in individual therapy. The analysis helps both client and therapist discriminate vulnerability factors, precipitating events, consequences, and key links in the chain. This allows the client (1) to gain greater insight into the key links in the behavioral chain that play a role in this behavior; (2) to generate potential solutions to help avert future suicidal behavior and/or NSIB; (3) to feel validated by the intense interest the therapist expresses through asking such detailed questions about a problem behavior; and (4) to experience a primary element of the DBT treatment during the assessment phase.

It also behooves the clinician to conduct a detailed assessment of the client's prior treatment history. This assessment should include both treatment successes and failures. Given the high rates of treatment noncompliance and dropout among suicidal multiproblem adolescents (see Chapter 1), the clinician needs to elicit what, if anything, contributed to the client's dropping out of any prior therapies. This information can potentially aid in keeping the client better engaged in the current treatment by anticipating and addressing the same pitfalls (i.e., therapy-interfering behaviors).

For example, Jessica (a fictionalized composite client) was a 15-year-old Hispanic female who was referred to Montefiore's outpatient DBT program by the personnel of a local emergency room, where she was brought by an ambulance and police. Jessica's mother had called 911 after Jessica threatened to kill herself with a knife following an altercation with her boyfriend. Jessica had been psychiatrically hospitalized twice before for medically serious suicide attempts in which she overdosed on her mother's prescription medications. She also had a history of self-cutting on her arms and legs, as well as occasional self-burning, although she had stopped the latter behavior 2 years ago. She had previously received the diagnoses of the following mental disorders: major depression, dysthymia, eating disorder not otherwise specified, alcohol abuse, and BPD. Her grandmother, mother, and older sister, with whom she lived, all had histories of depression and suicidal behaviors. Her brother was currently incarcerated for drug dealing and assault. Her parents were divorced, and although her father lived nearby, he had a rather cold and distant relationship with Jessica. Already on probation for poor grades during the last marking period, she was in the 10th grade at a local high school and was failing most of her classes. In addition to her boyfriend, she had two close female friends and numerous "acquaintances."

During the evaluation, Jessica reported disliking her prior therapist because "she told me what to do, even though she had no idea what it was like to be me." The clinician recognized that the client had felt invalidated; he asked, "Would it have been more helpful if the therapist got to know you better first before making suggestions about how to solve your problems?" Jessica answered in the affirmative. The therapist proceeded to highlight both ends of a dialectic and suggested a synthesis:

> "That makes sense on the one hand, and on the other, it seems to me that you're in a whole lot of distress at this very moment and need help. So we need to figure out a way for me to understand better what you're going through, and at the same time be able to make some suggestions to help you dig out of the hell that you feel like you're in. . . . So as we move ahead, Jessica, if you feel like I'm telling you what to do and I am missing what you're feeling, I want you to stop me in midsentence and say, 'Hey, you don't get it.' Then we can figure out how to proceed without you having to quit therapy. Deal?" [Jessica: "OK."] "Good. So let me hear you practice saying, 'Hey, you don't get it.' "

Once the clinician has conducted a detailed assessment of therapy-interfering behaviors, it is time to move on to quality-of-life-interfering behaviors. Not surprisingly, multiproblem adolescents typically present with multiple behaviors of this type. Prioritizing these behaviors in a meaningful way becomes one of the greatest challenges in the assessment and early phase of treatment; the challenge is even greater for those providers trying to deliver short-term treatment. Conducting a detailed assessment of quality-of-life-interfering behaviors allows the therapist to create an individualized subhierarchy of such behaviors that helps to organize the treatment (see Table 6.2). Without a detailed assessment, the clinician and the client typically resort to putting out "the fire of the week," and the treatment rarely has any meaningful continuity. For example, what does a clinician do if the client presents at intake with the following quality-of-life-interfering behaviors: depression, school truancy, binge-drinking episodes on weekends, ongoing conflicts with parents, intermittent breakups with boyfriend, and binge-eating episodes? It would be impossible to conduct detailed assessments of *all* these behaviors in the first or second session of the evaluation. To narrow the field, the clinician should assess whether any of these behaviors are functionally linked to either life-threatening or therapy-interfering behaviors. For example, if the binge-drinking episodes consistently precede a client's life-threatening behaviors, these episodes will be addressed while targeting suicide. If the behaviors are not functionally linked to higher-priority targets, the therapist and client attempt to base the subhierarchy on the client's own prioritization of what is important to him or her, while assessing the functional impairment caused by each of the behaviors. Often substance-abusing behaviors are placed at the top of the quality-of-life-interfering subhierarchy, given the adverse impact these behaviors typically have on adolescents' lives (including problems with sleep, mood, health, relationships, and the law), as well as the fact that they are a common link to and risk factor for suicidal behaviors. The subhierarchy is individualized to each client, and it may change as progress is made or as other problems worsen and take priority. Thus assessment needs to be woven throughout the entire treatment.

Target behaviors at the final priority level for Stage 1 (i.e., behavioral skills to be increased) are assessed less formally; however, clinicians must look for opportunities to evaluate their clients' skills repertoires and the context in which they can or cannot employ specific skills. For example, when conducting a detailed assessment of why a client dropped out of prior therapies, the clinician tries to elicit the adolescent's degree of awareness (mindfulness capacity) of his or her distress in the previous sessions, whether the adolescent attempted to employ any distress tolerance skills, and whether the client tried to use interpersonal effectiveness skills to express displeasure directly to his or her former therapists. This information allows the current clinician to judge the adolescent's skills capabilities and deficits in the context of therapy. It may be necessary to teach a new skill to the adolescent in that very session, or at least to be aware that the deficit will need to be addressed at some point. For example, with Jessica, the therapist taught the client to say, "Hey, you don't get it," if and when she felt invalidated in sessions. The therapist elicited Jessica's commitment to using the skill, and then

---

TABLE 6.2. Treatment Target Hierarchy, with Jessica's Individualized Subhierarchy of Quality–of–Life–Interfering Behaviors

1. Decrease life-threatening behaviors.
2. Decrease therapy-interfering behaviors.
3. Decrease quality-of-life-interfering behaviors.

   Jessica's individualized, collaboratively created subhierarchy:
   a. Reduce alcohol use.
   b. Reduce depression.
   c. Reduce school truancy.
   d. Reduce interpersonal problems with boyfriend and parents.
   e. Reduce binge eating.
4. Increase behavioral skills.

asked her to practice saying the statement to the therapist in session (behavioral rehearsal of the new skill).

STEP 3: ASSESSING FEASIBILITY OF DBT FOR THE CLIENT AND FAMILY

A frank discussion about the feasibility of delivering DBT needs to be conducted following the completion of Steps 1 and 2 of assessment. Several common feasibility questions are raised below, and Table 6.3 offers a feasibility checklist. When adolescents do not meet the inclusion criteria, the Montefiore program has the luxury of assigning them to other (non-DBT) treatment interventions offered within the larger outpatient program, or of referring them elsewhere. It's important to be able to offer noneligible clients alternative treatment resources.

Some adolescents and families are appropriate for DBT, but practical or logistical limitations prevent them from pursuing the treatment. For example, some clients have desperately sought out a DBT program, but live so far away from the clinic that it may not be feasible to have twice-weekly treatment. One solution may be to conduct the individual therapy on the same day as the skills training session, even though doing 3 hours of therapy in 1 day is far from ideal. In other rare cases, an adolescent is completely unwilling to consider decreasing suicide attempts and/or NSIB, and refuses to contract for safety even for 24 hours. This degree of risk without any commitment to change on the adolescent's part, despite massive efforts to employ all commitment strategies by the clinician, will preclude outpatient treatment from being conducted. In contrast, despite parents' reports, some teens minimize their problems and report, "I'm fine and I don't need treatment!" It is often necessary to spend several sessions in pretreatment to build a treatment alliance that will enable the adolescent to start identifying problems and goals. In the beginning, the therapist often approaches such a client in this way:

> "I hear that you feel like you're fine and you don't need treatment. . . . And, by the way, I wouldn't force you to come here if you did not want to. But it seems like your parents and

TABLE 6.3. Feasibility Checklist for DBT

- Is DBT the appropriate treatment? Does the adolescent meet inclusion criteria for the DBT program?
- Does the teen want to attend, and if so, can he or she get to the clinic or office regularly? (Is the adolescent willing and able to participate in a twice-per-week treatment program?)
- Is the adolescent willing to commit to making an attempt at working on the treatment targets, especially decreasing life-threatening behaviors?
- Do the parents endorse the DBT treatment program, explicitly acknowledging that the outpatient treatment is twice-weekly?
- Is at least one parent or another family member willing to participate actively?
- Can the adolescent and family commit to the duration of treatment (i.e., at least 16 weeks for outpatient treatment, 2 weeks for inpatient treatment, a minimum of 6 months for residential treatment)?
- Can the family afford the treatment financially?

your school guidance counselor think you need some kind of help. . . . What's going on that's gotten them all bent out of shape? Do you want some help figuring out how to get them off your back?"

It is often not feasible, and sometimes it is not clinically indicated, to involve family members actively in the inpatient, residential, and forensic DBT programs. In outpatient settings, however, we strongly urge parents to participate actively in all aspects of the treatment program. Even if parents are unable to take an active part in the multifamily skills training group (e.g., a parent is unable to take time off from work or does not speak English), the clinician wants at least to elicit a meaningful endorsement of the treatment and to engage them in collateral family sessions. Interestingly, Halaby (2004) recently found that adolescents' compliance with outpatient DBT is specifically associated with the parents' positive attitude toward the treatment and not necessarily with their active participation in it.

There are exceptions, however, in which the exclusion of parents from outpatient treatment is indicated. For example, if parents are psychotic, manic, coming to sessions under the influence of drugs or alcohol, or threatening, we do not want them attending a skills group. In one case, an adolescent male's mother was so chronically emotionally dysregulated that it was not feasible to have them together in the same room, due to repeated angry and violent episodes. In this case, the therapist conducted parallel skills training sessions for the parents while the adolescent attended the multifamily skills training group without his parents. Some parents require their own referrals to outpatient therapy or detox programs, and child protection services are periodically notified when concerns about abuse or neglect arise. Parental illiteracy may be another barrier; however, we have had some illiterate parents attend a skills group, with the understanding in advance that they will not be asked to read in front of the group.

STEP 4: DEVELOPING AN INITIAL TREATMENT PLAN

Developing an initial treatment plan that is clear to the treatment team, the adolescent, and his or her family is extremely important, as it forces the therapist to operationalize specific target behaviors, goals, and treatment objectives. This step should not be delayed too long, since the plan can always be altered as treatment proceeds. Within the first two sessions, the primary therapist should develop a treatment plan based on the identified target behaviors presented by the adolescent and family members. Special attention is paid to identifying specific problems, goals, and measurable objectives. Each of these needs to be reviewed to ensure agreement before all parties, including therapists, make a commitment and sign the document. In some settings, therapists must document these plans in each patient's chart, as per office of mental health requirements. Other settings (e.g., private practices, graduate school clinics), however, may not require this type of official documentation, and therefore this may not be written down or signed. Figure 6.1 is an example of a treatment plan developed for the fictionalized client Jessica and her family. Based on Jessica's intake assessment data, the primary therapist was able to formulate a preliminary treatment plan that matched Jessica's specific client behaviors with DBT targets and skills. The initial plan will inform the initial orientation and commitment phase, to be covered in Chapter 7. The plan itself is not formally introduced until the latter portion of this phase. Family orientation also takes place later in the orientation and commitment phase.

Target	Goal	Objective	Expected date
1. Decrease life-threatening behaviors: – Suicide attempts – NSIB (cutting) – Suicidal ideation	There will be no suicide attempts, NSIB, or suicidal ideation.	J. will utilize new behavioral skills and/or call primary therapist for coaching when in distress, and will not engage in any suicidal behavior and make every effort to not harm herself for 16 weeks. J. will report a 50% reduction in frequency and intensity of suicidal ideation.	5/16
2. Decrease therapy-interfering behaviors: History of poor tx. compliance	She will comply with entire treatment plan as prescribed and not drop out of treatment.	J. will attend all scheduled groups, individual sessions, and family sessions, and work collaboratively with all DBT providers.	5/16
3. Decrease quality-of-life-interfering behaviors: a. Alcohol use b. Depression c. School truancy d. Relationship problems with boyfriend and parents e. Binge eating	She will return to baseline functioning and no longer experience quality-of-life-interfering behaviors.	J. will (a) abstain from alcohol for the next 16 weeks; (b) report a 50% reduction in depressive symptoms as measured by the BDI-II; (c) increase school attendance to at least 80% of classes/week; (d) engage in no more than one argument per week with boyfriend and parents, and attend family sessions on an as-needed basis; and (e) reduce binge-eating episodes by 50% per week. J. will call primary therapist for coaching when she has difficulty controlling impulses and skills are ineffective.	5/16
4. Increase behavioral skills: – Emotion regulation – Interpersonal effectiveness – Distress tolerance – Mindfulness – Resolving parent-adolescent dilemmas	She will learn a new repertoire of behavioral skills.	J. will practice her DBT skills daily and complete her homework for skills group and ind. therapy during the next 16 weeks. She will report on her diary card using at least two DBT skills per day when experiencing any type of distress.	5/16

_____   _____
(Client's signature)   (Date)

_____   _____   _____   _____
(Parent's signature)   (Date)   (Skills trainer's signature)   (Date)

_____   _____   _____   _____
(Primary therapist's signature)   (Date)   (Skills trainer's signature)   (Date)

FIGURE 6.1. *Treatment plan (16 weeks) for Jessica.*

CHAPTER 7

Orienting Adolescents and Families
to Treatment and Obtaining Commitment

The pretreatment stage of orientation and commitment to DBT begins once suicide risk and diagnostic assessments are complete and the adolescent has been found to meet the inclusion criteria for the DBT program (see Chapter 6). As discussed in Chapter 3, the key goals of this stage are for the client and therapist to arrive at a mutually informed decision to work together and to make explicit their agreed-on expectations about that work. The process involves the primary therapist's helping the adolescent identify his or her long-term goals, orienting him or her to the treatment, and obtaining the teen's commitment to treatment. These therapeutic actions are considered "pretreatment targets." This chapter presents a set of strategies to use with adolescents and families to orient them and obtain their commitment. These are outlined in Table 7.1. In outpatient adolescent programs, an additional orientation to DBT often occurs in a multifamily skills training group format. (See Chapter 10 for orientation to skills training.)

Orientation and commitment to DBT begin with the adolescent alone first. Once the process has been initiated with the adolescent, the therapist can bring in the parents and/or other participating family members and repeat some of the key elements (this can occur late in the first session or in the second session). Even in more restrictive treatment settings (e.g., inpatient, forensic, and residential), we suggest following this same format, despite the fact that the adolescent may not have any choice whether to participate in the DBT program or not. It is important to foster some sense of control over the teen's participation. For example, the therapist might say,

> "We know right now that you do not want to be here. So you can remain miserable, stay in your room, not participate in DBT group or individual sessions, and keep talking to your friend— or you can try to get to know some new people, participate in the treatment, and maybe figure out what you need to do to build a life worth living outside of this place and we'll help you do it."

The development and maintenance of a therapeutic alliance with the adolescent are of critical importance in this initial stage and throughout treatment. Other key orientation tasks are (1) to introduce the treatment in terms of how it fits, and can help solve, the individual teen's problems; (2) to link work on Stage 1 treatment targets with the adolescent's long-term goals; and (3) to present an overview of the treatment and its requirements. Orientation is not simply a description of the treatment; rather, it aims to build motivation. It is a discussion of

TABLE 7.1. Orientation and Commitment Strategies for Adolescents and Families

1. Begin to establish a therapeutic alliance:
   a. Use friendly, egalitarian, down-to-earth, and open demeanor, while simultaneously earning respect and conveying credibility.
   b. Convey realistic degree of confidence in oneself as therapist, the client, and the treatment.
   c. Establish active stance while collaboratively setting the agenda.
2. Fold adolescent's specific problems into areas of dysregulation (and explain corresponding skills developed to address each problem area):
   a. Confusion about self
   b. Impulsivity
   c. Emotional instability
   d. Interpersonal problems
   e. Adolescent–family dilemmas
3. Define adolescent's specific problems as primary target behaviors:
   a. Life-threatening behaviors
   b. Treatment-interfering behaviors (based on prior treatment history)
   c. Quality-of-life-interfering behaviors
   d. Skills capabilities and deficits

4. Elicit client's long-term goals, and link these to work on Stage 1 targets.
5. Introduce the biosocial theory.
6. Introduce the treatment's format and characteristics.
7. Introduce DBT diary cards.
8. Review treatment agreements:
   a. Client agreements
   b. Therapist agreements
   c. Client–therapist relationship agreement
   d. Family agreements
9. Use commitment strategies with adolescent to obtain and strengthen commitment.
10. Use commitment strategies with family members to obtain and strengthen commitment.

what the particular teen can (and can't) realistically hope to get out of the treatment, and of how the treatment works to fulfill those hopes. The process clarifies the adolescent's specific goals and the specific DBT procedures used for reaching those goals. This becomes the basis for an explicit treatment agreement to which all parties are asked to commit themselves. Strategies for obtaining client commitment are discussed later in this chapter.

Jessica, the 15-year-old introduced in Chapter 6, is typical of adolescents in our outpatient clinic. When her assessments were complete, she met the criteria for the DBT program. She then met alone with the person who was to become her primary (individual) therapist. This began the orientation process.

ORIENTING ADOLESCENTS TO DBT

Beginning to Establish a Therapeutic Alliance

The primary task at the start of DBT is beginning to develop a collaborative relationship with the adolescent. This is crucial as well as difficult. Many adolescents presenting for treatment initially believe that they do not need it. Even those who have made a recent suicide attempt often minimize it as an impulsive act and state that they "feel better now." These adolescents often have had conflictual relationships with their parents as well as other adults. Being told that they must talk to a therapist, a stranger, because "something is wrong" makes many teenagers angry, resistant, and noncompliant. Given that up to 77% of suicidal adolescents either do not attend follow-up therapy appointments or drop out of treatment prematurely, it becomes important for therapists to equip themselves with a variety of techniques and strategies to engage such adolescents (Trautman et al., 1993).

A key strategy to working with adolescents involves conveying a down-to-earth, friendly, egalitarian, and open demeanor, while maintaining an understated degree of expertise and credibility. The challenge for therapists entails getting teens both to like and to respect them. In our experience, therapists who have had more experience with adult clients at times approach teenagers with an authoritarian, doctor-like, "one-up–one-down" stance. This approach consistently alienates adolescents. In working with an adolescent, it is also important to communicate a high level of confidence in one's own ability as a therapist, in the client's ability to improve, and in the efficacy of the treatment. Feigning confidence in oneself, in the client, or in the treatment will inevitably prove ineffective; a teenager will see through the act and disengage from the treatment. This may pose a challenge for a therapist who is new to the treatment and feels less competent. Thus the therapist should strive for a balance between genuinely communicating confidence in all three domains (self, client, and treatment) and not overpromoting them.

It is important to take an active stance in work with adolescents, especially early in treatment. Therapists who work within other treatment orientations often take a less active stance at the beginning of treatment and allow clients to choose freely what to discuss. In standard DBT, as well as in DBT with adolescents, the therapist uses these early sessions to get to know the client and to allow the client to get to know the therapist. This active stance is part of a dialectic, however, since one of the biggest mistakes that a novice DBT individual therapists tends to make is forcing an agenda on the client instead of letting the session unfold and skillfully weaving in the necessary components identified below. Thus taking an active stance involves the therapist's developing a plan for the session content with the client and then guiding the client through this content, as well as adhering to DBT principles. Setting an agenda at the beginning of the session is a customary part of most forms of CBT. Although DBT does not require agendas, it can often be helpful to lay out at the beginning of a session which tasks and topics need to be covered. It also gives the adolescent a chance to say what topics he or she wants to cover. In the first or second session, which may include assessment, orientation, and commitment, the therapist will set the agenda by stating, "Jessica, I want to get some history and hear what problems you may currently be having before we decide what is the appropriate treatment for you." Some beginning therapists feel compelled to tell clients everything they are supposed to cover in the first session, as opposed to skillfully weaving the material into the first couple of sessions.

One stylistic strategy in DBT is the use of irreverence—a style characterized by calling a spade a spade, as well as by using humor, sarcasm, or confrontation. Whereas some therapists are wary that being "too" irreverent early in therapy might alienate teens, we believe exactly the opposite. We recommend weaving irreverence into treatment immediately, since it functions to get adolescents' attention in a manner different from most others with whom they discuss their problems. For example, when Jessica nonchalantly discussed her suicidal behaviors and her ambivalence about discontinuing them, the therapist stated, "Jessica, you realize that this treatment will not work if you are dead." Irreverent communication strategies are discussed further in Chapters 3 and 8 as well as in Linehan's (1993a) text.

Folding Adolescent's Specific Problems into Areas of Dysregulation

The orientation session begins with asking for a recap of the client's problems. Hence it is important to validate the client's potential frustration at having to repeat his or her story to yet another mental healthcare provider. This is relevant only if the primary therapist is different from the initial evaluator. For example, the therapist might say,

> "Jessica, I know you already told a lot of this information to Liz, who spent 3 hours with you last week during the diagnostic evaluation. She did share much of that information with me; however, if I am going to be your individual therapist, I want to get to know you, your strengths, and your weaknesses, and I will probably be asking at least some of the same questions. So bear with me."

As the session proceeds, the therapist folds the client's problems into the five major problem areas identified on Figure 7.1. These problem areas correspond directly to the areas of dysregulation associated with BPD (i.e., emotional, behavioral, cognitive, interpersonal, and self; see Chapter 3). We describe the five problem areas as follows: (1) confusion about self, (2) impulsivity, (3) emotional instability, (4) interpersonal problems, and (5) teenager–family dilemmas. For example, if a teen identifies sudden and apparently baseless anger as a problem, the therapist might say,

> "Jessica, when you are feeling OK one minute and then angry for seemingly no reason, DBT therapists call that a 'problem with regulating emotion' or 'emotional instability' (Problem 3 on the handout). Since you don't know why your emotions shift sometimes, you probably experience some confusion about yourself (Problem 1 on the handout). If you then start cutting yourself or purging without thinking about the consequences, we consider that impulsive behavior (Problem 2 on the handout)."

The therapist will review the other problem domains if the adolescent does not raise them naturally during the first session. Typically, adolescents referred to our program endorse at least four out of the five problem areas.

> "Jessica, do you find that your relationships—with your boyfriend, your parents, your sister, your friends—run hot and cold? That is, even though you have friendships, do you find it hard to keep these relationships stable? Is it hard to get what you want from these relationships? If so, that would be Problem 4—interpersonal problems. And Problem 5 relates to teenagers who feel that they don't see eye to eye with their family members. Do you feel you're on one side of the Grand Canyon and your family members are on the other side, and it is difficult to understand one another and come to an agreement on issues, such as curfew, dating, homework, or body piercing?"

The DBT therapist then tells the teen that although having these problems may feel overwhelming, there is some good news:

> "For each of these problems, the skills group will teach you specific skills that will target and reduce your specific problems. For example, in regard to impulsivity, we are going to teach you distress tolerance skills so that you will learn how to distract and soothe yourself when you have urges to kill yourself, cut yourself, overdose, drink alcohol, or purge. When you say you have interpersonal problems, we are going to teach you a set of inter-

Dialectical Behavior Therapy

PROBLEMS (What to decrease)	SKILLS (What to increase)
I. Confusion about yourself (Not always knowing what you feel or why you get upset; dissociation)	I. Mindfulness
II. Impulsivity (Acting without thinking it all through)	II. Distress tolerance
III. Emotional instability (Fast, intense mood changes with little control; or, steady negative emotional state)	III. Emotion regulation
IV. Interpersonal problems (Pattern of difficulty keeping relationships steady, getting what you want, or keeping your self-respect; frantic efforts to avoid abandonment)	IV. Interpersonal effectiveness
V. Teenager–family dilemmas (Polarized thinking, feeling, and acting–e.g., all-or-nothing thinking)	V. Walking the middle path

FIGURE 7.1. *Handout on DBT for adolescents and family members.*

personal effectiveness skills in order to help you keep your self-respect; you're your relationships stable; and get what you want from your boyfriend, your girlfriends, and your parents. Do those skills sound helpful?"

In addition to what takes place in individual therapy, the skills trainer briefly reviews each problem area as it relates to each individual client and then describes the corresponding skills module, one by one. This review typically instills hope in the adolescent and family.

Defining Adolescent's Specific Problems as Primary Target Behaviors

The individual therapist (who may or may not be the same clinician as the diagnostic interviewer, as noted earlier) is responsible for eliciting the information relevant to the DBT Stage 1 targets. Much of this information may have already been gathered during the diagnostic evaluation. The therapist connects the client's specific problems with DBT's primary target behaviors. The therapist might say, "So those overdoses are considered life-threatening behaviors, and your depression, your bingeing and purging, your school problems, and your intense conflicts with your parents are what we call 'quality-of-life-interfering behaviors.' Is it your belief that these problems interfere in the quality of your life?" Reframing these problems in DBT language enables the therapist to explain how DBT will be able to target these problems, while also beginning (unobtrusively) to teach the client this language.

Once the primary target behaviors are identified, the DBT therapist is then able to review the Stage 1 treatment target hierarchy and informs the client that individual sessions will be organized accordingly from that day forward. To make this point clear, the therapist may draw a pyramid and list the client's problem behaviors from top to bottom in a fashion corresponding to the Stage 1 hierarchy (see Figure 7.2). It is explained to the adolescent that if in the past week there have been any self-injurious behaviors or increases in suicidal ideation, those behaviors will need to be analyzed first. The therapist goes on to explain that it does no one any good if the therapist and client spend the session talking about issues unrelated to the self-injury, since the client may intentionally or accidentally kill him- or herself by the next visit if they do not understand what is going on and how to deal with it differently. The remaining targets are then discussed, in hierarchical order.

Eliciting Client's Long-Term Goals, and Linking These to Reducing Stage 1 Target Behaviors

In obtaining a commitment to reducing such Stage 1 target behaviors as suicide and self-injury, drug use, and truancy, as well as increasing behavioral skills, it is critical for the therapist to link them to the adolescent's long-term goals. Thus it is always important to elicit these goals. Jessica's goals included graduating from high school and starting college, continuing her cheerleading activities, joining a band as a singer, getting married, having kids, and finding a high-paying job. Jessica agreed not to kill herself, but was initially reluctant to reduce her self-cutting, since the behavior helped distract her from her intense anxiety and sadness. The therapist then queried Jessica as follows:

THERAPIST: You mentioned that you are self-conscious about the marks on your arms and legs. If we could figure out a way for you to reduce your anxiety and sadness without leaving cuts and scars on your body, would you choose another method?

JESSICA: I don't know . . . I know this works.

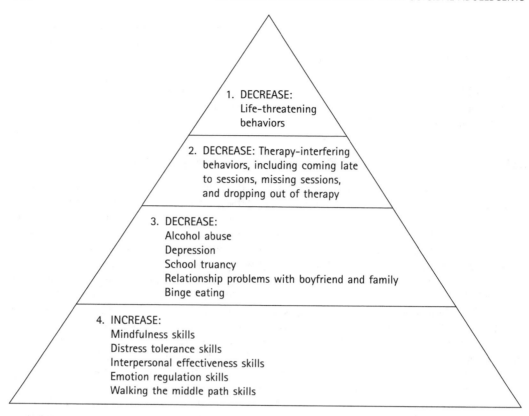

FIGURE 7.2. *Jessica's Stage 1 target pyramid drawn in session.*

THERAPIST: I get that . . . and if you want to continue your cheerleading next year, I imagine it may be hard to wear long sleeves and pants to cover those marks. And I also know that while you initially experience relief when you cut, you also often experience shame later. This becomes a vicious cycle for many people and makes them more vulnerable to cutting again . . . Does that happen to you?

JESSICA: Yes, I often feel worse. I know I have to work on this, but I am so scared to give it up.

THERAPIST: That makes perfect sense to me, given how effective this behavior has been for you in the short term at reducing certain negative emotions. I feel confident, though, that if I can teach you some new skills and we try them out, we'll find some of them will help you in similar ways to cutting, without leaving those marks or creating the negative emotions that perpetuate the problem as well.

Introducing the Biosocial Theory

Referring back to the five problem areas listed on Figure 7.1, the therapist asks the adolescent rhetorically, "How do you think you developed these types of problems?" Typically, the adolescent is baffled and somewhat demoralized by the rhetorical question. To help answer this question, we explain that Marsha Linehan, the originator of DBT, developed a theory that helps explain why some people have these types of problems (Linehan, 1993a; see Chapter 3 for a full discussion of the biosocial theory). Using visual aids such as a handout can help adolescents better understand this abstract theory. The therapist first reviews and defines the two components of the theory: "bio" and "social." "Bio," derived from the word "biology," involves the biochemistry of one's brain. The therapist might ask, "Jessica, have you ever experienced yourself as more emotionally sensitive, quicker to react, and slower in returning to your emotional baseline once you get upset than your siblings or friends?" Indeed, most of these adolescents admit that little things seem to "get under their skin easily" and affect them more than their peers. Moreover, they acknowledge that when they get upset, their emotional reactions are more intense and reactive (e.g., not just a little sad, but feeling very depressed; not mildly anxious, but having panic attacks; not merely irritated, but experiencing angry outbursts). The third characteristic—slow return to emotional baseline—is explained by drawing a graph on a piece of paper, with a line halfway up the bell curve to represent the adolescent's moderate to high level of emotional arousal. Instead of returning back to 0, the line remains elevated at this level for an extended period (sometimes hours or even days). Many teens endorse this characteristic as true of themselves as well. Jessica reported, "Sometimes when I get really angry, it takes me almost a whole day to chill."

The "social" part of the theory is described as the "invalidating environment." Once "validation" and then "invalidation" are defined, an example is provided immediately to help illustrate the concept of invalidation. The therapist attempts to use examples offered by the adolescent during the first session if possible:

> "Jessica, you told me that whenever you feel depressed and you feel you have less energy to do your chores in the house, your mother calls you a crybaby and tells you to snap out of it, or you'll get a beating. You also told me that when you travel with your father to visit your relatives in Puerto Rico, your father insists that you put on a smile even if you are not in a smiling mood. These experiences are examples of 'invalidation'—in other words, communications indicating that your thoughts, feelings, or actions are wrong, inappropriate, and invalid. . . . Who's to say how you should feel and act and what you should think? Those are your thoughts and feelings, not theirs!"

Jessica responded, "I'm so used to it, I guess I never thought of it that way." The therapist emphasizes that invalidation occurs frequently, to varying degrees, and can often be inadvertent. The therapist also explains the transactional nature of the biosocial theory (see Chapter 3), emphasizing a nonjudgmental and nonblaming attitude. For example, a mother and child may have different temperaments, as in the case of a quiet, shy, mellow toddler unmatched temperamentally with a gregarious, high-energy, demanding mother, or a highly emotional child with an emotionally controlled parent. Some teens tend to protect their parents in response to this explanation of an invalidating environment. The therapist can suggest that parents who invalidate often learned it as children from their own parents and do not know any way to communicate more effectively. If this is applicable, the therapist might state, "It makes perfect sense that your parents invalidate you, since that is what they learned growing up." The therapist then has an opportunity to point out the intergenerational transmission of invalidation. Aditionally, teens sometimes invalidate their family members as well.

Regardless of the intent, the therapist targets the invalidation experienced in the family, in order for the adolescent to feel better understood by the family and for the family members to feel better understood by the adolescent. (The biosocial theory review, like other aspects of orientation to treatment, typically occurs first with the adolescent alone and then is reported with the entire family.) The therapist then continues, "Here's the good news: Now is the time for you (and your family) to learn how to validate one another properly, and to put an end to the inadvertent invalidation that occurs in your household each day. You, Jessica, and each member of your family have to take responsibility for becoming more aware of this behavior and practicing the skill of validation."

For many adolescents, hearing the biosocial theory explained is the first time they understand why they act and feel the way they do. Some adolescents are literally moved to tears by the experience.

Introducing the Treatment's Format and Characteristics

The therapist reviews the treatment format next, consistently checking in with the client to ensure that he or she understands what is being said. Then the therapist attempts to obtain initial commitment to the various treatment modalities (see the later discussion of commitment strategies), using a conversational yet didactic style. A therapist would introduce the 16-week Montefiore program as follows:

> "Jessica, our DBT program is two sessions per week for 16 weeks.[1] The treatment consists of one individual session (for 60 minutes) and one multifamily skills training group (for 2 hours) per week. So since you live with your mom, and you and she have a lot of conflicts, I think it makes sense to invite her as the family member who will attend the multifamily skills group with you. Don't you agree? Also, the individual session is periodically divided in half, so that we can have some time to address family issues with your mom, your dad, and even your sister. How does that sound to you? The bottom line is that you and your family will be treated by a team made up of your individual therapist, two skills trainers, your prescribing psychiatrist, and other DBT therapists in our program.
>
> "The first phase of treatment lasts 16 weeks. When you finish that, you could be eligible for the graduate group, which involves a lot of fun activities and is only for people who graduate from the first phase. Another important component of the treatment is the telephone coaching. There are three reasons I would like you to call me. First, I want you to page me before you engage in a problem behavior, like cutting, overdosing, purging, or drinking. It doesn't help to call me afterwards, since you already decided how to handle that situation. Second, I want you to call me with good news. I love to hear good news— and you can leave a message on my machine and I will be thrilled to get it. Finally, I want you to call me if you feel that we have to repair our relationship [see Chapter 3 for further explanation]. Some teens have trouble with this pager idea . . . they say, 'I didn't want to call you and bother you on the weekend.' Jessica, let me be crystal-clear: I wouldn't be instructing you to call me if I thought it was a problem. If I am tied up with something else when you page me, I'll tell you so and let you know how soon I can call you back. Does that seem reasonable? Good. So I'd like to have you practice paging me this week, at some point when you're not in crisis, just to see how this whole thing works. Don't worry, I won't keep you on long—just to say hello. Can you we do a practice page on Tuesday night?"

The practice page helps the client add this new skill to his or her behavioral repertoire during an undistressed period, with the hope that he or she will be more likely to use it when actually faced with a stressor.

---

[1]The most important issue is to set a treatment time period (e.g., 16 weeks, 6 months, 1 year) for the client to commit to. The therapist and client can then either renew the agreement at the "initial" endpoint for a specified period of time, or consider referring the client to a different therapist or therapy if sufficient progress is not being made.

The therapist then says to the client enthusiastically, "If we work together as a team, I can help you solve your problems. There are several key points you need to understand as we move ahead." The therapist describes seven characteristics of DBT to the adolescent in the first or second individual therapy session. We list them below, with sample therapist descriptions for the client:

1. *DBT is not a suicide prevention program, but rather a life enhancement program.* Although the therapist acknowledges the client's misery and concedes that suicide provides one way out of suffering, he or she emphasizes that the alternative is to make life more livable. "The bottom line is that I cannot keep you from killing yourself if you are intent on doing so, but I can help you create a life worth living."

2. *DBT is supportive of clients' attempts to improve the quality of their lives.* "Jessica, I want to support you to achieve your goals in any way I can."

3. *DBT is behavioral.* "In order for you to change your life and achieve your goals, you are going to have to decrease some of your old problem behaviors, and begin to increase new skillful behaviors that you're going to learn in DBT. Given your depression and anxiety, I think you will find it interesting to know that by changing your behavior, you can actually change your emotions."

4. *DBT teaches skills.* "As you know from your cheerleading and piano lessons, it will take practice to get good at these new skills."

5. *DBT is collaborative.* "We're going to work as a team to help you achieve your goals. Clearly, you haven't been able to get there yet without help, and I know that I will not be able to help you if you don't pull some of the weight . . . so I feel confident that if we work together, we can do it."

6. *DBT employs telephone consultation.* In the first session, the therapist gives the client his or her phone number or pager number and explains the three reasons for phone calls in DBT (see above). To emphasize this point, the therapist can use the metaphor of a basketball player and coach. "Jessica, you're a basketball player [the therapist identifies Jessica's favorite player and calls her by that name]. You're dribbling down the court, your team is down by 1 point, and there are 20 seconds left. As you dribble past half-court, the other team sets up a defense, and you feel stuck. What do you do? You call a time out and check in with your coach to figure out how to get unstuck, instead of getting trapped and turning the ball over. Similarly, in life, when faced with a very tough or unfamiliar situation, I want you to call a 'time out' and call your coach—that's me—so that I can help you get out of sticky situations without making things worse."

7. *DBT is a team treatment.* "Here's more good news: I am not treating you alone. I have a team I talk to every week. The team is made up of me, your individual therapist; the skills trainers; and other DBT therapists who work in this program. Their job is to make sure I deliver the best possible treatment to you. You've got me to help you, and I have the team to help me."

Introducing DBT Diary Cards

Introduction of the diary card (see Figure 7.3) typically occurs at the end of the first session or during the second session. (The two-page card can be photocopied and trimmed down to fit on one 8½ × 11 page.) The client is told that the diary card is a crucial component of the therapy, and that he or she is expected to complete it and return it to the therapist each week. The therapist explains the rationale for the diary card by explaining its several extremely important functions.

Dialectical Behavior Therapy **Adolescent Diary Card**	First name					Filled out in session? Yes/no		

Date	Self-harm		Suicidal		Alcohol		Drugs		Meds
	Urge	Actions	Thoughts	Actions	Urge	Use amount/ type	Urge	Use amount/ type	Taken as prescribed
	0–5	Yes/no	0–5	Yes/no	0–5		0–5		Yes/no

*USED SKILLS

0 = Not thought about or used
1 = Thought about, not used, didn't want to
2 = Thought about, not used, wanted to
3 = Tried but couldn't use them

4 = Tried, could do them, but they didn't help
5 = Tried, could use them, helped
6 = Didn't try, used them, didn't help
7 = Didn't try, used them, helped

Instructions: Circle the days you worked on each skill.

Core Mindfulness	1. Wise mind	Mon	Tues	Wed	Thur	Fri	Sat	Sun
	2. Observe (Just notice what's going on inside)	Mon	Tues	Wed	Thur	Fri	Sat	Sun
	3. Describe (Put words on the experience)	Mon	Tues	Wed	Thur	Fri	Sat	Sun
	4. Participate (Enter into the experience)	Mon	Tues	Wed	Thur	Fri	Sat	Sun
	5. Don't judge (Nonjudgmental stance)	Mon	Tues	Wed	Thur	Fri	Sat	Sun
	6. Stay focused (One-mindfully: in the moment)	Mon	Tues	Wed	Thur	Fri	Sat	Sun
	7. Do what works (Effectiveness)	Mon	Tues	Wed	Thur	Fri	Sat	Sun
Emotion Regulation	8. Identifying and labeling emotions	Mon	Tues	Wed	Thur	Fri	Sat	Sun
	9. PLEASE (Reduce vulnerability to emotion mind)	Mon	Tues	Wed	Thur	Fri	Sat	Sun
	10. MASTER (Building mastery, feeling effective)	Mon	Tues	Wed	Thur	Fri	Sat	Sun
	11. Engaging in pleasant activities	Mon	Tues	Wed	Thur	Fri	Sat	Sun
	12. Working toward long-term goals	Mon	Tues	Wed	Thur	Fri	Sat	Sun
	13. Building structure // time, work, play	Mon	Tues	Wed	Thur	Fri	Sat	Sun
	14. Acting opposite to current emotion	Mon	Tues	Wed	Thur	Fri	Sat	Sun

FIGURE 7.3. *Adolescent diary card.*

How often did you fill out this section? ___ Daily ___ 2–3x ___ Once		Date started	

How often did you use phone consult? ___

Other				Emotions									Notes:
Cut class/ school	Risky sex			Anger	Fear	Happy	Anxious	Sad	Shame	Misery	Skills*		
Yes/no	Yes/no			0–5	0–5	0–5	0–5	0–5	0–5	0–5	0–7		

Rating scale for emotions and urges (above):

0 = Not at all   1 = A bit   2 = Somewhat   3 = Rather strong   4 = Very strong   5 = Extremely strong

Urge to quit therapy: _____   Misery index: _____

Instructions: Circle the days you worked on each skill.

Interpersonal Effectiveness	15. DEAR MAN (Getting what you want)	Mon	Tues	Wed	Thur	Fri	Sat	Sun
	16. GIVE (Improving the relationship)	Mon	Tues	Wed	Thur	Fri	Sat	Sun
	17. FAST (Feeling effective and keeping your self-respect)	Mon	Tues	Wed	Thur	Fri	Sat	Sun
	18. Cheerleading statements for worry thoughts	Mon	Tues	Wed	Thur	Fri	Sat	Sun
Distress Tolerance	19. ACCEPTS (Distract)	Mon	Tues	Wed	Thur	Fri	Sat	Sun
	20. Self-soothe (Five senses)	Mon	Tues	Wed	Thur	Fri	Sat	Sun
	21. Pros and cons	Mon	Tues	Wed	Thur	Fri	Sat	Sun
	22. Radical acceptance	Mon	Tues	Wed	Thur	Fri	Sat	Sun
Walking the Middle Path	23. Positive reinforcement	Mon	Tues	Wed	Thur	Fri	Sat	Sun
	24. Validate self	Mon	Tues	Wed	Thur	Fri	Sat	Sun
	25. Validate someone else	Mon	Tues	Wed	Thur	Fri	Sat	Sun
	26. Think dialectically (not in black and white)	Mon	Tues	Wed	Thur	Fri	Sat	Sun
	27. Act dialectically (walk the middle path)	Mon	Tues	Wed	Thur	Fri	Sat	Sun

141

First, filling out the diary card daily requires the client to self-monitor target behaviors, emotions, and skills. In and of itself, this is an intervention that may help reduce problem behaviors while also serving as a consistent mindfulness skills practice exercise. Second, the card functions as a general overview of the client's week, so the therapist and client have a "week at a glance." This helps reduce the risk of overlooking any primary target behaviors. Third, the card functions as a "diary," in that it helps keep a more accurate record of the adolescent's daily emotions and behaviors than would the adolescent's memory alone, especially 7 days later. Fourth, the diary card enables the client and therapist to perceive potential links between emotions and maladaptive as well as adaptive behaviors. Fifth, the diary card is the primary tool used at the beginning of every individual session to help focus the session content. The therapist states,

> "I really hope we can figure out a way for you to remember to complete and return your diary card each week . . . because if you forget your diary card, I will have to ask you to fill out a blank one in session, and then we'll have to figure out what interfered in your ability to complete and return it. That will take up a good portion of our session time, and I would much rather use your time to discuss other issues happening during the week. Wouldn't you?"

In order for the adolescent to learn how to complete the diary card, the therapist asks the client in session to remember the previous day and to rate any maladaptive behaviors and emotions listed on the card, starting from left to right. The therapist clarifies the difference between "self-harm urges and actions" and "suicidal thoughts and actions" by highlighting the presence of suicidal intent as the sole criterion. Typically, the adolescent is instructed to complete only a portion of the diary card for the subsequent week. This helps the adolescent avoid feeling overwhelmed by the fairly complex card and potentially helps to build mastery. Moreover, the door-in-the-face commitment strategy (see below) is effectively used around this issue. Expecting an objection, the therapist first tells the adolescent to complete the entire card for the following week. When the teen states that it is too much work, the therapist makes a deal and says, "how about completing just half the card for this week?" Usually the adolescent sees this as a bargain. Furthermore, it constitutes a relatively easy homework assignment and thus provides the therapist with something to positively reinforce at the beginning of the next session.

In addition to standard behaviors, such as suicide attempts, NSIB, and risky sexual behaviors, the diary card for adolescents should also include age-appropriate targets and should be tailored to each individual client. Hence we have added to the adolescent diary card a "Cut class/school" column, along with some blank columns. For some teens, we track binge and purge urges and behaviors. For other teens, we track assaultive urges, dissociative behaviors, and/or invalidating statements toward self and others. When teens rate these behaviors (and emotions) on a 0–5 scale, they are instructed to rate the "most intense" urge or affect, instead of the "average." Often, for example, the average anger on a given day might fall at about 3 on the 0–5 scale, and it becomes difficult to assess those days when anger was clearly most intense. For those clients who report high urges and emotions all day nearly every day (5's), the therapist might encourage the client to track the "average" as well as the "most intense" rating each day, in order to differentiate one day from another.

A common mistake made by a new DBT therapist is forgetting to troubleshoot after obtaining initial commitment that the adolescent is going to fill out the diary card during the week. The therapist should say something like this:

> "Jessica, now that you have agreed to complete the diary card, what might interfere with your getting it done and then bringing it back here next week? Let's think about some

potential obstacles. . . . For starters, what time of the day do you think you might fill it out? Where will you keep it each day and night? How will you remember to leave home with it next Wednesday, so that you can bring it to our session?"

We often suggest to teenagers who do not have an opinion that filling out the diary card before bed, and leaving it in a place near the bed or desk, is a good idea. Also, we suggest that they write a note and leave it on the refrigerator or bathroom mirror so that they cue themselves to (1) fill out the diary card each day and (2) bring the diary card to therapy.

Many teens exhibit initial noncompliance with completing their diary cards. Common reasons for this noncompliance include, but are not limited to, (1) not understanding the rationale for the diary card; (2) not understanding how to fill out the diary card properly; (3) feeling as though they do not have the time to complete the diary card; (4) feeling angry about having more "homework"; and (5) worrying about their parents' sneaking a peek at their diary cards (which are supposed to remain confidential). Understanding what is interfering with completion of the diary card is crucial.

Because some teens have initial difficulty with completing the diary card, therapists must remember to employ the principle of shaping. Getting the teens to bring in a portion of the diary card filled out is a good start. For those who have trouble with that, sometimes simplifying the diary card is indicated. In addition, it is often necessary for a therapist to ask a client after a week or two of noncompliance, "Remind me again why I am assigning this work for you to do at home. Am I doing this to be a pain in your neck, or are there other reasons?" A more thorough behavioral analysis may be indicated at this point to assess the function of the noncompliance. Therapists must be careful not to be shaped by their clients' noncompliance into not asking for and obtaining a diary card each and every week! It is equally important for therapists to remember that clients may feel shame when they do not complete the diary card, just as they may experience shame when they do—since completing the diary card "forces" them to acknowledge certain behaviors and emotions that they have been trying to avoid.

Reviewing Treatment Agreements: Client, Therapist, Client–Therapist Relationship, and Family Agreements

Orientation cumulates in a set of agreements that spell-out the responsibilities and goals for all parties involved, including families. Client, therapist, and family agreements are typically presented and discussed during the second or third session. Client agreements, which may overlap with but are not necessarily the same as addressing the specific target behaviors identified on the treatment plan, are made orally and include the following: (1) to enter and stay in therapy for a specified length of time (e.g., 16 weeks, 6 months, or 1 year, depending on the program); (2) to attend both individual therapy and group skills training (the therapist should review the attendance policy); (3) to work on reducing specific life-threatening, therapy-interfering, and quality-of-life-interfering behaviors that have been identified during the initial assessment and orientation, while increasing behavioral skills; and (4) to page the therapist for coaching as needed.

Implicitly and explicitly, the therapist agrees (1) to make every reasonable effort to be effective; (2) to act ethically; (3) to be available to the client (both for sessions and by pager); (4) to show respect for the client; (5) to maintain confidentiality, with the exceptions of (a) suicidal or homicidal ideation with plan and intent (to be reported to the clients' legal guardian) and (b) suspected physical or sexual abuse or neglect (to be reported to child protective services as mandated by state law); and (6) to obtain consultation as needed from supervisors and colleagues attending the therapist consultation team meetings.

The client–therapist agreement with adolescents is introduced by dialectically highlighting omnipotence and impotence:

> "Jessica, I know as a DBT therapist that I am pretty darn good. However, I am not perfect. I make mistakes. I am confident, therefore that I will do something during treatment that will bother you, piss you off, and maybe even cause you to question continuing in therapy. Now let's be clear: I expect you will make mistakes, you may do things that piss me off, and so on. The point I am making here is that if you are going to get the help you need, we *both* need to be sure that we keep the therapeutic relationship strong. That requires both of us to be honest with the other if we feel there is a problem. If one of us upsets the other (even accidentally), we have to say to the other person, "Hey, when you said that, you pissed me off," or "Hey, why didn't you call me when you said you would?"

Given that suicidal adolescents typically drop out of treatment at very high rates, it is imperative for the therapist to raise these relationship issues on Day 1, and to obtain commitment from the teen and demonstrate personal commitment to attend to them as the treatment progresses.

Lastly, when families are involved in DBT, it is equally important to review agreements pertaining to them as well. We develop an oral agreement with family members that includes the following (1) to attend and actively participate in a multifamily skills training group (or family skills training); (2) to participate in family therapy sessions on an as-needed basis; (3) to facilitate transportation for the teen, either by driving him or her to scheduled appointments or by providing money for public transportation; and (4) to observe rules of confidentiality by not asking the primary therapist to provide specific information gleaned from individual sessions. Parents are told that they can feel free to leave messages on the primary therapist's answering machine or speak to the therapist directly to *give* relevant information. Parents are also reminded about conditions for therapists to break confidentiality. At times, the therapist may choose to tell the client that the parents left a message and share the contents of that message, especially when there is a serious concern (such as a suicide attempt, suicidal ideation, or increasing depressive symptomatology). When less dire messages are left, the therapist uses his or her judgment concerning whether to bring that information into the session or not. We provide further discussion of handling confidentiality between teens and their parents in Chapter 9 (see especially Table 9.4).

OBTAINING COMMITMENT TO TREATMENT WITH ADOLESCENTS

In our experience, inadequate commitment by the client, therapist, or both leads to many therapy failures and early terminations. The client may make an insufficient or superficial commitment in the initial stages of the change process—or, more likely, events both within and outside of therapy may conspire to reduce strong commitments previously made. This last point particularly relates to working with adolescents, since they are usually residing in their invalidating environments and often feel hopeless about any improvement in their situations. Client commitment in DBT serves as both an important prerequisite for effective therapy and a goal of the therapy. Thus a therapist does not assume a client's commitment. DBT views commitment as a behavior itself, which can be elicited, learned, and reinforced. The therapist's task thus includes figuring out ways to help this process along. When working in a clinic in which treatment is potentially short-term, the therapist must figure this out quickly (Miller, Nathan, & Wagner, in press).

In-session behaviors that are inconsistent with an initial degree of commitment and collaboration include refusing to work in therapy, avoiding or refusing to talk about feelings and events connected with target behaviors, and rejecting all input from the therapist or attempts to generate alternative solutions. At these moments, the commitment to therapy itself should be targeted and discussed, with the goal of eliciting a recommitment. The therapist cannot proceed further without it. Remember, problems other than commitment may underlie these behaviors; thus, a behavioral analysis is indicated.

Strategies for Obtaining Commitment

Often adolescents have not come voluntarily for treatment. They may be forced into treatment by parents or schools (which may not allow the adolescents to return if they are not in therapy), or treatment may be mandated by courts or child welfare agencies. Thus obtaining a commitment can be a particular challenge; however, without it treatment cannot begin.

Eliciting commitment necessitates a certain amount of salesmanship. The product being sold is new behavior and sometimes life itself. When treatment is mandated by the courts or by an adolscent's parents, sometimes the therapist's only course of action is to say, "OK, I know you don't want to be here. Would you feel any better if we could figure out a way to get the court [or your parents] off your back? Yes? Great. So what has to happen before they get off your back? Let me help you with that." Although we hope to obtain a full, enthusiastic commitment to any and all target behaviors, we often settle for a partial commitment to one or two target behaviors, with the hope of obtaining a deeper and broader commitment as the treatment progresses. It is useful here to remember a key DBT maxim: "DBT therapists get what they can take and take what they can get."

To obtain commitment to DBT, the therapist needs to be flexible and creative while employing one or more of the following commitment strategies: (1) selling commitment: evaluating pros and cons; (2) playing devil's advocate; (3) the foot-in-the-door and door-in-the-face techniques; (4) connecting present commitments to prior commitment; (5) highlighting freedom to choose and absence of alternatives; and (6) cheerleading (Linehan, 1993a).

Selling Commitment: Evaluating Pros and Cons

In evaluating the pros and cons of proceeding with treatment, the therapist wants (1) to review the advantages of the decision to proceed, as well as (2) to develop counterarguments based on reservations that are likely to arise later, when the client is alone and has no help in diffusing doubts. For example, the therapist might say,

> "Jessica, by making a commitment to treatment, we will work together to help you achieve your goals of reducing your suicidal and self-injurious behaviors; reducing your drinking, depression, bingeing, and purging; decreasing your problems with your boyfriend and parents; and helping you stay in school so that you can graduate. Now let's think together about the cons of making this kind of commitment. It is going to take a huge effort to change some of your long-standing behavioral patterns. Plus the time commitment necessary for group and individual sessions, as well as therapy homework assignments and phone consultations, may be too much for you right now . . . so we should think about both the pros and cons before you make a final commitment. Whenever I have to make an important decision, I try to weigh the pros and cons."

Often therapists start with the cons and then identify the pros, since many teens are already starting from the "con" side of participating in treatment. The therapist may want to highlight cons to treatment if the adolescent has forgotten some standard ones, such as having less free time, doing homework for therapy, and stirring up intense emotions. It is important for the therapist to highlight the short- and long-term nature of each pro and con, since participating in treatment often looks less compelling in the short term. Many teens have trouble considering the "long term." Some teens are unable to visualize their lives 2 or 3 years from now; therapists may have to help such clients "stretch" their imaginations to weeks and months, and visualize the pros and cons from that vantage point.

Playing Devil's Advocate

In the devil's advocate approach, the therapist poses arguments against making a commitment to treatment, with the intent that the client will make his or her argument for participating in treatment. The therapist might say, "Jessica, this treatment requires a huge time commitment and a good deal of work . . . and I am not sure that you are up to it right now" or ". . . wouldn't you rather be in a treatment that wasn't so demanding?" This technique becomes quite useful with teenagers who are more likely to offer simplistic "blanket" agreements, such as, "Oh, yeah, I definitely want to do this therapy . . . And, yes, I will never cut myself again." Therapists want adolescents to argue for the therapy by building a strong case for themselves: "I do want therapy now, because my life is a wreck, my parents are going to kick me out of the house, I am already on probation at school, and my drug problem is getting really out of control. I don't know if I'll have another chance before it's too late. I gotta get help and get it now."

Foot-in-the-Door Technique

The foot-in-the-door and door-in-the-face techniques are well-known procedures from social psychology that enhance compliance with requests. In the foot-in-the-door technique (Freedman & Fraser, 1966), the therapist makes a request that seems easy, followed by a more difficult request. For instance, a therapist first got a client with social phobia to agree to attend group skills training. Then the therapist said, "OK, now that you are there, can you volunteer to report on your homework, or at least read something from the skills notebook when the skills trainers ask for volunteers?" Here is another example: In the first session, after the therapist gets the adolescent to commit to participate in treatment and work on all target behaviors, the therapist then says, "Oh, by the way, there's one more little thing I would like you to do for next week . . . it's called a diary card." At that point, the therapist reviews the card.

Still another example of the foot-in-the-door technique involves maladaptive behaviors that the client does not want to address. One therapist said to a suicidal adolescent with alcohol abuse and marijuana use, "OK, I understand you do not think marijuana is a problem for you. I am not clear one way or another. So let's not have you try to reduce it. How about if you merely track your use on the diary card like you do your alcohol use, which we agree you *are* trying to reduce. OK?" As previously discussed, self-monitoring is the first step to ultimately reducing any behavior.

Door-in-the-Face Technique

In the door-in-the-face technique (Gialdini et al., 1975), the therapist first makes a harder request, and then solicits a more easily performed behavior. This strategy proves helpful in obtaining early commitment to treatment and to reducing suicidal behavior and NSIB. For example, with one teen who was angry about being "dragged to a shrink," this strategy was helpful: the therapist slowly reduced the length of his commitment from 16 weeks to 2 weeks, and it was agreed that treatment would focus on "how to get your parents off your back." Regarding a commitment to stop suicidal behavior, Jessica would not agree to stay alive for the entire length of the program (i.e., 16 weeks), but she could make a commitment not to end her life for the next week. The therapist said, "Jessica, how about if you agree to stay alive this week, and we will reevaluate next week to see if you are willing to renew your agreement?"

Another example of the door-in-the-face technique is often used with the diary card (see Figure 7.3). This strategy can also be useful in the skills training group as well. For example, one afternoon one of the group members entered the group room 2 minutes early—but he chose to sit away from the table (where everyone else sits), looking agitated, with the hood of his jacket covering his face. The skills trainer asked, "Alan, would you please come sit at the table, pull your hood off your face, and lead us in a mindfulness exercise?" Alan said, "I ain't doing all that!" The therapist seemingly relented by saying, "How about if you just come to the table and lower your hood, then?" The client said, "All right." In this case, the therapist never expected the client to agree to all of those requests and lead the mindfulness exercise. But making an additional, more challenging request at first led to increased compliance when the therapist then asked Alan for less.

Connecting Present Commitments to Prior Commitments

When the therapist has a sense that the commitment is fading, or when the client's behavior is incongruent with previous commitments, the therapist can remind the client of commitments made previously. For instance, when Jessica threatened at one point to use laxatives again, the therapist said, "But I thought you were going to try your best not to do that ever since you made that commitment 6 weeks ago? That's one of the commitments you made upon entering therapy with us."

Highlighting Freedom to Choose and Absence of Alternatives

The strategy of highlighting freedom to choose and absence of alternatives is particularly useful for working with all teenagers, but especially for those who are in treatment involuntarily or who are not particularly interested in treatment at this point. The idea behind this strategy is that commitment and compliance are enhanced when people, especially adolescents, believe that they have chosen freely and when they believe there are no alternatives to reach their goal. Hence the therapist should enhance the feeling of choice, while at the same time stressing the lack of effective alternatives. For example, in developing or redeveloping a client's commitment to stop attempting suicide, the therapist may emphasize that the client is free to choose a life of coping by suicide—but that if he or she makes that choice another treatment should be found, since DBT requires reduction of suicide attempts and NSIB as a goal. When using this strategy to strengthen commitment to the treatment program, the DBT therapist attempts to list in graphic form all of the problems the teen is currently experiencing and then says,

> "Jessica, you can try to manage your suicidality, depression, substance use, disordered eating behaviors, school problems, and huge conflicts with your boyfriend and parents on your own as you have been doing. The other option is to try this therapy twice per week and see if we can get these problems under control, so that you can stay alive, get

your parents off your back, and remain at home and school instead of being sent to residential treatment. . . . Of course, it's totally your choice, since this is your life! What do you think?"

Cheerleading

The purpose of cheerleading is to generate hope. One of the major problems confronting suicidal adolescents with BPD or borderline features is their lack of hope that they can effect change in their lives. In cheerleading, the therapist encourages the client, reinforces even minimal progress, and consistently points out that the client has the qualities needed to handle his or her problems. For example, Jessica was raised in a family in which the primary coping and problem-solving style was to attempt suicide. This became a learned response that seemed to be passed from generation to generation. Another client was raised by an emotionally abusive, alcoholic father who continued to demean and insult her. Both of these clients needed extensive amounts of cheerleading and encouragement to help build a sense of hope that they could actually change themselves and alter (somewhat) their oppressive home environments.

Instilling hope is intimately connected to getting an initial commitment to treatment and recommitment when needed. Cheerleading may also be required when the devil's advocate technique falls flat. With Jessica, the therapist aggressively employed the devil's advocate technique by saying, "This does not seem to be the right time for you to work on these problems . . . maybe you can recontact the program when you feel more ready to work on all of your problems." Jessica started to agree with the therapist and looked dejected. The therapist quickly responded with "You know, however, I do get the impression that when you do put your mind to something you can do extremely well, as you used to do in school, choir, and cheerleading. Is that true? If so, then if you really and truly put your mind to working at this treatment, like you do in other areas of your life, I bet you will start to feel better. What do you think?" Jessica was buoyed by these last comments and was more able to make a firm commitment to the treatment program. The devil's advocate technique and cheerleading can be used in a dialectical fashion to build commitment.

The periodic and intense hopelessness of these clients can overwhelm a therapist. At these times, the therapist consultation meeting becomes critical in helping the therapist reestablish commitment, perspective, and balance. Many therapist teams make good use of cheerleading to enable their weary colleagues to continue treatment effectively.

ORIENTATION AND COMMITMENT WITH FAMILY MEMBERS

After orienting and obtaining commitment from the adolescent, the therapist invites the family members in for the latter portion of the first session (or a portion of the second section) to begin orientation and commitment with them as well. First, the therapist reviews the handout illustrating the five problem areas and corresponding skills modules (Figure 7.1), and asks the adolescent to identify which of the five problem areas applies to him or her. Then, in order to instill hope in the family members just as was done with their child, the therapist makes the connection between the problem areas and the corresponding skills modules specifically developed for those behavioral problems and taught in skills sessions (e.g., multifamily skills group, family skills training, individual skills training). Depending on the particular family issues as well as time remaining in the session, the therapist may choose to ask the parents whether they believe the skills being taught in the multifamily skills training group may be helpful to them as well (see Chapter 9 for an extended discussion), especially given the heightened stress in the household. In many cases, identifying parents' own current and/or past problem areas occurs in the family skills training sessions.

The therapist then orients the family members to the treatment format, including the modes of treatment. Parents are strongly urged to participate in the 2-hour multifamily skills training group for the duration of treatment. Exceptions are made when certain employment and language barriers exist. If a parent is at risk of losing his or her job if time is taken off even after a medical letter is provided, we will make an exception. In addition, exceptions are made for parents who are monolingual in a language other than English, since we cannot translate the entire skills group content in a 2-hour time period. In either of these cases, parents unable to attend the skills group are expected to spend extra time in family sessions reviewing skills and having their own child teach them some of the content when appropriate. The other modes of treatment are briefly reviewed: weekly individual therapy, family therapy as needed, telephone consultation, and the therapist consultation/supervision group. Permission is obtained from the parents at this point for their adolescent to use the telephone to page the primary therapist for skills coaching as needed. Parents are told that they too can receive skills coaching when they need it by paging the multifamily group skills trainer. Also, the DBT therapist informs parents of the adolescent diary card and kindly requests that they do not ask to look at or ask their teens to share the contents of the card, since the card is intended for the therapist only. Again, the therapist attempts to preempt any intentional or inadvertent breaches of confidentiality or pressure from the parents.

Addressing issues of confidentiality is an important part of orienting the family to the DBT program. A DBT therapist typically explains the rules of confidentiality to the adolescent alone first, and then repeats them with the parents present. Although variations exist, many practitioners apply similar "rules" for breaking confidentiality: (1) if the adolescent informs DBT staff that he or she has a specific suicide plan and intent; (2) if the adolescent informs DBT staff that he or she has a specific plan and intent to harm someone else; and (3) if the adolescent suggests that any physical or sexual abuse or neglect is occurring.[2] It is explained that the therapist will encourage the client to tell the parents about any of these aforementioned situations (with the possible exception of abuse/neglect if it is occurring in the household); however, the therapist will not hesitate to notify the parents if the adolescent does not.

One of the more sensitive confidentiality issues involves the issue of NSIB and whether to report that to families. Our recommendation is that DBT therapists validate parents' concerns regarding the behavior, while at the same time saying they will not notify them of such behaviors unless they become life-threatening. The rationale for this is that adolescents may be less likely to disclose the very behaviors that bring them to treatment if they believe their parents will be notified. Many families understand this dilemma and comply with the confidentiality regarding NSIB. The exception is that if a client's self-injury becomes increasingly dangerous and nonresponsive to DBT interventions, a therapist will break confidentiality. Other sensitive issues include substance use and sexual activity. Unless these behaviors are apparent at the outset, confidentiality about them is maintained (i.e., they are not discussed explicitly with families). Although some families probe the primary therapist for this information, we employ the same rationale for maintaining confidentiality regarding these behaviors as we do regarding NSIB. The exception also remains the same: "If I believe that your daughter [or son] is doing anything that puts her [or him] at grave risk, I will certainly let you know."

---

[2]Mental health professionals are mandated by state law to report any suspicion of child abuse or neglect.

Finally, the same commitment strategies used with the adolescent are used with the family members as needed. Typically, fewer commitment strategies are necessary to engage families in the DBT program. There are times, however, when family members exhibit insufficient commitment by suggesting that the treatment providers need to "fix" their kid without their participation, or state hopelessly that "nothing can help" the adolescents. In these cases, as well as others that are less obvious, the therapist validates the family members by suggesting how concerned and frustrated they must be to say those things. In addition, it is apparent that these problems are affecting everyone in the family. The therapist can mention recent data suggesting that those adolescents whose parents maintain a positive attitude about their treatment are more likely to have a more positive outcome (Halaby, 2004). In addition, at some point in the orientation, it behooves the therapist to mention the wealth of DBT effectiveness data for suicidal multiproblem adults and the promising pilot data with adolescents (Rathus & Miller, 2002).

When parents express their unwillingness to participate actively in the treatment, the therapist must first assess the reason. If it is not a logistical problem that needs to be solved, but rather a psychological one, the therapist may need to employ several of the commitment strategies discussed earlier. If the parents are still unwilling or unable to participate, the therapist should discuss with the consultation team how to proceed. There are times, unfortunately, despite the therapist's and the team's best efforts, when a family does not actively participate and an adolescent is treated alone. To date, we have no empirical data to suggest that these outcomes are necessarily any worse. Clinically, it is important for the therapist to validate the adolescent's feelings of disappointment and rejection, while at the same time cheerleading the teen and conveying the belief that he or she can do this treatment with the therapist's help, even if it must be done without the family's participation.

Anecdotally, whether a client remains in treatment beyond the first session depends largely on how effective the therapist applies the orientation and commitment strategies. Although we describe these strategies here in the early phase of treatment, most clinicians need to refer back to the majority of them, because the client's motivation and commitment inevitably wax and wane as the treatment progresses. The next three chapters—describing individual therapy, family work, and skills training, respectively—also make use of these orientation and commitment strategies.

CHAPTER 8

Individual Therapy with Adolescents

This chapter is organized around the conduct of an individual therapy session. We cover strategies for beginning sessions, for targeting Stage 1 treatment priorities, for carrying out those treatment priorities in midsession, and for ending sessions. Later in the chapter, we also describe how individual therapists conduct telephone coaching with their clients. All DBT strategies are employed in individual therapy, making this modality the most challenging to deliver competently. Good training in DBT, individual supervision, and intermittent observation of tapes by one's consultation team or individual supervisor all help to ensure adherence to the treatment model.

The individual therapist is the primary therapist in outpatient DBT. He or she is responsible for increasing the adolescent's motivation, inhibiting maladaptive behaviors, increasing the adolescent's skillful behaviors, and generalizing them outside the therapy setting. In settings where there may not be an individual therapist (such as juvenile justice), one staff person needs to be designated the primary therapist and to be responsible for conducting behavioral analyses and for making the final decisions about the treatment plan; hence all other modes of treatment (e.g., skills training, family therapy, pharmacotherapy) revolve around the primary therapist.

One of the biggest challenges for the individual therapist is that many multiproblem suicidal adolescents have emotion phobia. Thus they tend to avoid content that induces affect in session in a variety of ways, including shutting down, attacking the therapist, or not coming to sessions in the first place. These therapy-interfering behaviors can make individual therapy with an adolescent extremely challenging. Once the teen arrives, however, the individual therapist employs a variety of strategies.

SESSION–BEGINNING STRATEGIES

Initially, many adolescents dread coming to sessions. They fear that they will get reprimanded for "bad" behavior or will be "forced" to talk about painful events; either, they believe, will inevitably make them feel worse. Moreover, they do not believe that their problems can be solved, especially by adults whom they barely know. Starting sessions in a fairly routine fashion fosters a predictable structure for an adolescent and helps reduce anxiety and fear. The following is a useful sequence of strategies for beginning a session: (1) greeting the client; (2) reviewing the client's diary card and/or handling diary card noncompliance; (3) discussing the plan for the session; (4) recognizing and, if necessary, targeting the client's current emotional state; (5) reviewing individual therapy homework assignments (if given); and (6) checking progress in other modes of therapy.

Greeting the Client

With any client, but particularly with an adolescent, the therapist must communicate early in the encounter a feeling of warmth and caring toward the client. Whether this is done with a genuinely warm smile and a "Hello," a "Hey, what's up?", or some variation of a handshake (e.g., a high-five), the therapist must make the client feel welcomed each week—even when the therapeutic relationship has been strained by therapy-interfering behaviors. Adolescents often carry the expectation that if a problem with an adult has developed, it is unlikely to be resolved. The therapeutic relationship is no different until proven different. Even when a client has missed the last session, the therapist may want to comment on how good it is to see the client again before discussing the agenda and determining what interfered with his or her attending the last appointment.

Reviewing the Diary Card

After greeting the client, the therapist asks for and reviews the diary card (as described in Chapters 6 and 7). Frequently, after the first few weeks of the therapist's asking, "Do you have your diary card?" the client becomes conditioned and generally hands over the diary card without being asked. A common mistake by DBT therapists is waiting too long to ask for the diary card or forgetting to ask for it altogether. When this happens, therapists inadvertently communicate that the diary card is not important. Hence they should train themselves and their clients to review the diary card immediately following the greeting. The diary card informs the remainder of the session. If a client fails to bring in the diary card or has not completed it, the therapist asks the client to fill out a blank card in session or complete the unfinished one. The therapist's message is clear: "We cannot continue the therapy session until we have a completed diary card in hand." Potentially serious problems arise when the therapist forgets or chooses not to attend to the diary card early in the session. For example, imagine the scenario of a therapist's focusing on employment issues, only to discover—with 5 minutes left in the session and another patient waiting—that the client engaged in life-threatening behavior yesterday.

Handling Diary Card Noncompliance

The first time the client fails to turn in the diary card, the therapist responds nonjudgmentally and asks, "What happened?" Regardless of the response, the therapist is likely to say, "Remember, we cannot proceed in the individual therapy session without a completed diary card. So I am going to ask you to fill out this blank one, and we'll talk when you are done." The therapist should then start doing some deskwork and refrain from interaction with the client as he or she fills out the card. If there is a specific question about how to fill out the card, the therapist should respond accordingly. However, if the client wants to talk through issues that are being noted on the diary card, the therapist should encourage the client to complete the diary card before the two of them engage in any further discussion. At the start of therapy, however, the therapist often helps the client fill out the card. Sometimes clients are unable to fill out the card when they are acutely suicidal or emotionally overwhelmed.

If the client fails to bring in the diary card a second time, the therapist treats this as therapy-interfering behavior, conducts a detailed behavioral chain analysis and solution analysis, and may also choose to apply a slight aversive consequence. For example, when the client acknowledges that he or she forgot the card, the therapist hands a blank card to the client, turns away from the client, gets involved in some deskwork, and says, "Let me know when you're done." This makes continued interaction contingent upon filling out the card. Yet, behavior analysis is a crucial step for understanding the factors that may be interfering.

Another approach is the therapist's use of DEAR MAN interpersonal effectiveness skills (see Table 4.2 and Linehan, 1993b). Obviously, it is most effective when the client has been exposed to this skill set in group already, but it can be effective nevertheless if the therapist asks the client to turn to this skill in his or her notebook and they review it together for a moment. For example, one DBT therapist chose to use DEAR MAN skills with one of his adolescent clients whose history included dropping out of high school 2 years earlier, never doing her homework when she attended school, and (after 5 weeks of DBT) exhibiting consistent noncompliance with her diary card. He said, "T., I am not sure what else to say or do right now. I feel as though we have exhausted all problem-solving strategies to get you to bring in your diary card each week, and nothing seems to work. So I am going to use my best DEAR MAN skills and hope that I can get you to change your behavior this way." The therapist then went through the DEAR MAN sequence as follows:

- Describe: "T., for the past 5 weeks you have not been able to bring in your diary card. I know you never liked doing homework at school, and from what you have told me, in some ways the diary card feels the same to you. Unfortunately, without the diary card, I am limited in my ability to help you, and it really interferes in our ability to work on other things that you want to work on."
- Express: "I feel disappointed and frustrated, because I feel unable to convey to you the importance of completing and returning the diary card each week. I actually begin to feel less effective as a therapist, and I am worried that the treatment will not be successful."
- Assert: "So, I really want you to do everything in your power to make the diary card a top priority—not for me, but for yourself."
- Reinforce (reward): "You have told me that coming to therapy has already started to help you, and I am so glad to hear that. I can tell you are dedicated to helping yourself feel and do better, and I respect and admire you for that. T., I really have enjoyed working with you, I like you, and I truly feel like we could work so much better together if you could jump this hurdle that has begun to block your progress. I want to be able to trust you when you tell me, 'OK, I will definitely do it this week.' "
- Mindful Stay: In this step, a therapist should stay focused on the issue, repeating whatever is necessary like a broken record; if the client brings up other issues that may divert the conversation, the therapist consistently brings the conversation back to the issue at hand. This was what T.'s therapist did.
- Appear confident: This step is self-explanatory.
- Negotiate (if necessary): "What do you think? Does this make sense? Does it seem reasonable?" If a client says it is too difficult, a therapist should negotiate the issue appropriately. "Then what if you completed the top portion of the diary card this week, and filled it out completely the following week?"

The therapist's effective application of DEAR MAN skills worked with T., and it has influenced other adolescents who until a certain point in treatment had not brought in their diary cards. It helped that this therapist had already known this client for 5 weeks and had already established a strong alliance. Trying DEAR MAN after only one or two sessions might have proven less effective.

In some special cases, exceptions to reviewing the diary card are made—at least in the beginning of treatment. For example, one of us conducted an entire therapy around diary cards with an 18-year-old client. The client's "noncompliance" with the diary card was emblematic of most other aspects of her life in which she was unable to get herself to do things that were new and difficult. Thus, instead of requiring her to fill out the diary card in session, the therapist conducted behavioral analyses and addressed the emotions and skills deficits that impeded her functioning.

Discussing the Plan for the Session

With an adolescent, it is critical for the therapist to discuss the agenda early in the session, albeit in a relaxed and flexible manner. This ensures that sufficient time is allotted to discuss the higher-priority issues. Many multiproblem suicidal adolescents appear relieved to have a flexible outline of topics to be discussed. This helps alleviate some anxiety as to whether specific topics will or will not be addressed and why. To help organize what could otherwise be a chaotic and disorganized session, a therapist follows the DBT Stage 1 target hierarchy. As discussed in earlier chapters, this hierarchy starts with decreasing life-threatening behaviors, followed by decreasing therapy-interfering behaviors, decreasing quality-of-life-interfering behaviors, and increasing behavioral skills (in that order). If the client refuses to cooperate with the topics' being discussed according to the target hierarchy, this refusal is considered therapy-interfering and is addressed accordingly. Therapists who do not flexibly adhere to the DBT target hierarchy for whatever reason are not adhering to DBT and need to present this problem in the therapist consultation meeting as "therapist treatment-interfering behavior." For both the client and therapist, the issue here is not so much the *order* of discussion as it is the importance of addressing certain topics during the session.

To organize the agenda, the therapist reviews the diary card aloud while mentioning which target behaviors appear to warrant discussion. If the client does not volunteer any items for the agenda, the therapist should ask in a collaborative tone whether the client has any other items to put on the agenda. This fosters a sense of openness and mutuality, in that each member's agenda is known to the other, and therefore each one knows what will be discussed and in what order. As the therapist reviews the diary card aloud, he or she offers positive reinforcement for any target behaviors that are diminishing, while also highlighting any target behaviors that appear to have worsened and putting them on the agenda to be discussed next in hierarchical order. Jessica's diary card, some weeks into treatment, is seen in Figure 8.1. The therapist reviewed it aloud as follows:

"Jessica, I am so glad you completed your diary card this week before coming to session. That will leave time for some other things you've been wanting to discuss with me, like your relationship with your boyfriend, your sister, and school stuff. So let's take a look at your card. . . . I see you had low urges to use alcohol except on Friday, when you wrote down a 5. The really good news is you didn't let your urges control your behavior, since it appears you had nothing to drink that night, right?" [Jessica: "That's right."] "Great! So let's make sure we talk about those increased urges for today, and let's also take note how you managed *not* to drink when your urges were that high. . . . I see at the bottom of your diary card that on Friday you used pros and cons, as well as the ACCEPTS skills, and rated them a 5. That is, you thought about the skills, you used them, and they helped. Were those skills used to manage your urges?" [Jessica: "Yes."] "Great work! I also see you were compliant with your antidepressant medications. Now you also had low self-harm urges with the exception of Thursday, when you wrote down a 4, and I see you harmed yourself that night (*therapist's tone becomes neutral*). What did you do?" [Jessica: "I cut myself."] "With what?" [Jessica: "My razor blade that I keep in my room."] "Well, this will be the first thing we discuss this evening. Let's finish reviewing the diary card

Dialectical Behavior Therapy **Adolescent Diary Card**	First name *Jessica*					Filled out in session? Yes (no)		
Date	Self harm		Suicidal		Alcohol		Drugs		Meds
	Urge	Actions	Thoughts	Actions	Urge	Use amount/ type	Urge	Use amount/ type	Taken as prescribed
	0–5	Yes/no	0–5	Yes/no	0–5		0–5		Yes/no
Mon 2/1	3	No	2	No	1	None	0	None	Yes
Tues 2/2	2	No	0	No	1	None	0	None	Yes
Weds 2/3	2	No	0	No	1	None	0	None	Yes
Thurs 2/4	4	Yes	2	No	2	None	1	None	Yes
Fri 2/5	3	No	2	No	5	None	2	None	Yes
Sat 2/6	1	No	2	No	2	None	0	None	Yes
Sun 2/7	1	No	0	No	2	None	0	None	Yes

*USED SKILLS

0 = Not thought about or used
1 = Thought about, not used, didn't want to
2 = Thought about, not used, wanted to
3 = Tried but couldn't use them

4 = Tried, could do them, but they didn't help
5 = Tried, could use them, helped
6 = Didn't try, used them, didn't help
7 = Didn't try, used them, helped

Instructions: Circle the days you worked on each skill.

Core Mindfulness	1. Wise mind	(Mon)	(Tues)	(Wed)	(Thur)	Fri	(Sat)	Sun
	2. Observe (Just notice what's going on inside)	(Mon)	(Tues)	Wed	Thur	Fri	(Sat)	(Sun)
	3. Describe (Put words on the experience)	(Mon)	(Tues)	Wed	Thur	Fri	(Sat)	(Sun)
	4. Participate (Enter into the experience)	Mon	(Tues)	Wed	Thur	Fri	Sat	(Sun)
	5. Don't judge (Nonjudgmental stance)	Mon	Tues	Wed	Thur	Fri	Sat	Sun
	6. Stay focused (One-mindfully: in the moment)	Mon	(Tues)	Wed	Thur	Fri	Sat	(Sun)
	7. Do what works (Effectiveness)	Mon	(Tues)	Wed	Thur	Fri	Sat	(Sun)
Emotion Regulation	8. Identifying and labeling emotions	(Mon)	Tues	Wed	Thur	Fri	Sat	Sun
	9. PLEASE (Reduce vulnerability to emotion mind)	Mon	(Tues)	Wed	Thur	Fri	(Sat)	(Sun)
	10. MASTER (Building mastery, feeling effective)	Mon	(Tues)	Wed	Thur	Fri	Sat	Sun
	11. Engaging in pleasant activities	(Mon)	Tues	Wed	Thur	Fri	Sat	Sun
	12. Working toward long-term goals	(Mon)	(Tues)	Wed	Thur	Fri	(Sat)	(Sun)
	13. Building structure // time, work, play	Mon	Tues	Wed	Thur	Fri	Sat	Sun
	14. Acting opposite to current emotion	(Mon)	Tues	Wed	Thur	Fri	Sat	(Sun)

(cont.)

FIGURE 8.1. *Jessica's diary card.*

How often did you fill out this section? _X_ Daily ___ 2–3x ___ Once **Date started** 2/1
How often did you use phone consult? ___

Other				Emotions								Notes:
Cut class/ school	Risky sex	Urge to argue with boyfriend	Argued with boyfriend	Anger	Fear	Happy	Anxious	Sad	Shame	Misery	Skills*	
Yes/no	Yes/no	0–5	Yes/no	0–5	0–5	0–5	0–5	0–5	0–5	0–5	0–7	
No	No	4	Yes	2	3	1	3	3	2	3	5	
No	No	2	No	3	3	3	3	3	2	2	4	
Yes	Yes	4	Yes	4	2	4	4	4	4	2	5	
No	No	5	Yes!!!	5	5	2	5	5	4	5	3	
No	No	4	Yes	5	5	2	4	2	5	5	5	
No	No	3	No	4	3	3	2	1	4	2	5	
No	No	2	No	3	2	1	3	1	3	1	5	

Rating scale for emotions and urges (above):

0 = Not at all   1 = A bit   2 = Somewhat   3 = Rather strong   4 = Very strong   5 = Extremely strong

Urge to quit therapy: __1__   Misery index: __4__

Instructions: Circle the days you worked on each skill.

Interpersonal Effectiveness							
15. DEAR MAN (Getting what you want)	Mon	(Tues)	Wed	Thur	Fri	Sat	Sun
16. GIVE (Improving the relationship)	Mon	(Tues)	Wed	Thur	Fri	Sat	Sun
17. FAST (Feeling effective and keeping your self-respect)	(Mon)	Tues	Wed	Thur	Fri	Sat	Sun
18. Cheerleading statements for worry thoughts	Mon	Tues	Wed	Thur	Fri	Sat	Sun

Distress Tolerance							
19. ACCEPTS (Distract)	Mon	Tues	Wed	Thur	(Fri)	Sat	Sun
20. Self-soothe (Five senses)	Mon	(Tues)	Wed	Thur	Fri	Sat	Sun
21. Pros and cons	Mon	(Tues)	Wed	Thur	(Fri)	Sat	Sun
22. Radical acceptance	(Mon)	Tues	Wed	Thur	Fri	Sat	Sun

Walking the Middle Path							
23. Positive reinforcement	Mon	Tues	(Wed)	Thur	Fri	Sat	Sun
24. Validate self	(Mon)	Tues	(Wed)	Thur	Fri	Sat	Sun
25. Validate someone else	Mon	Tues	Wed	Thur	Fri	Sat	Sun
26. Think dialectically (not in black and white)	Mon	(Tues)	Wed	Thur	Fri	Sat	Sun
27. Act dialectically (walk the middle path)	Mon	Tues	Wed	Thur	Fri	Sat	Sun

FIGURE 8.1 *(cont.)*

first. I see you had low suicidal urges all week. I'm glad to see there were no suicidal behaviors, though. The incident with the razor blade was not suicidal?" [Jessica: "Right,
that was my usual self-harm."] "You cut school on Wednesday, and you had risky sex that
day as well. As I look at your emotions, it seems like you were not particularly angry until
Wednesday. On Thursday you had a lot of sadness and anxiety. And then on Friday, you
wrote 5 for shame. We will see if some of these emotions triggered some of these behaviors, or whether they were consequences of the behaviors, or both. . . . Is there anything
else you want to put on the agenda before we start?" [Jessica: "No, that's plenty for today."] "OK, so let's start by doing a behavioral analysis of your self-harm."

Therapists must also remember to insert into the agenda any therapy-interfering behaviors that have occurred in the past week, such as coming late to sessions (either individual
therapy or skills training) or forgetting to bring in the diary card. For example, in the subsequent week's individual session with Jessica the therapist stated while setting the agenda:
"Jessica, I'm glad to see that you didn't engage in any self-harm this week, nor did you use any
alcohol. The problem is that you were 20 minutes late today, so we need to start with that so
we can get you here on time. I do want to hear how you're using these skills and coping with
your problems differently. Also, since you were late, I hope we have time left to talk about
your conflict with your boyfriend."
    As highlighted by the statement "since you were late, I hope we still have time left to talk
about . . . ," the therapist makes use of an opportunity for contingency clarification. Also, by
reviewing the diary card out loud, the therapist reminds the client of the target hierarchy and
the customary order in which problem behaviors need to be addressed.

Recognizing the Client's Current Emotional State

It is helpful to recognize the client's current emotional state when discussing the agenda at
the beginning of the session. Some adolescents report that they have nothing to add to the
session agenda, but their affect indicates otherwise. The therapist may suggest to such a client, "you look upset. If there is something on your mind, it may be something to place on the
agenda." Placing items on the agenda does not mean there will always be time to address
them, however. Especially in the early stages of therapy, a client's quality-of-life-interfering
behaviors (e.g., bingeing, alcohol use, interpersonal problems) inevitably get less attention
than life-threatening and therapy-interfering behaviors do.
    Sometimes an adolescent's negative emotional state is related to a problem in the thera-
peutic relationship. As with the other relationships adolescents have, the therapeutic relationship is not exempt from challenges and strains. As a result, it is crucial that the therapist be
sensitive to problems that arise within the relationship and, with few exceptions, attempt to
repair the relationship early in the session before engaging in other work. Without a stable
therapeutic alliance, the "therapy" is moot. Of course, relationship repair should not replace
targeting high-priority behaviors within the session, which may inadvertently reinforce the
client's discussing problems in the therapeutic relationship. If the therapist is upset or having
negative feelings about the client and is unsure how to broach them, sometimes it is necessary
for the therapist to use the consultation group first to discuss those feelings before airing them
to the client. The dialectical bottom line is this: Therapists should target the current emotional state, if necessary, and then shift back to the other target behaviors as quickly as possible.

Reviewing Individual Therapy Homework Assignments

Individual therapists sometimes assign their own homework (in addition to the diary card) beyond that assigned weekly in the multifamily skills training group. The job of the individual therapist is to drag out new behaviors, and relevant exercises function to achieve that goal. These exercises are typically assigned at the end of the prior session and must be reviewed at least briefly at some point during the next session. These questions and answers may take as little as 20 seconds and often not more than a couple of minutes. In contrast to the predetermined practice exercises assigned in the skills training group, homework in individual therapy is based on the particular client's issues arising in a particular session. For example, when Jessica reported poor sleep hygiene during the past week, the therapist assigned her to practice her PLEASE skills during the upcoming week and report back next session. The S in PLEASE represents sleep, which implies employing good sleep hygiene (e.g., going to bed and waking at regular times, not drinking caffeinated beverages, stopping naps, and engaging in a relaxing activity before bed). For a client who may regularly engage in self-invalidation, the therapist may ask the client to track self-invalidating thoughts on his or her diary card for homework. Another therapist may assign an anxious client the task of practicing diaphragmatic breathing or engaging in specific exposure exercises, such as initiating a phone call with an acquaintance. At still other times, the assignment may involve problem solving or talking to Mom about an important issue. The point here is that an individual therapist should assign practice exercises that are relevant to a specific client at a specific moment in time in order to drag out new behaviors each week, if not each day. As in all behavior therapies, the DBT therapist must remember to ask about the previously agreed-upon homework assignments during the session. Not asking communicates that no real importance is attached to doing the homework. Thus the therapist (1) decreases the likelihood that the client will do the next homework assignment and (2) can assume more of the responsibility for the client's noncompliance.

Checking Progress in Other Modes of Therapy

Because the individual therapist is the primary therapist, this therapist must oversee all other modes of therapy. In DBT, clients can only have one primary therapist, and they cannot be in other forms of treatment simultaneously (e.g., psychodynamic psychotherapy) in which they have "another" primary therapist. In each session, the individual therapist should briefly check progress in the other modes of treatment. The individual therapist often asks about the multifamily skills training group (including the homework assignments), medication appointments, and so forth. If the client is having trouble completing skills training homework, the therapist examines the problem. If it is a matter of the client's not understanding the skills sufficiently, the therapist teaches the skill in more depth, linking the skill to the client's current life. If the client is feeling dissatisfied with skills training and unmotivated to practice the skills outside of group, the individual therapist reviews commitment strategies and helps the client recommit to change (see Chapter 7).

The individual therapist must always consider the timing of targeting specific issues. For example, if during a behavioral analysis regarding self-cutting it comes up in an unrelated way that the client went to skills training group but did not understand the material taught, the therapist may merely highlight that there needs to be further discussion regarding skills, but that they will address it later. However, if during a behavioral analysis regarding self-cutting the client mentions she did not understand the distress tolerance skills being taught in group, the therapist might take the opportunity while weaving in the solution analysis to teach a brief lesson on a distress tolerance skill (e.g., distract with ACCEPTS; see Linehan, 1993b) and ask the client to practice that skill during the next week. In this case, the skills deficit is relevant in dealing with the life-threatening behavior being discussed. The client's not attempting to complete her skills training group homework is considered a therapy-interfering behavior. The therapist might conduct an independent behavioral analysis of the therapy-interfering behavior once the life-threatening behavior has been analyzed.

By failing to ask about progress in other modes of treatment, the therapist communicates to the client that the other modes are not as important. If the client fails to attend or cooperate in other modes, it is the responsibility of the individual therapist to treat the behavior as therapy-interfering and analyze the problem. In particular, having an ancillary psychopharmacologist can become problematic with noncompliant teens; thus it may be helpful to construct the contingency that the attendance policy is the same for their medication visits as it is for skills training. The therapist can argue that both modalities are intended to enhance the client's capabilities. By only adhering to the attendance policy with regard to skills training and individual therapy, the treatment program staff may inadvertently communicate to clients that their medication compliance is less important.

MIDSESSION STRATEGIES FOR TARGETING STAGE 1 PRIORITIES

Setting the agenda, as described earlier, is a method to identify high-priority target behaviors and so determine the individual session's focus. The problem is that many adolescents do not want to discuss these target behaviors, and this forces a therapist to "toe the line" against a client's wishes. The therapist must believe in attending directly to high-priority behaviors and resist the client's pressure to attend to other topics. This avoids the risk of inadvertently reinforcing the client's dysfunctional behaviors (e.g., refusing to speak, attacking the therapist verbally, throwing a tantrum, etc.). We recommend that the therapist focus on long-term gain rather than short-term peace during the session. This may require the therapist to use his or her own crisis survival skills. The key is to continue moving the adolescent toward discussing the high-priority behaviors while simultaneously validating and soothing his or her discomfort as the therapist proceeds. In one case, after a client stated she would rather not discuss her recent suicide attempt during session, the therapist responded with the following:

> "I know you'd rather not talk about your suicide attempt, since you mentioned that it stirs up a lot of negative emotions, and who *wants* to talk about such difficult things [validation at Levels 2 and 3; see Chapter 3]? You also remember, though, that any time someone has engaged in life-threatening behavior, it takes priority over other issues. How could it be otherwise? We have to figure out what happened last week that resulted in your trying to hang yourself. Any problem that leads you to want to die is a really serious problem! If you end up dead, what point would there be in our talking about any other problems you want to discuss? I'd like to be able to discuss other things as well that will help you build a life worth living. But first we have to be sure you have a life to build on."

Over time, the client learns there is no way to avoid discussing these target behaviors, and either the resistance behaviors eventually remit or the client becomes more willing to discuss them in session.

The "meat" of the session begins as the therapist addresses the agenda item with the highest priority. For Jessica in the session described earlier, this meant addressing her self-injurious behavior identified on her diary card at the beginning of the session (see Figure 8.1). Adolescent dysfunctional behaviors, including suicide attempts and NSIB, are considered faulty solutions to problems in living (Linehan, 1981); thus problem-solving techniques are the core DBT change strategies (see Table 8.1). However, without therapist acceptance strategies such as validation of those problems in living, the adolescent will have no hope or motivation to change. To be effective, DBT requires the individual therapist to weave together acceptance and change strategies throughout all treatment sessions. With change comes acceptance, and with acceptance inevitably comes change. The therapist must also utilize dialectical, stylistic, and case management strategies with adolescents to help keep the therapy palatable and moving.

If an incident of self-injury is a faulty solution, the first challenge for the therapist is to help the adolescent clearly articulate the problem that occasioned the "solution" of self-harm. This is the first step of the problem-solving process outlined below. Behavioral chain analysis, together with validation, is used to build awareness and acceptance of the problem. The second step is for the therapist is to determine which solutions and change procedures should be

TABLE 8.1. Midsession Problem–Solving Strategies in Individual DBT

Phase 1

Task: Identification and acceptance of the problem
Primary method: Behavioral chain analysis

1. Identify the problem.
2. Describe the problem in behavioral terms.
3. Reconstruct the sequence of environmental and behavioral events (variables) leading up to the problem, co-occurring with it, and following it:
   • Vulnerability factors
   • Precipitating event(s)
   • Each emotion
   • Each thought
   • Each action
   • Each environmental event
4. Pinpoint the actual prompting event(s). For suicidal behaviors, these are likely to be intense or aversive emotion states; they may also involve a lack of behavioral skills or of dialectical thinking.
5. Identify the environmental and behavioral consequences (contingencies). (Where are the reinforcers?)
6. Foster insight by highlighting recurrent patterns, and by pointing out contingencies and reinforcements.
7. Construct and test hypotheses about what generates and maintains the problem behavior. Where are the links that could break the chain? Where are the targets for intervention?
8. Provide brief didactic instruction on relevant topics as needed.

Phase 2

Task: Generating alternative solutions
Primary method: Solution analysis

1. Identify points of interventions.
2. Brainstorm solutions. Encourage long-term versus short-term solutions.
3. Evaluate solutions in terms of expected outcomes.
4. Choose the solution most likely to be effective.
5. Troubleshoot solutions.
6. Obtain commitment to practice new solution.

applied to this specific client, at this moment, for this particular problem. That process too is outlined below.

It is important to note that these problem-solving "steps" are not always done in sequence. In fact, as a clinician becomes more facile at conducting these analyses, as well as more familiar with the client's behavioral patterns, these "steps" can be woven together. In the next section, we describe behavioral chain and solution analyses, using another example from Jessica's treatment.

Problem–Solving Phase 1: Building Awareness and Acceptance of the Problem

Strategies: Behavioral Chain Analysis (Interwoven with Validation) and Others

The first step in changing problematic behavior in DBT is to identify the variables that control the behavior. If more than one instance of the target behavior has occurred, then the most severe and best-remembered instance is chosen. The therapist and the client then develop a complete account of the chain of events that led to and followed the problematic behavior. As the behavioral chain analysis[1] proceeds, the therapist looks for controlling antecedent and maintaining variables. He or she also tries to identify each point at which an alternative behavior could have kept the problem behavior from occurring. The detail obtained in a good chain analysis is similar to that of a movie script. In other words, the description of the chain provides enough detail that one would be able to visualize it sufficiently to replicate and reenact the sequence of events. Table 8.2 offers guidelines for a behavioral chain analysis.

As an example of a behavioral chain analysis, we present the work done by Jessica and her therapist on an incident of self-cutting that had actual suicidal intent (not the NSIB in Figure 8.1). The therapist began by stating, "I see you made a suicide attempt on Saturday. As we have done before, let's review what happened—including things that may have made you vulnerable, what may have precipitated this behavior, and the thoughts and feelings that are potential links in the chain that led to your suicide attempt. And, of course, we have to review the consequences of your behavior." Jessica reported that two days before her suicide attempt, she had had a conflict with her boyfriend that resulted in a near-breakup (vulnerability factor). She reported already having sleeping problems previously and then being awake all night in a distressed state (vulnerability factor). One day later (Friday), Jessica's best friend, Tanya, had told Jessica that she had to choose between Tanya and her boyfriend. Jessica was shocked and hurt that her so-called "best friend" was putting her in this predicament (vulnerability factor). The therapist, listening intently, responded, "Wow, what a situation! What did you say? [Level 1 validation]?" Jessica responded to Tanya with anger: "No, I wont do that!" She wanted to discuss Tanya's actions with her boyfriend, but he "blew me off to go out with his friends instead."

Jessica felt rejected and alone. She reported trying to indirectly obtain support from her mother and father (who had dropped by the house for a visit) by spending time with them in the kitchen. Her father reportedly told her that because of her declining academic performance, he was not going to buy her the special shoes in Puerto Rico that she had requested. While Jessica began to "contribute" (DBT distraction skill) by cleaning the dishes, her mother became extremely critical of her less-than-thorough dish cleaning. Jessica reported in a shameful posture and tone, "When my mother turned on me and started criticizing me for no reason, I wanted to kill myself because I felt upset, like no one loved me any more." The therapist asked, "Can you define 'upset'?" Jessica stated, "I don't know, just upset." The therapist

---

[1]The chain analysis differs from the traditional behavior-analytic strategy of functional analysis in that it assesses a *particular* sequence of events controlling a specific instance of a targeted behavior, rather than assessing *classes* of controlling variables for repeated instances of a targeted behavior.

TABLE 8.2. Guidelines for a Behavioral Chain Analysis and Solution Analysis

1. Describe the specific *problem behavior* (e.g., throwing a chair, cutting, hearing voices, dissociating, not coming to a therapy appointment)
   a. Be very specific and detailed. Avoid vague terms.
   b. Identify exactly what you did, said, thought, or felt (if a feeling is the targeted problem behavior).
   c. Describe the intensity of the behavior and other characteristics of the behavior that are important.
   d. Describe the problem behavior in enough detail that an actor in a play or movie could recreate the behavior exactly.

2. Describe the specific *precipitating event* that started the whole chain of behavior.
   a. Identify the environmental event that started the chain. Always start with some event in your environment, even if it doesn't seem to you that the environmental event "caused" the problem behavior. Here are some possible questions to get at this:
      1. When did the sequence of events that led to the problem behavior begin? When did the problem start?
      2. What was going on the moment the problem started?
      3. What were you doing/thinking/feeling/imagining at that time?
      4. Why did the problem behavior happen on that day instead of the day before?

3. Describe the *vulnerability factors* happening before the precipitating event. What factors or events made you more vulnerable to a problematic chain? Areas to examine include the following:
   a. Physical illness; unbalanced eating or sleeping; injury.
   b. Use of drugs or alcohol; misuse of prescription drugs.
   c. Stressful events in the environment (either positive or negative).
   d. Intense emotions, such as sadness, anger, fear, or loneliness.
   e. Previous behaviors of your own that you found stressful.

4. Describe in excruciating detail the *chain of events* that led up to the problem behavior.
   a. What next? Imagine that your problem behavior is chained to the precipitating event in the environment. How long is the chain? Where does it go? What are the links? Write out all links in the chain of events, no matter how small. Be very specific, as if you are writing a script for a play.
      1. What exact thought (or belief), feeling, or action followed the precipitating event? What thought, feeling, or action followed that? What next? What next?
      2. Look at each link in the chain after you write it. Was there another thought, feeling, or action that could have occurred? Could someone else have thought, felt, or acted differently at that point? If so, explain how that specific thought, feeling, or action came to be.
      3. For each link in the chain, ask yourself: Is there a smaller link I could describe?

5. What were the *consequences* of this behavior? Be specific. (How did other people react immediately and later? How did you feel immediately following the behavior? Later? What effect did the behavior have on you and your environment?)

6. Describe in detail different *solutions* to the problem.
   a. Go back to the chain of your behaviors following the prompting event. Circle each point or link where, if you had done something different, you would have avoided the problem behavior.
   b. What could you have done differently at each link in the chain of events to avoid the problem behavior? What coping behaviors or skillful behaviors could you have used?

7. Describe in detail a *prevention strategy* for how you could have kept the chain from starting by reducing your vulnerability to the chain.

8. Describe what you are going to do to *repair* important or significant consequences of the problem behavior.

paused to consider whether it made sense to pursue further questioning on clarifying her emotion, and then decided to continue: "And when did the thought 'No one loves me any more' occur? Before or after you felt upset?" "Before," she said. The therapist went on, "Do you think you felt sad?" "Yes," Jessica replied. The therapist reflected, "Sounds like after your best friend and your boyfriend blew you off, and then your mother and father became critical, you really felt sad and thought of yourself as unloved by everyone [Level 2 validation]. I can imagine most people would feel really sad, and even disappointed or angry, after a series of interactions like you had with the closest people in your life [Levels 3 and 5 validation]." The therapist then asked whether this was the first moment Jessica thought about suicide, and the client acknowledged that this was the precipitating event. Although she was unable to clearly identify her emotion in the moment, other than "upset," the critical link (to her suicide attempt) in the chain appeared to be the thought "No one loves me any more." Jessica reported the urge to flee the situation and to kill herself. The therapist stated, "We know from your past behavioral analyses that for you, thinking you are unloved is intolerable, and you desperately try to escape it even if it means killing yourself [Level 4 validation]."

At this point in the incident, Jessica immediately left the kitchen and chose to go to the bathroom, where she kept her razor blades. She locked the bathroom door, began to cry, and reached for the razor blade in the shower, which she then used to cut her arm several times. She immediately experienced some sense of relief (negative reinforcing consequence) after she began to cut herself. She got into her bed, where her arm left bloodstains on the sheets. In the morning, her mother went to wake her up and found her bloody sheets. Alarmed, her mother asked what had happened; Jessica replied, "No one loves me." Jessica's mother proceeded to tell Jessica, "I love you very much! How about after school today you and I will go shopping?" (positive reinforcing consequence for cutting and for leaving blood on the sheets). Jessica smiled and agreed to go. When she went to school and saw her boyfriend later that morning, Jessica told him what had happened. Her boyfriend expressed his love to her and asked her to go out that night, which Jessica happily agreed to do (positive reinforcing consequence). During the school day, Jessica experienced increasing amounts of shame for cutting herself; she was very ambivalent about the "love" she was receiving after the incident, but did not say or do anything about it. The therapist commented, "It sucks that you receive the most love and affection from your boyfriend and mother *after* you attempt to kill yourself instead of *before*. They have no idea that they are positively reinforcing your suicidal behavior. I'd think you'd be a lot better off if we could switch the order around, don't you [Level 6 validation]?"

In sum, the individual therapist skillfully weaves problem-solving and validation strategies together in constructing a behavioral chain analysis. Figure 8.2 illustrates the chain analysis of Jessica's suicide attempt.

Hypothesis Testing and Problem Definition

The therapist generates and tests hypotheses about potential controlling variables as the chain analysis is conducted, and summarizes these in a problem definition that makes it clear how the behavior/event is dysfunctional with respect to the client's long-term goals:

> "Jessica, did you first think about cutting yourself when you had the thought 'No one loves me any more?' " [Jessica: "Yes."] "That thought—'No one loves me any more,'—is clearly a problematic thought, don't you think? We are going to spend some time teaching you how to challenge that thought when it pops into your head, so that it doesn't lead you down the path to self-harm. I'd also like to work with you on ways to tolerate the intense distress set off by that remark without trying to kill yourself."

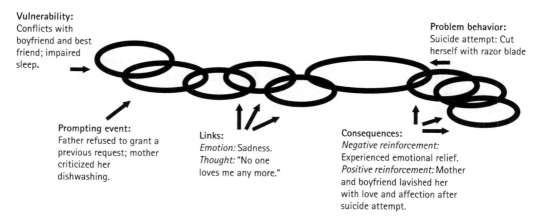

Vulnerability: Conflicts with boyfriend and best friend; impaired sleep.

Problem behavior: Suicide attempt: Cut herself with razor blade

Prompting event: Father refused to grant a previous request; mother criticized her dishwashing.

Links: *Emotion:* Sadness. *Thought:* "No one loves me any more."

Consequences: *Negative reinforcement:* Experienced emotional relief. *Positive reinforcement:* Mother and boyfriend lavished her with love and affection after suicide attempt.

FIGURE 8.2. *Behavioral chain analysis of Jessica's suicide attempt.*

In addition, reminders of contingencies are helpful at this point. For example, the therapist might say to Jessica,

> "Cutting yourself to the point that you are being hospitalized is screwing up your entire life, even though, unfortunately, cutting yourself is really effective at reducing your intense emotional pain [Level 5 validation]. Unfortunately, at the moment you can't resist these impulses and stop this behavior, because you don't yet have the necessary emotion regulation and distress tolerance skills to accomplish the task [Level 4 validation]."

Insight and Highlighting Strategies

Some strategies are used to highlight recurrent patterns across instances of targeted problem behaviors. The therapist observes and describes recurrent patterns, and comments on the implications of the client's behavior. For example, Jessica had a general pattern of cutting when she thought she was being rejected or was "unloved." The other problem pattern was receiving positive reinforcement from her loved ones after she cut herself. Jessica needed to receive validation and support *before* she harmed herself; instead, Jessica would often get the most love, attention, and affection *after* engaging in self-harm. This pattern was openly discussed in session. At other times, the DBT therapist may highlight a problem during session without addressing it further in the moment. For example, it became clear during the behavioral analysis that a problem with Jessica's best friend needed to be addressed at some point. Instead of continuing in that direction at that moment. the therapist chose to highlight it briefly instead and said, "Wow, Jessica, I can see why you felt so hurt in response to Tanya's ultimatum [Level 5 validation]. Your relationship with her has always been very intense. We'll come back to that later. OK, keep going. . . ."

Didactic Strategies

Didactic strategies include presenting information (research findings or psychological or biological theories) to the client or her family. The purpose is to counter self-blaming morality- or mental-illness-based explanations of problem behaviors. This may happen briefly during the chain analysis or afterwards. For example, after determining that sleep disturbance was a vulnerability factor in Jessica's chain analysis, the therapist provided a brief didactic lesson on sleep hygiene (Williams, 1993), oriented her to the potential benefits of beginning such a program, and then obtained a commitment to try it during the upcoming week. Jessica was quickly instructed to stop napping during the day, to decrease her caffeine intake, to create a soothing bedtime ritual that included reading, and to wake up and go to sleep at regular times each morning and night. She agreed to attempt her new sleep routine and wrote down the assignment.

Problem–Solving Phase 2: Generating, Evaluating, and Implementing Alternative Solutions

Strategies: Solution Analysis, Change Procedures, Orienting, Commitment, and Troubleshooting

Solution Analysis

The second phase of problem solving requires the therapist and client to generate possible solutions for the difficulties pinpointed by the behavioral analysis as described above. Together, the therapist and client must ask, "What solutions other than the target behavior could be applied to the problem at hand?" More specifically, the therapist looks for different points in the behavior chain to intervene, and there are many possible places to intervene. For example, solutions can target any potential vulnerability factors (such as the sleep factor mentioned above); the precipitating event; key links such as specific cognitions, emotions, and behaviors; and specific contingencies that may be maintaining dysfunctional behavior, as well as extinguishing or punishing adaptive behavior. The therapist helps the client generate alternative solutions, encouraging the use of long-term over short-term solutions.

Change Procedures

Alternative solutions to the client's problem, and the tools to implement them, can usually be found among a variety of empirically validated technologies. The most common of these change procedures fall into four categories: (1) skills training, (2) exposure, (3) cognitive modification, and (4) contingency management. When conducting a solution analysis, the therapist must consider all change procedures available. One of the many challenges for the individual therapist is to prioritize these possible strategies quickly, from most to least relevant to the target behavior. Tips for selecting change strategies are offered in Table 8.3.

Based on information obtained from Jessica's behavioral chain analysis, the therapist selected strategies from all four main types of change procedures (see Figure 8.3). In addition, the therapist felt that a family therapy session was warranted. Jessica first felt rejected, abandoned, sad, and hurt by her best friend and her boyfriend, only to feel disappointed by her father and criticized and hurt by her mother. That precipitated the thought "No one loves me any more." Jessica and the therapist identified the cognitive link "No one loves me any more," and further identified the emotions of sadness as leading to her first thought of suicide. A review of the four change procedures follows below.

Skills Training: Emotion Regulation and Distress Tolerance

Skills training strategies are called for when a solution requires skills that are not currently in the client's behavioral repertoire, or when the client has the components of a skilled response but cannot integrate and use them effectively in the moment they are needed. Skills

TABLE 8.3. Tips for Selecting Change Procedures for Problem Solutions

Change procedure	Useful when:
Skills training	Client lacks skills needed to solve the problem or doesn't know how to use them effectively.
Exposure	Client's emotions and associated action tendencies interfere with effective use of coping skills.
Cognitive modification	Client's faulty beliefs and assumptions inhibit effective coping abilities.
Contingency procedures	Client lacks motivation despite knowledge of skills.

were deemed useful in targeting one of Jessica's vulnerability factors (lack of sleep) and the precipitating event (i.e., her reaction to her mother's criticism) as identified in the behavioral chain analysis. It was determined that when Jessica was in distress, she had two options: (1) She could avoid her mother, given her mother's tendency to invalidate her; or (2) she could directly express her feelings to her mother, so that her mother would know that she was in distress. The problem with the latter option was that Jessica was often unaware of what she was feeling. Thus the recommended solution for Jessica was to practice identifying and labeling emotions when she was not in distress, in order to prepare her for future episodes of emotion dysregulation: "Jessica, before you can choose a coping strategy, you need to know what you are feeling." In addition to this emphasis on mindfully identifying and labeling emotions, Jessica and the therapist identified adaptive skills that could be used to achieve a sense of relief, such as distraction and self-soothing. For example, Jessica agreed to watch her favorite comedy video or take a soothing bubble bath when she was feeling abandoned or "like no one loves me."

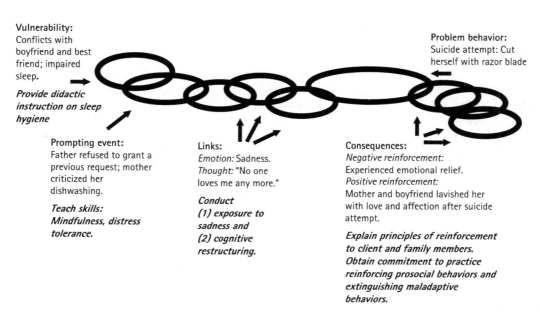

FIGURE 8.3. *Solution analysis of Jessica's suicide attempt.*

Exposure-Based Procedures: Reducing Sensitivity to Shame and Sadness

Although most exposure therapies target fear as the primary emotion (e.g., in treating specific phobia, PTSD, or panic disorder), DBT expands the list of targeted emotions to include shame, guilt, anger, sadness, and other emotions that are experienced as aversive and interfere in the client's life and/or treatment through avoidance of those emotions. In particular, shame may play a key role in suicidal behavior in women with BPD (Brown & Linehan, 1996). It is often a target for informal exposure in DBT sessions. Linehan (1993a) notes that the natural action tendency associated with shame is hiding; thus the DBT exposure procedure involves directing the client to discuss the shameful experience while not hiding (both literally and through postural expressions).

For example, with Jessica, before beginning exposure to feelings of sadness, the therapist chose to address the feeling of shame that she displayed as she recounted her suicide attempt in session. The therapist encouraged actions opposite to shame by being persistent and soothing; he also reminded Jessica as needed to look the therapist in the eye, to sit up straight, not to mumble, and not to change the topic. Often during informal exposure, a client will begin to discuss what is shameful and then interrupt him- or herself. One metaphor (dialectical strategy) Jessica's therapist used to try to get her to stop such interruptions was that of jumping off a high diving board:

> "Telling me something you're ashamed of is like a novice diver walking slowly to the edge of the high diving board 20 feet up in the air and looking down. . . . What happens? The diver becomes afraid and wants to turn around and climb back down the ladder. The only way that the diver is going to feel comfortable up there is to run off the board without looking down. The same thing is true for you: Keep telling me your story without stopping and 'without looking down.' I will have you tell it to me again and again until you can just spit it out without stopping and without your body getting into the 'ashamed' body posture (*briefly mimics Jessica's body posture*) it gets into when you feel that way."

After this targeting of shame, the next intervention with Jessica was to conduct formal exposure exercises to her sadness. Jessica's sadness often precipitated impulsive behaviors and distorted cognitions. "Jessica, it is important for you to be able to experience sadness as not dangerous and requiring escape. The better able you are to sit mindfully with your sadness, the less likely you will be to turn to your maladaptive coping strategy of suicide and self-injury." These exposure exercises took place during significant portions of the subsequent three sessions. Exposure is a very important part of treatment used with a variety of target behaviors. For example, with a client whose eating is disordered, the therapist might bring tempting foods into session and have the client watch urges to binge or purge. For a client who is apparently unable to tolerate high anxiety and panic, the therapist teaches the client to mindfully observe and describe the anxiety until the client habituates to the emotion and no longer feels the urge to escape from it. Often in DBT sessions, the therapist asks the client, "Where in your body are you feeling an emotion? Now just observe it."

Cognitive Modification: Changing Dysfunctional Beliefs

One important distinction between DBT and cognitive therapy is DBT's emphasis on functional, effective thinking rather than on rationally or empirically based thinking (Linehan, 1993a). If an adolescent thinks, "Nobody wants to date me," there may be some truth to it— but the thought may lead to dysfunctional behaviors that make it self-fulfilling, such as overeating or assuming postures that convey shame. Cognitive modification may involve helping the client change her thinking to "I haven't been dating, and many of the things I do contribute to that. I will have to start working on some of these things."

Jessica's automatic thought "No one loves me any more" was an example of emotional reasoning ("I feel like no one loves me; therefore it's true") and all-or-nothing thinking ("Either everyone loves me or no one loves me") (Burns, 1989). The therapist helped Jessica recognize that although her parents, boyfriend, and best friend were not actively expressing love in their respective interactions in those moments, they were all known to express love at other times. And even if it were true that her boyfriend did not love her like he used to, did that mean that *no one* else loved her? The therapist helped Jessica generate some rational responses to these distorted cognitions, such as "Although they're not expressing it right now, I know they love me because they've expressed it at other times," and "Even though I'm not sure about my boyfriend's feelings for me right now, I know I am loved by my family." At the same time, Jessica learned that these thoughts contributed to certain dysfunctional behaviors that she could address. She might be better able to experience loving interactions with the people in her life if she reduced her irritability, was more overtly reinforcing and loving toward them at appropriate times, and was less avoidant when conflicts arose. After spending the remainder of the session on cognitive restructuring, the therapist oriented Jessica to the fact that they would continue to check on her work in this domain.

Contingency Management Procedures

Typically, one of the most effective and powerful reinforcers for clients with BPD, and for adolescents in general, is the therapeutic relationship. The therapist explicitly uses the relationship as reinforcement for in-session target-relevant adaptive behaviors, by expressing appropriate warmth, attachment, approval, care, concern, and interest. With adolescents, the use of between-session phone contact is often reinforcing, but not always. It is essential to identify reinforcers for each particular client, rather than assuming that something is reinforcing. One way we address this potential problem is by inviting our adolescent clients to "practice-page" us in the first week of treatment. This allows an adolescent to have a brief, benign contact with a therapist, which helps disconfirm the notion that the call will be aversive when a problem arises. Jessica was asked to practice-page her therapist during the following week when she was not in distress:

> "Jessica, as you said, your suicide attempt was an impulsive act. We need to help you slow down enough that you can identify your distress, recognize your need for help, and generate alternative solutions. If you have trouble doing that in the beginning, which you may, I want you to page me for coaching. This way we can work together as a team. Therefore, I want you to practice-page me on Tuesday night when you are not in crisis, so that calling becomes more comfortable and automatic."

Once a client feels attached to the therapist, the therapist's emotional responses to the client—warm or cool—can become a powerful contingency. At times, these are the only powerful contingencies a therapist has control over. It is important that the therapist respond to client behaviors strategically, remaining well aware of the potential power of his or her response. It is also critical that the therapist assess the potential impact of his or her behaviors. With one client, very slight coolness of affect may be all that is needed to punish unwanted behavior; with another client, it may be necessary to express strong disappointment; with still another, it may be necessary to take a "time out" from a session. The DBT therapist may use the therapeutic relationship as an aversive contingency (i.e., through response cost) in certain specific circumstances: when all other response options have been unsuccessful; when the reinforcing consequences of a high-priority target-relevant maladaptive behavior (such as drug use or promiscuous sexual behavior) are not under the therapist's control; or when the maladaptive behavior interferes with all other adaptive behaviors.

After 6 weeks of treatment, Jessica started calling the therapist frequently and at the same time acting as though the calls were not helpful, not attempting to try the therapist's suggestions for using skills, and sometimes not talking when the therapist attempted to end a phone call.

> THERAPIST: Jessica, I have something I want to talk to you about. You're pushing my limits on phone calls. When you call me every day, act as though none of my suggestions are helpful, and then either hang up or refuse to get off the phone, I don't feel like talking to you on the phone [Level 6 validation]. I could make a rule such as "one phone call per week," but instead of having a rule, let's say we have a problem that we need to address. I am also wondering if I am missing something else that we should be addressing. What do you think? Doesn't it seem like you are asking for more phone contact than you used to?
>
> JESSICA: (*Looking out window*) Do you know that I had a 102-degree temperature yesterday [diverting]?
>
> THERAPIST: What do you think is going on with these phone calls? What is it that you need that you are not getting right now?
>
> JESSICA: (*Silent, then:*) Fine, I won't call you.
>
> THERAPIST: I thought that instead of having a rule, we could have a conversation and problem-solve together. Rules give *me* all of the control. Let's figure out how to get your behavior under *your* control and help you get what you need without pushing my limits [highlighting both ends of the dialectic].

In the example above, the therapist explained that Jessica's behavior was pushing the therapist's personal limits. The therapist used self-involving self-disclosure (a reciprocal communication strategy) to explain how he felt when Jessica acted that way. He oriented Jessica to the problem, attempted to problem-solve, and used contingency clarification (i.e., if this behavior was not extinguished, the therapist would have to employ consequences, such as "rules" to change the behavior). The fact that a therapist has personal limits needs to be communicated ahead of time, usually during the orientation process.

Clients can apply contingency management techniques to their own lives outside of sessions. Clients are taught to reward themselves for taking small steps in the right direction. For example, one client who had stopped going to classes, and thus stopped doing any schoolwork, chose to buy herself a new compact disc by her favorite artist after the first week of having gone back to school and done her homework. Another contingency management technique taught to clients is to structure their environment in such a way as not to reinforce their own maladaptive behaviors. For example, one client agreed to have no contact with her boyfriend at all during the hours of multifamily skills training group sessions, whether she attended the group or not. This contingency was effectively implemented so that contact with the boyfriend could not serve as a reinforcer for her *not* attending group, which it had in the past.

In Jessica's behavioral chain analysis, it became clear that Jessica's boyfriend and parents inadvertently reinforced her suicidal behavior by lavishing her with affection and offering her gifts *after* such incidents rather than before. Changing these reinforcement contingencies for Jessica involved the use of DBT case management strategies—specifically, consultation to the client and environmental intervention. In the role of consultant, Jessica's therapist encouraged and coached her to speak with her boyfriend and her parents about their inadvertent reinforcement of her suicidal behavior. Jessica had initially requested that the therapist do it for her. The coaching happened in the context of role playing with the client beforehand. If Jessica deemed it too difficult to discuss this issue outside of session, or if her parents were unresponsive to her, the therapist mentioned the possibility of having her speak to her parents in a family session.

The environmental intervention of a family session is typically used only as a last resort in DBT with adults. But, obviously, working with adolescents requires mental health professionals to intervene in the environment more often than with adult clients. If an adolescent is at high risk for suicide, the therapist must contact the client's relatives, asking them to remove any available means of suicide from the home, and in some circumstances must admit the client to a hospital. Also, at times, the therapist is required for legal and practical reasons to become less of a consultant to the client and more of an advocate. For example, mental health professionals are mandated reporters of child abuse and neglect. Thus, for clients under the age of 18, therapists must call child protective services when there is a suspicion of abuse or neglect, even when an adolescent does not want the call to be made.

When Jessica attempted to discuss the issue of inadvertent reinforcement at home, her parents were distracted and unable to comprehend the important message she was trying to deliver. It then became necessary for her therapist to present the issue to her parents in a family session. With the therapist's encouragement in session, Jessica acknowledged to them that her suicidal behavior also functioned as a method of escaping her emotional pain (i.e., negative reinforcement) and was effective to that end in the short term. However, she also admitted to feelings of shame that she had to resort to this extreme life-threatening behavior to achieve a sense of relief. These feelings of shame ultimately outweighed the short-term benefit of escape that the suicidal behavior provided.

We discuss general family session procedures in Chapter 9.

Orienting and Commitment Strategies

Once alternative solutions and change procedures have been identified, the client needs to be motivated to use them. Therefore, the orienting and commitment strategies we have discussed in Chapter 7 are also woven into problem solving as needed. For example, Jessica's therapist assigned her four major tasks as homework, knowing she would protest: (1) Follow sleep protocol; (2) track automatic thoughts when she was feeling emotional; (3) discuss with her boyfriend and family the positive reinforcement she received from them after self-harming; and (4) practice-page the therapist. This was an example of the door-in-the-face strategy, and the therapist received the reaction he expected: Jessica said, "That's too much. I can't do that much homework for therapy when I am behind on my schoolwork!" The therapist replied, "OK, how about choosing the two assignments that you can commit to practicing this week? We'll work on the others after that." Jessica experienced this as somewhat of a bargain, and the therapist saw this as an accomplishment by getting her to practice two behavioral assignments instead of the usual one, while simultaneously strengthening her commitment by having her choose which two she was going to practice.

Troubleshooting Possible Solutions

With every possible solution generated there is potential trouble. When the client and therapist have evaluated several possible solutions to a problem, it is imperative that the therapist help the client troubleshoot each solution. That is, the client and therapist must consider potential obstacles to these solutions and figure out how these obstacles can be overcome to ensure that the solution works. Since Jessica chose to practice her sleep hygiene protocol and talk to her boyfriend and parents about their inadvertent reinforcement of self-harm, the therapist asked, "Jessica, what might interfere in your following your sleep protocol? And what might interfere in your discussing this problem with your boyfriend and parents? Let's take the possible difficulties one at a time." First, Jessica revealed that she did not have an alarm clock and thus relied on her family members to wake her up each morning. She also anticipated that it might be hard to stay off the Internet at night, since she would often e-mail her friends until the early morning hours. Jessica agreed that she would purchase an alarm clock immediately after the therapy session. In addition, she estimated that she would be able to extricate herself from her computer if she designated a specific time (10:30 P.M.) and had another activity to engage her (i.e., reading a book). Finally, she agreed to call her therapist at midweek if she found herself unable to follow this plan.

Troubleshooting the second solution revealed Jessica's fear of her parent's reactions. She expected a critical reaction to her raising the issue of their reinforcement of her suicidal behavior. She and her therapist decided that she would only discuss this issue with her boyfriend during this week, since they had just role-played it during session and she had much less apprehension about discussing this subject with him. Once she had an opportunity to "practice" this discussion with him, and then report back in therapy, Jessica and the therapist could decide how to proceed with her parents.

The important message here for all of us as clinicians is while we encourage, push, and sometimes drag new behavior out of our multiproblem adolescents, we often get even more mileage when we can successfully troubleshoot solutions and remember the principle of shaping. New DBT therapists rarely devote enough time to troubleshooting the solutions. As a result, they often have poorer compliance with their assignments, and thus worse outcomes.

TARGETING IN-SESSION DYSFUNCTIONAL BEHAVIOR

Similar to out-of-session dysfunctional behaviors, the therapist must attend to in-session dysfunctional behaviors. There are several payoffs for treating in-session behaviors. First, learning takes place "in the fire," where it is most relevant and with the therapist present. In addition, the therapist can explicitly link in-session learning with relevant natural contexts. For example, when Jessica became ashamed while discussing her self-harm during the behavioral analysis, she began to shut down and tried to avoid discussing the problem behavior. The therapist was able to target this emotional response immediately, point out the adverse consequences of avoiding, and establish commitment to begin exposure to this emotion, which would then allow them to target the feelings of abandonment and sadness that preceded the self-harm.

Unfortunately, therapists often fail to address in-session dysfunctional behaviors because of several factors: failure to recognize behaviors as dysfunctional; removal of cues that provoke the in-session dysfunctional response (e.g., stopping the discussion of a topic that makes the adolescent angry); the therapist's own dysfunctional cognitions ("If I bring this topic up with my client, she'll get angry and storm out, so I better not"); the therapist's own skills deficits (recognizing a problem behavior but not knowing how to address it, such as by orienting and then conducting exposure to shame); the therapist's own emotional avoidance (e.g., the therapist has difficulty tolerating sadness or anger, and consequently avoids discussing topics with the client that may elicit those emotions); and contingencies operating on the therapist (e.g., the therapist receives smiles and laughs from the client when discussing nontarget behaviors, and receives verbal attacks and noncollaboration when discussing in-session dysfunctional behaviors).

Some important guidelines for treating an in-session dysfunctional behavior include staying dialectical, identifying and naming the problem behavior, trying not to remove cues, regulating one's own emotions, linking in-session behaviors with out-of-session behaviors, and demanding and getting new behavior in session.

Several sessions into Jessica's treatment, whenever discussion of therapy-interfering behaviors became necessary, she became increasingly sad, noncollaborative, and passive by stating, "I don't know, I don't care." The therapist made use of a DBT protocol to target this in-session dysfunctional behavior (Linehan, 1995). Table 8.4 lists the essential steps for targeting such behaviors.

THERAPIST: Jessica, I notice a problem that we have here: Every time we discuss a therapy-interfering behavior, you get sad, passive, and noncollaborative [observing]. I realize that this problem comes up in your other relationships, too. When you feel like someone is critical of you or pointing out a problem in the relationship, you get sad and withdrawn. In here, when you get passive and withdraw, I feel like we're not working as a team; I can tell you are upset [Level 3 validation]; and I feel frustrated [self-involving self-disclosure, Level 6 validation]. It's like you feel and act "blah." Do you know what I am talking about?

JESSICA: Yes. . . . I never thought of it that way before, but you're right (*sigh*).

THERAPIST: This "blah" approach to solving interpersonal issues is your mortal enemy. You avoid solving the problem, and you don't learn how to work through issues with other people—which often lead to a variety of problems, including suicidal behavior. If you have the urge to withdraw when you're feeling sad, you have to fight it as hard as you can. What skills can you use when this happens [eliciting a skillful response or opposite action]?

JESSICA: (*Hesitates*) I don't know . . . and I really don't know; I am not just saying that.

THERAPIST: Listen, when this "blah" shows up, first you have to be mindful. That is, you

TABLE 8.4. Essential Steps for Targeting In-Session Dysfunctional Behaviors

1. Observe a dysfunctional behavior/event.
2. Describe the behavior/event as dysfunctional: "This behavior/event is your mortal enemy."
3. Elicit a coping response or opposite action.
   Is the skill a good one, the best one can hope for in the real world? If so, skip to 5.
   If the skill is not useful, or if the client gives no response or says, "I don't know," go to 4.
4. Instruct (teach) client what to do: "Listen, when this behavior/event shows up or threatens, do this thing [or simple set of things]."
5. Orient the client to the importance of the new behavior: "This new behavior must be done to save your life."
6. Get the client's commitment to do it: "Are you willing to do that?"
7. Have the client practice the new behavior in session (at least once): "OK, imagine that the problem behavior/event shows up. You do . . ."
8. Troubleshoot (elicit or teach what will interfere): "Now what can we count on to go wrong and interfere with your being skillful?"
9. Move to next topic.

need to observe it, describe it, and not judge it. Next you have to do your best to be effective and participate in the session as best you can. That may involve telling me what you're feeling in words . . . or it may be noticing the blah feeling, letting it wash over you, and then participating in the session by the acting opposite of your current emotion without further discussion of the blah [instructing].

When clients are in distress, it is not always immediately apparent to them why they should use a specific skill in a specific situation and/or how they can use it effectively. To make use of a metaphor, it can be like telling a person in a burning, smoke-filled kitchen to run through the burning living room to get outside, since that is the only way to get to the door. You may see it's the only way out, but the person inside might not. The therapist must make it vivid and impress upon the client as highlighted above how treatment tasks and rationales clearly relate to the client's goals, especially when the client is in intense emotional pain that the therapist and client are unable to alleviate quickly. The aforementioned metaphor is one example of a dialectical strategy used with clients in distress in order to facilitate movement (behaviorally, emotionally, and/or cognitively) when they are "stuck."

THERAPIST: You have to try this new approach to save your life. Seriously, not only does it slow us down in here, but it dramatically affects your relationships outside of here. I think it also connects to your life-threatening behavior [orienting]. Are you willing to use your mindfulness skills (and possibly act opposite) [commitment]?

JESSICA: Yes, I'll try it, but it's going to be hard.

THERAPIST: Of course it will be difficult [Levels 4 and 5 validation]. If it were easy, you'd be doing it already [irreverent communication]. . . . OK, let's practice it. Imagine that we start discussing your lateness to session, and that the "blah" feeling comes over you again. What do you do [practice]?

JESSICA: I have to observe and describe my blahness.

THERAPIST: Good [positive reinforcement]. What else?

JESSICA: I can say, "Dr. M., I am feeling sad and I am starting to feel blah."

THERAPIST: Perfect. Then I might say, "Jessica, try to participate fully and nonjudgmentally by throwing yourself back into the problem-solving discussion about your lateness. I am not criticizing you when we discuss this . . . I just want to figure out what is interfering in your getting here on time and come up with a solution, so that we have more time to discuss the other things you put on the agenda."

JESSICA: OK. I know I was late because my boyfriend wanted to fool around after school and I lost track of time.

THERAPIST: That makes sense [Level 5 validation]. And good work, Jessica, throwing yourself back into the discussion of therapy-interfering behavior! . . . Now what can we count on to go wrong and interfere with your using these skills next time it comes up in session? How are we going to handle *that*?

Dialectical strategies permeate the entire treatment and are used heavily in individual therapy. They emphasize the tensions elicited by contradictory emotions, cognitions, and behavior patterns, both within the individual and between the individual and the environment. Within the therapeutic interaction, the therapist consciously monitors the balance of change and acceptance, flexibility and stability, challenging and nurturing, and other dialectics, in order to maintain a collaborative working relationship in the moment-to-moment interactions with the patient. The therapist also highlights for the patient the dialectical contradictions of the patient's own behavior and thinking by opposing any term or proposition with its opposite or an alternative. The point is that either extreme of a dialectic is an unhelpful place to be, so the patient is helped to find the middle way by moving from "either–or" to "both–and." For example, when discussing with Jessica her maladaptive telephone calling behavior that was pushing his limits, the therapist said, "Let's figure out how to get your behavior under *your* control *and* help you get what you need without pushing my limits."

SESSION-ENDING STRATEGIES

As mentioned earlier, many suicidal multiproblem teens experience intense emotions during their therapy sessions. Some clients are worried about "opening up" because they are concerned that they will have insufficient time to get themselves "back together" if they do. Thus one of the most important aspects of ending a session is allotting enough time to wrap up. The client needs to know that the therapist is considerate and sensitive to the issue of intense emotion; this increases the likelihood that the adolescent will "open up." The therapist does not want the client to walk out of the office in an unadulterated state of emotion mind (e.g., panic, sadness, hopelessness) and resort to self-harm. Since each client is different and may require different amounts of time to wind down, each client and therapist dyad should discuss this issue together as it becomes apparent, so that the appropriate amount of time is left for closure. Closure time may include (1) agreeing on (and troubleshooting) homework for the upcoming week; (2) summarizing the session, including (when appropriate) cheerleading, soothing, and reassuring the client; (3) troubleshooting the client's emotional reactions; (4) giving the client a tape of the session; and (5) engaging in an ending ritual. For example, many teens find engaging in a mindfulness exercise helpful in reorienting themselves at the end of an emotionally dysregulating session.

Agreeing on (and Troubleshooting) Homework for the Upcoming Week

During the session, the client and therapist have usually identified certain problem areas the client needs to work on during the upcoming week. At the end of the session, the therapist and client collaboratively review what has been discussed and determine whether any of these areas should serve as homework assignments during the upcoming week. Once the assignment is identified, the therapist should troubleshoot any potential difficulties that may arise for the client when he or she tries to use these skills later in the week. As mentioned earlier, Jessica agreed to practice her sleep hygiene and discuss the issue of inadvertent reinforcement of her self-harming behavior with her boyfriend. Before she went off to use her interpersonal DEAR MAN skills with her boyfriend, Jessica and her therapist considered all possible outcomes. These included which emotions were likely to result from the different outcomes, and which distress tolerance skills could be employed if the outcome was less than desirable. In addition, they decided that Jessica would purchase an alarm clock to help her with her sleep protocol.

Summarizing the Session, Including Cheerleading, Soothing, and Reassuring the Client

It is sometimes useful to review the major points addressed in the session, especially when numerous issues have been discussed in a session. When this has been done, the therapist should give a one- or two-sentence summary in an upbeat manner, which highlights any new insights gained during the session as well as any accomplishments or progress made. For example, "Jessica, you did a wonderful job resisting the urge to use drugs this past week by using your ACCEPTS skill to distract yourself. Let's keep that up and recommit to doing the same with your self-harm." Most session time is spent on analyzing dysfunctional behaviors, and so it is important at the end to validate the client's experience of the difficulty of changing these behaviors. At the same time, the therapist needs to cheerlead and encourage the client onward: "You did a great job role-playing the conversation you want to have with your boyfriend. It may be difficult to initiate it, but I think when you get rolling, you'll do a fine job."

Given that most adolescent clients have tremendous difficulty reaching out for help, it is important for the therapist to reassure the client that the therapist is available to call for coaching before a crisis is reached. With Jessica, the therapist reassured her by encouraging her to call for coaching if she wanted it before she spoke to her boyfriend. Letting clients know that their therapists are available to them outside of session time is extremely valuable in its capacity to soothe and reassure them that they are not alone and that help is just one phone call away. Some clients have told us that being told they could call any time had an immediate impact on lessening their suicidal ideation.

Troubleshooting the Client's Emotional Reactions at the End of the Session

It is a good rule of thumb for therapists to anticipate that emotional reactions will linger after sessions. Even when a client reports feeling "OK" at the end of a session, it is wise for the therapist to anticipate reactions that may result, troubleshoot those reactions, and determine what distress tolerance and emotion regulation skills the client can use to avoid engaging in maladaptive behavior.

Giving a Tape of the Session

Some clients who need or want an audiotape of a session are more than welcome to take the tape home with them and listen to it during the week. This is especially useful for many of our clients, who become profoundly emotionally dysregulated during sessions and have difficulty recalling anything that happened afterward. Also, for clients who want to have more contact with the therapist, listening to the tape can sometimes achieve that goal.

Engaging in an Ending Ritual

For some clients and therapists, developing an ending ritual can make leaving the session easier. With one male client, the male therapist engaged in a particular "street" handshake that conveyed a level of intimacy. For other therapists and clients, a goodbye hug might be used. For some, a mindfulness exercise is employed. At a minimum, the therapist should walk the client to the door and convey the expectation that they will see each other again soon.

TELEPHONE CONSULTATION STRATEGIES

The individual therapist is responsible for the treatment mode of telephone consultation with the adolescent on an as-needed basis. As described in Chapter 4, telephone calls with the therapist between individual sessions enable the therapist to provide skills coaching and emergency crisis intervention, enable the client to report good news, and help both to repair ruptures in the therapeutic relationship. Our emphasis in this section of the chapter is on the first two of these functions (skills coaching and emergency crisis intervention) in the context of self-injurious behavior.

In keeping with the principle of not reinforcing suicidal behavior, an adolescent client should be emphatically encouraged to contact the therapist *prior* to any such behavior. Adult clients in DBT are not allowed to call their therapists for 24 hours *after* a self-harm act (unless the injuries are life-threatening). This rule is not appropriate for adolescents, for several reasons. Since adolescents are minors, it is unwise to entrust them with handling the aftereffects of suicidal behavior. They may not be aware of, or have access to, resources for help (e.g., emergency phone numbers). They are less able than adults to determine the level of lethality of their behavior, and their parents may not know what has occurred. Therapists should, however, explain to adolescents the futility of contacting them afterward and use commitment strategies from the outset of treatment toward this end. Here is how Jessica's therapist oriented her to the guidelines for this type of phone call:

> "Jessica, when you have an urge to harm or kill yourself, I want you first to attempt to use skills you are learning in group. However, if those do not help, I want you to page me for coaching before you harm yourself. It does no good to call me afterward, since you already decided how to solve your problem in that moment, and there is nothing I can do at that point, right?" [Jessica: "I guess so."] "You see, if you recognize your distress early enough and call me before it gets too intense, we can work together at identifying some alternatives besides self-harm or suicide."

In this example, the therapist did not formally employ the 24-hour rule; rather, he strongly discouraged calling afterwards by pointing out its ineffectiveness. And although we recommend that therapists should not employ a policy against contact following a suicide attempt or NSIB by adolescents, they should make every effort not to reinforce such behavior if clients do contact them afterward.

Responding to a Suicide Attempt or NSIB That Has Already Occurred

Earlier in this chapter, we have shown how a primary therapist handles an adolescent who reports during a therapy session that he or she has already engaged in suicide attempts or NSIB. On the phone, however, the main goals are more narrowly defined: to assess the medical lethality of the act, to ensure that the adolescent receives any needed medical attention, and (when possible) to inform a family member, while trying hard not to reinforce the self-injurious behavior. Issues of confidentiality with adolescents regarding suicidal behavior are discussed in Chapter 9.

One week after Jessica's therapist instructed her to call before engaging in any self-injurious behavior, Jessica called her therapist at 1 A.M. The call followed an episode of self-cutting, and the conversation went as follows:

THERAPIST: Hello?

JESSICA: Hi, Dr. M., it's me Jessica.

THERAPIST: Hi Jessica, what's going on?

JESSICA: Well, Jason [boyfriend] really pissed me off because we planned to spend the weekend together, and then he came over, we had sex, and then he told me he was going to hang out with his friends tomorrow. . . .

THERAPIST: So, Jessica, what are you calling about right now?

JESSICA: Well, I cut myself a few minutes ago.

THERAPIST: Oh, I see (*withholding warmth*). So where did you cut yourself, and with what?

JESSICA: I cut my ankle with a pin.

THERAPIST: Are you bleeding?

JESSICA: Yeah, but not that bad . . . it's basically stopped.

THERAPIST: Well, I can tell you had a fight with Jason, which made you upset. But since you already cut yourself, there is nothing I can do at the moment. Are you having more urges to cut now?

JESSICA: No . . . I am just angry.

THERAPIST: OK, then we'll talk about the situation when I see you on Thursday. Remember, if you have new urges, call me *before* you hurt yourself, OK?

JESSICA: OK.

THERAPIST: So what are you going to do now?

JESSICA: I guess I can go out into the living room and talk to my friend Elaine.

THERAPIST: Sounds like a good idea. That should help decrease your anger. Good night.

In this situation, the therapist was careful not to reinforce the client for calling afterward. Consequently, he withheld warmth and conducted a quick assessment of the NSIB's medical severity. Once he heard it was not severe, and that the client had a plan to help herself deescalate further, he clarified the phone-calling principles and said goodbye.

If Jessica had engaged in intentional suicidal behavior, the phone call might have gone as follows:

THERAPIST: Hello?

JESSICA: Hi, Dr. M., it's Jessica.

THERAPIST: Hi, Jessica, what's going on?

JESSICA: Well . . . I had such a big fight with my boyfriend, and I feel like I want to die . . . and I just took some pills.

THERAPIST: You took pills? What did you take, and how many?

JESSICA: I just swallowed a whole bottle of my mother's imipramine [known by medical professionals to be lethal in overdose]. I just want to go to sleep, and I don't ever want to wake up.

THERAPIST: Jessica, how many pills were in the bottle?

JESSICA: I don't know . . . a handful. I just took them all.

THERAPIST: How long ago did you take them?

JESSICA: Just now . . . right before I called you. Jason [boyfriend] said I'm a bitch, and I just walked out and went to the bathroom and there they were . . . right in the medicine cabinet. I hung up on him and I hate him and . . .

THERAPIST: Listen—I know you must be really upset, and we will talk about all of this later, but what we need to do right now is to get you medically evaluated. Are you willing to do that?

JESSICA: I don't know; I guess so.

THERAPIST: Is your mother at home now?

JESSICA: Yeah, but she's sleeping.

THERAPIST: I want you to go wake her up and tell her that you took the pills and that you have to get to a hospital—either go to the emergency room or call an ambulance.

JESSICA: I can't tell her I took her pills! She'll be so mad and so freaked out!

THERAPIST: I know she might be upset, but you need to tell her right away. Take the phone to her room, and I will listen as you tell her.

JESSICA: OK . . . I guess . . .

THERAPIST: Go ahead. You can do this. I'll be right here with you.

JESSICA: OK. (*Therapist hears Jessica tell her mother. Mother anxiously agrees to call 911.*)

THERAPIST: Good. Now can you let me speak with her for a minute, so I can be sure she's clear on what's going on?

JESSICA: OK.

MOTHER: Hello? Dr. M.?

THERAPIST: Hi. Just checking in that we're clear about the plan, given what just happened.

MOTHER: Yes, she told me she took the pills, and I'm gonna get her right to the hospital.

THERAPIST: OK, good. You can tell the EMS personnel and the doctor at the ER that she told me that she overdosed on your bottle of imipramine. Please feel free to have the ER doctor page me to discuss the situation further, and I will speak to you later as well.

Here, the therapist quickly determined that there was high medical risk and immediately focused on ensuring that the client would get medical attention. He not only asked Jessica to inform her mother, but also confirmed himself that the mother was aware of the situation and in agreement with the plan. If the mother had not been present, the therapist would have either had to stay in close touch with Jessica as she called an ambulance for herself (and followed up to be sure), or himself sent an ambulance to her residence. For these occasions, it is always important for a therapist working with a suicidal client to have the client's home address and phone number easily accessible at all times, in case the client hangs up or in case an ambulance needs to be sent to the client's home.

Regardless of whether a client engages in NSIB or makes a suicide attempt, the therapist should conduct a detailed behavior analysis in the following session, being sure to include an analysis and problem solving regarding why no contact with the therapist was initiated *prior* to the suicidal behavior or NSIB (this lack of contact would be considered not only a life-threatening behavior, but a therapy-interfering behavior).

Responding to Imminent Suicidal Behavior

When an adolescent calls, as instructed, *before* any act of self-injurious behavior, the therapist is reinforcing (e.g., brighter affect, verbally reinforcing the client for calling in advance) and willing to stay on the phone longer to carry out suicidal crisis intervention strategies. These steps begin with *assessing the risk of suicide or self-harm*. A risk assessment involves obtaining information about the risk factors listed in Table 8.5.

Once a risk assessment has been conducted and it has been determined that there is a genuine threat, the therapist removes or convinces the client to remove lethal items; emphatically instructs the client *not* to engage in self-injury or commit suicide; maintains that suicide is not a good idea; generates hopeful statements and solutions; keeps contact and keeps to the treatment plan; anticipates a recurrence of the suicidal urges; and reminds the client of the limits on confidentiality (see Chapter 9). Treatment planning will then need to occur, as outlined in Table 8.6. Regardless of the mode, it is important to determine whether the suicidal behavior is operant or respondent to inform the intervention (Linehan, 1993a), and these points are relevant for phone calls as well. These guidelines can be summarized as follows:

Behavior is respondent when it is automatically elicited by a situation or specific stimulus event. The behavior is under the control of the preceding events, not of the consequences. With respect to suicidal behavior, the behavioral paradigm is that of escape learning. That is, suicidal responses are viewed as escape behaviors elicited by aversive conditions, such as traumatic events or physical or emotional pain. When Shneidman (1996) proposes that the universal precipitant of suicidal behavior is unbearable perturbation, he is proposing that suicidal behavior should be conceived of as respondent. Suicidal ideation and urges elicited by extreme hopelessness and by serious depression are examples here.

When the suicidal behavior is operant, it is under the control of the consequences. Operant behaviors function to affect the environment. When suicidal ideation and threats function to get others actively involved—for instance, to get help, get others to take one seriously, get

TABLE 8.5. Assessment of Imminent Risk for Suicidal Behaviors: Factors to Consider

Direct indices

Suicide threats
Suicide planning and/or preparation
NSIB in the last year
Suicidal ideation

Indirect indices

Client belongs to a high-risk group for suicide or NSIB
Recent disruption or loss of interpersonal relationship
Negative environmental changes in past month
Indifference to or dissatisfaction with therapy; elopements and early pass returns by hospitalized
    clients
Current hopelessness, anger, or both
Recent medical care
Indirect references to own death; arrangements for death

Circumstances associated with suicidal behaviors and/or NSIB in the next several hours/days

Alcohol consumption
Suicide note written or in progress
Methods available or easily obtained
Isolation
Precautions against discovery or intervention (deception or concealment about timing, place, etc.)
Recent media publicity about a suicide[a]
Recent suicide in school or neighborhood[a]

Note. Adapted from Linehan (1981). Copyright 1981 by Routledge Publishing Inc. Adapted by permission.

[a]The phenomenon of copycat suicides is an adolescent but not an adult risk factor (Velting & Gould, 1997).

TABLE 8.6. Treatment Planning for Suicidal Behaviors

If suicidal behavior is respondent:

Stop eliciting events; teach skills for preventing events, teach skills for coping with events.

If suicidal behavior is operant:

Respond with slightly aversive, natural contingency; do not reinforce; pull for improved behavior before intervening; do not actively intervene to prevent self-injurious behavior unless medical risk is high.

Be flexible in considering response options.

Be more active when suicide risk is high.

Base nonconservative response on failure of conservative responses.

Be honest about reasons for responses.

Note. Data from Linehan (1993a).

others to solve problems, gain admission to a hospital, and so on (assuming that these outcomes are not neutral)—the behavior is functionally operant. The notion of suicidal behavior as a "cry for help" popularized by Farberow and Shneidman (1961) is an example of such behavior as operant. It is extremely important for the therapist not to *assume* suicidal behavior is operant or respondent. Assessment is crucial.

The two transcripts below provide examples of how to handle a phone call made prior to suicidal behavior.

THERAPIST: Hello?

JESSICA: Hi, Dr. M., this is Jessica.

THERAPIST: Hi, Jessica, what's going on?

JESSICA: Well, my mother is being critical of me again, and I am feeling so bad about myself, I want to die. I told my mom how I was feeling, and she told me to call you. I was thinking about taking my father's gun to shoot myself. . . .

THERAPIST: Jessica, have you found the gun yet?

JESSICA: No, it's at my father's house. I decided to call you. . . .

THERAPIST: Jessica, I am glad you decided that . . . especially when you are obviously in emotion mind. What did your mother do when you told her how you were feeling?

JESSICA: She said she was sorry and that she would try not to be so critical.

THERAPIST: That's good news. Were you able to try any skills yet?

JESSICA: No (*starts crying*).

THERAPIST: OK, so what's happening right now that is causing you to feel suicidal?

JESSICA: My mother's pissed off at me, since I don't help around the house and I'm screwing up in school. . . . She tells me I am ruining her life!

THERAPIST: OK, obviously you and your mom are having some problems, and that can't feel good to have your mom saying those things to you. And it doesn't help that she says she is sorry just after you tell her you want to kill yourself! We will have to work on getting her to say that when you are using your skills. So what skills have you learned to help you cope with a crisis?

JESSICA: I don't know, like some distress tolerance skills?

THERAPIST: Exactly. Which ones do you remember?

JESSICA: Umm, like ACCEPTS or self-soothe?

THERAPIST: Very good! You have used ACCEPTS skills to distract yourself before, and they seem to have helped. Do you remember?

JESSICA: Yes. One time I called a friend, another time I went online, and last time I went outside and played basketball.

THERAPIST: Did they all help distract you from your distress long enough that you didn't try to hurt or kill yourself?

JESSICA: Yes.

THERAPIST: OK, so can you try one of those you just mentioned?

JESSICA: Well, I feel like crap and don't want to play basketball.

THERAPIST: OK, what else?

JESSICA: I guess I could call my friend Elaine and talk to her . . . she's usually very supportive.

THERAPIST: What if she's not available, or you still have urges after you talk to her?

JESSICA: I could go online and instant-message some of my other friends who I know are always on their computers.

THERAPIST: Good. What else?

JESSICA: I could watch a funny movie. My sister has a few DVDs I could watch.

THERAPIST: Jessica, excellent job. I know you are upset about your mother, and we obviously will discuss this more when I see you, but right now I want you to avoid your mother, and first call Elaine. Then, if you need to or want to, go online and e-mail your other friends. And if after that you need to or want to watch a movie, go for it. If after you try all of those things and you are still feeling suicidal, feel free to page me again. OK? And, lastly, will you commit to not seeking out the gun or any other means to harm yourself until I meet with you?

JESSICA: Yes, I promise.

THERAPIST: So is that a plan?

JESSICA: OK. Let me call Elaine right now. Thanks.

In the example above, Jessica's suicidal urge appears to have been operant (e.g., expressing her urge to her mother softened her). The following approaches were emphasized: The therapist assessed the consequences of Jessica's telling her mother she was feeling suicidal, pointed out that the mother was reinforcing suicidal behaviors, took extra care to refrain from reinforcing the urge, and strongly reinforced Jessica's mention of other alternatives. The therapist might also have highlighted the potential negative consequences, and might have applied a slight aversive (withholding warmth while discussing the suicidal thinking, yet still balancing this with warmth and other reinforcement with regard to her reaching out before engaging in the behavior).

The next example illustrates a very dangerous situation, in which a client has a definite plan for suicide and a high-lethality means is readily available.

THERAPIST: Hello?

JESSICA: Hi, Dr. M., this is Jessica.

THERAPIST: Hi Jessica, what's going on?

JESSICA: Well, my mother is being critical of me again, and I am feeling so bad about myself. She started yelling at me, and I just want to go away and not be here any more.

THERAPIST: What do you mean, "not be here any more"?

JESSICA: Well, you know.

THERAPIST: Are you thinking of suicide?

JESSICA: Well, I have my father's gun on my bed, and I want to use it. I know I promised to call you before I did anything. So I want to tell you goodbye. You won't be mad at me, will you?

THERAPIST: Jessica, is the gun loaded?

JESSICA: Yes, of course.

THERAPIST: Where are your parents now?

JESSICA: Oh, my father is over at his house, and my mother is watching TV. She doesn't even care that she has ruined my life (*crying*).

THERAPIST: Are you in your room?

JESSICA: Yeah. Oh, Dr. M., I just can't stand it any more, I just can't. I don't fit in this family. They would all be better off without me. No one loves me and . . .

THERAPIST: Jessica, I want to help, you but it is hard to do that when you are sitting there with a loaded gun on your bed that could kill you. How about taking the gun down to your mom and . . .

JESSICA: *No!* I'm going to shoot myself right now if you make me take it to my mom.

THERAPIST: OK, Jessica, how about putting it down on the floor just outside of your room, just while we talk? Are you willing to do that?

JESSICA: Why? What if my mother sees it?

THERAPIST: Well, it is hard for both of us to focus on figuring out what to do to make things better if you are sitting there with a gun right next to you.

JESSICA: Why does it matter exactly where the gun is when I am talking to you?

THERAPIST: Well, you could pick it up impulsively when that is not even what you necessarily want to do. Putting it outside your room gives us some space to work on what is going on right now with you. You wouldn't want to accidentally die, would you? (*Long pause*) That's pretty serious. (*Long pause*) Don't you think it would be a good idea to give yourself some time to be sure that's what you want to do?

JESSICA: I guess so. But I don't want my mother to see the gun.

THERAPIST: So put a shirt or something on top of it, and then put it outside your room while we talk.

JESSICA: OK. (*A pause while she takes the gun and shirt outside the door*)

THERAPIST: Did you put it outside your room?

JESSICA: Yes. You aren't calling Mom on another line, are you? Like your cell phone or something? My mom would get really mad.

THERAPIST: No, but, Jessica, you know that if you are having such serious problems with your mom, she would want to know about it. She would not want you to die.

JESSICA: Yes, she would. She doesn't even care. No one does (*crying*).

THERAPIST: Well, first of all, I care a whole lot. Second of all, even though your parents piss you off a fair amount, my gut tells me they love you . . . even if they don't always know how to show it to you effectively.

JESSICA: Whatever . . .

THERAPIST: Third of all, I know many of your friends love you dearly and would be devastated if you killed yourself. So let's correct that thought that "no one" cares about you, OK?

JESSICA: I really feel like that a lot!

THERAPIST: I know you do, but just because you feel that way does not mean it is necessarily true. Remember last week we discussed how when you get into emotion mind, you believe things to be facts when they are really just passing thoughts or emotions without actual data to back them up?

JESSICA: Yeah, I remember (*sounding slightly less dysregulated*).

THERAPIST: You've told me before you want to become a psychologist or a lawyer in order to help kids. So let's start now by remembering what you can do to help yourself when you're in emotion mind. You're going to need these skills later to help those kids with their own emotions. OK, so how do you get into wise mind?

JESSICA: I know, I know. . . . I have to observe and describe what I am feeling without being judgmental.

THERAPIST: So let's do it.

JESSICA: I feel sad, I feel angry . . . I hate those feelings, and I hate my mother.

THERAPIST: Yes, and you need to remember those are *feelings*. Although they are painful, they come and go. If you stay judgmental toward your mom, you will keep yourself in those emotions.

THERAPIST: How intense would you rate those emotions on a scale from 1 to 10?

JESSICA: About 5 for sadness and 6 on anger.

THERAPIST: OK. Remember one of the DBT assumptions is that people are doing the best they can, right? That includes me, you, and your mom. So even though she is pissing you off, can we assume she's doing the best she can in the moment . . . just as you are?

JESSICA: I guess so . . . I assume she's not intentionally trying to piss me off. She just becomes so critical, and she doesn't appear aware of it.

THERAPIST: Nice use of your skills. You're describing and not judging.

JESSICA: She talks that way to everyone, so I guess I shouldn't take it so personally.

THERAPIST: Right. I'm very impressed with the way you are already helping yourself return to wise mind right now. Wow!

JESSICA: Me too . . . I am already a little less upset.

THERAPIST: So are you feeling like you want to stay alive right now?

JESSICA: Yes. Boy, when I get upset, I get a little crazy.

THERAPIST: That's something we still need to work on together. Rest assured, you're going to get a whole lot better at managing your emotions more effectively. In the meantime, however, I'd like you to take your phone, take the gun, and tell your mother you were having a suicidal urge. Tell her you had enough control to contact me for coaching, which you have used extremely effectively. Then you need to tell her and your father (when he returns) that he needs to take the gun so this doesn't happen again. Finally, I'd like you to invite them in for a family session at our usual time tomorrow to discuss this issue in more depth. OK, I'll listen while you walk downstairs and explain this to her. Before you do, however, can you do two things? First, can you commit to safety until I see you again tomorrow?

JESSICA: Yes.

THERAPIST: Good. Second, are we correct in assuming that your mother might be surprised and concerned, and that it may come across as anger, when you walk downstairs and show her the gun?

JESSICA: Yes. Oh, I can't deal with that.

THERAPIST: It's difficult, but you can do this. I'll be listening in, and if she gets upset and you can't deal with it any further, pass the phone to me and I will speak with her. Later today, if you are getting upset, remember to use some of your preferred ACCEPTS and self-soothe skills and, if need be, page me again.

JESSICA: OK, I will. (*Therapist overhears Jessica describe the situation to her mother. Her mother starts yelling, "What were you thinking? I can't believe you are acting this way!" Therapist asks Jessica to put her mother on the phone.*)

THERAPIST: Hi, Mrs. L. I know this is upsetting to see your daughter with the gun that she was briefly considering using on herself. While her suicidal impulses are very concerning, she did an excellent job paging me for coaching. She has calmed down, and although I know you are upset, I would ask that you try *not* to become judgmental and angry at her, as that will discourage her from expressing her feelings or asking for help when she needs it . . . as she does now. She assured me she was going to keep herself safe until we meet tomorrow. I ask two things: First, can you and Jessica's father join the session tomorrow, so that we can discuss this situation in more depth? Second, can you promise me that you will ask Jessica's father to figure out another place to keep the gun, since, as we discussed previously, it is extremely dangerous for Jessica to have access to it when she is still depressed and intermittently suicidal?

MOTHER: Yes, Dr. M., I promise we will do something with it today. I have been telling Jessica's father, but he hasn't listened. I think today he'll do it. . . . I'll do my best to make sure of it. And we'll both be there tomorrow. Thank you for your concern and help. Goodbye.

THERAPIST: Of course. May I just say a quick goodbye to Jessica? Thank you.

In this second example, Jessica's suicidal urges appear to have been more respondent in nature, although this is not absolutely clear from the transcript. The therapist still had to be careful not to reinforce the behavior, as well as to make sure that the parents did not start reinforcing it; this was possible, now that the parents knew that Jessica's suicidal intent was more serious than they thought. Remember, respondent behavior can quickly become operant. Further clarification of whether Jessica's suicidal behavior was operant, respondent, or both could be obtained from a behavioral analysis conducted during the next individual therapy session.

During this call, the therapist worked with Jessica to help her cope with the distress, actively supporting her in identifying viable coping skills (some of which he knew she had previously used effectively). In addition, the therapist clearly reinforced Jessica for contacting him prior to engaging in suicidal behavior. Note that the therapist did not get into any depth regarding the precipitant of the suicidal ideation, other than validating that her mother's comments were hurtful. Instead, he briefly assessed the problem and moved swiftly into problem solving. Clearly, the problem solving here involved coping with the crisis at hand rather than trying to solve the family conflict with her mother. This latter problem would be addressed in more depth at the next individual or family session.

Taking phone calls from individual clients is an important and challenging aspect of DBT, in that the therapist is on call 24 hours a day, 7 days a week. Some programs elect to have a designated on-call phone coach available other than the primary therapist. Although this may be necessary in certain programs (e.g., due to union regulations), it is our strong recommendation that the primary therapist serve this function. In consulting with experts on treatment of suicidal behaviors, we have not found one who does not accept after-hours calls from suicidal clients. This is particularly important with adolescent clients. They are not always comfortable calling or paging their primary therapist for coaching, much less contacting a therapist for coaching whom they do not know. Although the primary therapist has to observe reasonable personal limits on phone calls after hours, getting a call at an inconvenient time and saving a life is obviously preferable to getting a call saying that a client has committed suicide. Even for a nonsuicidal client, not taking after-hours calls can adversely affect an important function of this modality—skill generalization. In addition to suicidal behaviors, DBT therapists offer coaching for other target behaviors as well (drug use urges, binge–purge urges, assaultive urges, etc.).

Individual therapists working with suicidal adolescents must mindfully employ case management strategies as described in Chapter 3. Given the high-risk nature of this client group, coupled with the tendency for therapist burnout, we emphasize the importance of consultation-to-the-therapist strategies.

CONSULTATION-TO-THE-THERAPIST STRATEGIES

Supervision and consultation with other therapists are integral aspects of DBT, since delivering effective treatment to suicidal clients with BPD or borderline features is so difficult. Just as a therapist applies DBT to a client, the consultation team applies DBT to the therapist. For example, the team members dialectically balance the therapist by helping him or her remain inflexible in certain circumstances and flexible in other circumstances. Through cheerleading and support, the team also helps the therapist problem-solve and generate empathic explanations of clients' and family members' behavior. In Jessica's case, the therapist, Bill, expressed his frustration to the consultation team about "Jessica's stubborn, oblivious parents." Recognizing that this comment reflected a judgmental attitude toward the family, the other team members came to Bill's assistance. One colleague asked, "Why do you think her parents are acting in this apparently uninterested way about their role in her self-injurious behavior?" Bill replied in a frustrated tone, "I don't know; they are oblivious!" The same colleague asked, "Don't you think if they could do better, they would?" "Yes," Bill replied. "OK, then. Didn't you tell me that the older sister and the mother herself had a history of suicidal behavior? And when the mother was growing up, how was that behavior handled in the family?" The discussion provided a larger context in which to evaluate how this behavior was learned and maintained in an intergenerational pattern. This discussion also helped Bill become more empathic toward the mother, who was reinforced in her family of origin for the same behavior. The team discussion enabled Bill to interact more effectively with Jessica and her family.

DBT therapists desperately need consultation, since treatment can often be arduous, slow, and stressful because of clients' frequent suicide threats and other challenging behavior. Clients can inadvertently reinforce their therapists for engaging in ineffective therapy, and punish the therapists for engaging in effective therapy. Clients often avoid analyzing their life-threatening or therapy-interfering behaviors, since they would rather have an unstructured discussion about something less emotionally aversive. It takes a lot of hard work for therapists to keep their clients and the treatments on track, especially in the face of clients' direct criticism. The consultation team sometimes has to work equally hard to support the therapists and motivate them to continue through the difficult times.

CHAPTER 9

Including Families in Treatment

Family work is important because the contingencies in the home environment often play an important role in an adolescent's dysfunctional behavior. Working with the teen's family enables the therapist to gain insight into the transactional nature of the problem behaviors and directly address the interactions among fa mily members; recognizing and highlighting these transactional relationships are crucial. The therapist also encourages parents to employ the same skills their teen is being asked to use, and ultimately to alter the ways in which they respond to their adolescent's behaviors. Through the use of various interventions, the family members are recognized as partners rather than targets in treatment; hence the family feels more connected to and supported by the therapist, through ample amounts of validation and consistent family sessions.

WORKING WITH FAMILIES WITHIN A DBT FRAMEWORK

Modes of Family Work

Family members can participate in various modes of DBT when an adolescent child is the primary client. First, family therapy sessions provide a context for the family members and the adolescent to interact in the presence of the therapist, who can offer coaching to help address current problems and conflicts. This offers a strong opportunity for skill strengthening and generalization.

Second, the skills training mode (conducted either in the multifamily skills group format or individually with a family) allows family members to learn skills simultaneously with the adolescent. This enables them not only to serve as coaches, but to acquire skills themselves that are essential to productive interactions with their child, such as regulating emotions and communicating effectively. Note that although the multifamily skills group format is typically conducted in outpatient settings, some inpatient and residential treatment settings have begun offering skills training groups for families as well. Another means of teaching family members skills is a program that teaches family members DBT skills independently of their adolescent children. In one model of such a program, the group teaches family members DBT skills and then has graduates of the program train other family members in the skills (e.g., the Family Connections program; Hoffman, 2004). In a similar program, Porr (2004) runs the skills group with family members and coteaches with her own graduates. Similar programs exist around the United States.

Sometimes it is not possible to have family members participate in a multifamily skills training group, a parents-only skills training group, or even skills training with their own individual family members (single-family skills training). In these cases, therapists might find it useful at least to orient family members to the treatment, the biosocial theory, and the skills training, through such means as one-time orientation groups, parent workshops, or support groups for family members.

Third, telephone consultation with family members helps them further with skills generalization and provides a forum for helping them through crisis situations. Again, this mode mostly applies to DBT conducted with adolescents in outpatient settings, where ongoing parent–adolescent interactions spark conflict or crisis that needs immediate intervention.

Because the skills training mode is described in depth in Chapter 10, including ample attention to familial issues, we do not describe it here. Instead, we focus in this chapter on family therapy sessions, phone consultation with family members, and handling adolescents' suicidal crises with family members; we also briefly address how to handle issues of confidentiality. First, however, we emphasize the importance of taking a nonpejorative stance toward both adolescents and their family members in all modes of family treatment.

The Nonpejorative Stance toward Adolescents and Families

It is important to assume a nonpejorative, nonblaming stance with family members as well as with adolescent clients themselves (Miller et al., 2002). Parents or caregivers of multiproblem suicidal teens often experience intense feelings of shame and failure (Miller et al., 2002). They have intense fears for the safety of their children and guilt about their role in the adolescents' difficulties. Parents who experience strong negative emotions are more likely to communicate irritation and dysphoria if they believe they are incompetent (Clarkin et al., 1990). Reducing parental emotional vulnerability may not only increase treatment compliance, but also strengthen parental capacity for learning new behavioral skills. Therefore, it is important to remember that well-meaning family members can invalidate a teen for various reasons, and that DBT assumptions for the client also apply to the family, as we will see in Chapter 10. For example, the family members are doing the best they can, and they want to do better. Moreover, parents and other family members may not in fact constitute the only or even the primary invalidating environment; school, peer, neighborhood/community, and/or cultural contexts may all play central roles in adolescents' lives and be a major source of invalidation (see Chapter 3). High levels of invalidation in these settings can have an impact on an emotionally vulnerable teen, especially if parents provide relatively low levels of validation and so do not offset them,

In addition, families often bring a history of prior treatment failures or experiences of being blamed by therapists for their adolescents' problems. Using terms such as "poorness of fit in temperaments" may facilitate a family's perception of greater acceptance. Labeling *behaviors* as invalidating, rather than labeling *families* as invalidating environments, may also reduce pejorative implications. This not only allows for a simultaneous focus on teaching adolescents to validate their families, but also may help to reduce parental perceptions of global incompetence. Observing family interactions allows the therapist to avoid blaming the parents and to develop a more synthesized and empathic view of the family behavioral patterns. Seeing the adolescent interacting within the family system fosters the therapist's understanding of the teen's emotional reactions, skills deficits, and capabilities, while concurrently understanding the family members' perspectives, skills deficits, and capabilities.

FAMILY THERAPY SESSIONS

When and Why Should Family Sessions Be Scheduled?

Family sessions are typically scheduled on an as-needed basis. In inpatient, day treatment, or residential settings, family sessions may be scheduled at regular intervals or as deemed useful, and may be the only involvement the family members have with the adolescent's treatment.

In such cases, the family therapy sessions are typically adjunctive to the adolescent's individual therapy sessions and do not replace them.

In contrast, given the fact that in most outpatient contexts the adolescent is typically receiving two sessions per week already (i.e., individual therapy and skills training), it is difficult for many families to make it to treatment for a third (family) session during the week, given time and financial constraints. One solution is to schedule a 60- to 90-minute individual session, divide it in half, and conduct the family session during the latter half. This allows the adolescent and therapist to review the diary card privately and conduct brief behavioral analyses of any target behaviors before preparing for the family session. This preparation might entail identifying any relevant target behaviors that involve the family (see below), as well as anticipating some distress and then coaching the teen to use DBT skills during the family session.

Family sessions may be indicated for various reasons: orienting parents to DBT, including psychoeducation; working to facilitate communication between the adolescent and one or more family members about an important issue; conducting a behavioral analysis of a target behavior; or handling a crisis. As a general guide, Table 9.1 lists situations in which a family session is indicated.

Who Should Be Included?

Another factor to consider in holding family sessions is which family members should be involved. Typically, primary caregivers such as biological parents or stepparents participate in family sessions and skills training. However, other primary caregivers, such as grandparents, might be included. With an adolescent client, even siblings may at times be included in the family sessions, depending on the extent of the siblings' involvement with the client and on the focus of the family therapy. As Santisteban, Muir, Mena, and Mitrani (2003) point out, younger siblings are at risk for similar behavior problems, and there is important preventive work to be done by improving the functioning of the family. They further point out that highlighting the urgency of altering the environment for the younger children can be a strong motivator for mobilizing disengaged parents. With other clients, older siblings may be included—perhaps in the role of guardians to the clients, perhaps to address sibling discord related to the clients' target behaviors, or perhaps to help to expand the clients' support network.

Addressing Stage 1 Targets of Treatment for the Family

The Stage 1 targets for treatment of individuals can be modified for family treatment. One of the most common precipitants to suicide attempts among adolescents is interpersonal conflict (Miller & Glinski, 2000). In these situations, the primary target is to *decrease family interac-*

TABLE 9.1. Indications for Scheduling a Family Session as Part of Individual Therapy with an Adolescent

1. A family member is providing a central source of conflict; the adolescent needs intensive coaching or support in attempting to resolve this conflict.
2. A crisis erupts within the family.
3. The case would be enhanced by orienting one or more family members to or educating them about a set of skills, treatment targets, or other aspects of treatment.
4. The contingencies at home continue to reinforce dysfunctional behavior or punish adaptive behavior.

tions that contribute to the adolescent's life-threatening behaviors. When a DBT therapist conducts a behavioral analysis of an adolescent's self-injurious behavior, there is often a link in the chain that relates to familial relationships, or to attitudes or beliefs within the family. This seems to be the case more often for adolescents than for adult clients.

DBT sessions also target *reduction of family or parent behaviors that interfere with the treatment.* To target only the adolescent's therapy-interfering behavior without considering the parents' therapy-interfering behavior ignores the reality that parents often have a great deal of power over the adolescent's capacity to participate in treatment. For example, parents sometimes refuse to drive or give bus fare to their adolescent, or contribute to scheduling conflicts, preventing him or her from getting to individual sessions. It is certainly worthwhile to coach adolescents in interpersonal effectiveness skills to get what they need from their parents, but if this is not effective, a more active environmental intervention should be used (i.e., the issue should be directly discussed in the next family session).

The third target is to *reduce family interactions that interfere with the family's quality of life.* The focus is on helping the family as a group function in a more effective, respectful, and loving manner. Among the most common quality-of-life targets are family communication problems. Over time, many families become chronically emotionally dysregulated. Such a family may present as continually angry or with the sense that members are continually walking on eggshells. As a result, members tend to avoid direct communication with one another for fear of aversive consequences. A DBT family therapy session must often first address skills training in validation (see below) to set the stage for future behavioral and solution analyses regarding specific family problems. Because family members are often eager to start problem solving, it is important to orient families to the rationale for teaching validation and interpersonal effectiveness skills before problem solving begins. Anecdotally, this has been one of the most important discoveries we have made in conducting DBT family sessions.

The fourth target, which is related to the first three, is to *increase the family's behavioral skills*—particularly in terms of validation, direct communication, and finding a "middle path" for parent–adolescent dilemmas. For example, the standard DBT interpersonal effectiveness skills can be taught to the entire family. It might also be helpful for the parents to have training in specific parenting skills, such as how to develop house rules or use effective reinforcement and punishment. It has been our experience that teaching family members how to validate one another is the most crucial interpersonal skill for improving their relationships; thus, in addition to teaching it in the Interpersonal Effectiveness module, we highlight it in the Walking the Middle Path module. Role plays and family homework assignments help families to practice and generalize this invaluable part of the treatment. Note that if family members participate in skills training (in group or individual-family format), they will learn the DBT skills, but family sessions provide a forum for additional skill strengthening through coaching and *in vivo* practice.

Dialectical Dilemmas and Secondary Treatment Targets

Dialectical dilemmas (see Chapter 5) abound in work with suicidal adolescents and their families, because of the transactional nature of relationships and the resultant development of certain dysfunctional behavioral patterns. Highlighting a dialectical framework not only serves as a treatment strategy, but provides the foundation for a common language that is learned and regularly employed in sessions.

Once a dialectical dilemma or polarizing behavior pattern is identified and labeled, the challenge is often "What do we do now?" Finding a synthesis to these behavioral extremes, known to clients and families as "finding the middle path," is the task at hand. As described in

Chapter 5, each dialectical dilemma has corresponding treatment targets. For example, consider the extreme behavior pattern of excessive leniency versus authoritarian control with regard to the case of Jessica, discussed in earlier chapters. Jessica and her mother experienced conflict over Jessica's repeated violations of her curfew. Jessica believed that the curfew times were unreasonable, and stated that they prevented her from spending time with her friends. Her mother found herself vacillating: She was sometimes overly restrictive with the curfew (e.g., having Jessica come home immediately after school), but at other times she felt guilty and wished to avoid relationship tension, and thus she allowed Jessica to break curfew with no consequence or even to abandon the curfew altogether. This vacillation gave Jessica the message that the curfew was arbitrary and not to be taken seriously.

To help the family achieve a middle path, the therapist helped the family with the targets of (1) increasing authoritative (not authoritarian) discipline while decreasing excessive leniency, and (2) increasing adolescent self-determination while decreasing authoritarian control. In Jessica's family session, the therapist first used simple terms to clarify the dialectic (i.e., "being too loose" vs. "being too strict") and the tension it caused. Next the therapist elicited the perspectives of both Jessica and her mother, and modeled contextualizing and validating both viewpoints and sets of feelings (i.e., "Jessica, it is perfectly understandable that you want to hang out with your friends, and it is also reasonable that your mom wants to know that you are safe"). The goal here was then to get Jessica and her mother to validate each other directly. In this case, the DBT therapist coached both Jessica and her mother in interpersonal effectiveness skills so each could clearly express her feelings and wishes, make their viewpoints understood, and then validate the other's feelings, The ultimate goals with any polarized behavior pattern are to (1) help the parents and adolescent increase their problem-solving skills so they can find a synthesis between their opposing viewpoints, and (2) help the individual vacillating between extremes to find an effective middle ground that allows for more consistency in behaviors. So, for example, Jessica's therapist provided psychoeducation regarding parenting skills (e.g., consistent rules and consequences), suggested the use of positive reinforcement when Jessica came home on time, and encouraged flexibility in the curfew if and when Jessica acted more responsibly.

In sum, the original targets of standard DBT can be modified for family sessions, with the first priority always being the adolescent's life-threatening behaviors. However, the emphasis of the family targets is on the interactions between family members, rather than on individual behavior. It is important to note that while family interactions can contribute to the problem behaviors, family relationships can also be a source of strength and change that can help the adolescent cope with dysregulated affect.

The Family Behavioral Analysis

As a general rule, a family behavioral analysis provides a tool for highlighting both adaptive and maladaptive patterns of family interactions and determining potentially effective change strategies. Such an analysis is conducted when a family member is directly involved in an adolescent's life-threatening, therapy-interfering, or quality-of-life-interfering behavior (Miller et al., 2002). A behavioral analysis with a family involves eliciting the emotions, thoughts, and actions of family members that relate to an adolescent's targeted behavior. Conducting a behavioral analysis during a family session requires input from every family member present, to help elucidate the links in the chain of the behaviors that lead to or reinforce the adolescent's problem behavior This is not to say, however, that every family session requires a *formal* behavioral analysis. Sometimes a brief assessment of the interaction patterns is sufficient, and the remaining time can be spent on *in vivo* skills coaching.

Prior to the family session, it may be especially helpful for the therapist to prepare and coach the adolescent on being effective during the session, including anticipating what is likely to go wrong and how to handle it. The first time a behavioral analysis takes place with a family, the therapist should orient the family members to the procedure and its purpose. It can be confusing to elicit a detailed story from two or three people at once. Ground rules can be established, such as the following: Others may chime in to add a detail, but such chiming in should not cut someone off or otherwise be done in a rude manner; descriptive remarks are condoned, but derogatory or hostile remarks should be avoided; everyone will get a chance to comment and offer his or her viewpoint; offering an alternative viewpoint should be seen as a clarification and opportunity for understanding rather than a provocation. The therapist should then collaboratively establish, based on the hierarchy above, the target for the family behavioral analysis, and can ask one family member whether he or she wishes to start; often this person will be the adolescent. The process then proceeds similarly to an individual behavioral analysis (see Chapter 8), except that the family members in the room each share their perspectives or experiences of the various links. Note that observation of family interactions in session during the chain analysis can also help the therapist confirm or disconfirm contingent interactions.

For example, to begin a discussion of events antecedent to her self-harm behavior, Jessica told her father how upset she had been about an argument with her boyfriend. Her father, in an attempt to soothe her, had inadvertently said something that she experienced as invalidating ("Don't worry, you'll get over it"). Jessica then ruminated about how misunderstood she felt, which intensified her anger. Later in the evening when her father spoke with her, she cursed at him. In his mind, her angry response seemed to come from "out of the blue." He screamed back at her, and so on, until Jessica cut herself in order to numb her intense feelings of anger and frustration at feeling misunderstood.

The therapist would first identify the transactional nature of family interactions in this chain. Then, among other things, the therapist might work with the father to help him realize the strong impact this type of invalidation had on his daughter. He might work with Jessica to help her modify her assumption that parents "should" always understand her. He might work with both of them to increase their validating comments to one another. He might also have family members use interpersonal effectiveness skills to communicate without resorting to screaming matches, and apply distress tolerance skills to tolerate their frustration without acting impulsively on it. Role plays are an excellent means of achieving mastery over these new approaches.

The consequences of the target behavior are equally important to highlight in a family behavioral analysis. During the course of such an analysis, one therapist discovered that an adolescent client would stomp around, scream, and hit her father—who would then grab her, go up to her room, get her Kleenex, and sit by her, holding her hand and helping her process her troubles. Similarly, another adolescent would cut herself and spill blood all over the bathroom and bedroom, and then her mother would clean it up. In both of these examples, the well-meaning parents were reinforcing strongly maladaptive behaviors.

In such a case, the therapist needs to work out a plan with the parents in which they either reduce attention to the destructive behaviors or respond with slight aversive consequences, while communicating to the adolescent that they will attend positively to adaptive behaviors (i.e., contingency clarification). Contingency management skills need to be highlighted for the family members, so that they can learn how not to reinforce problem behaviors. In general, these skills include positive and negative reinforcement, extinction, shaping, and effective punishment. Note that it is impossible for parents to completely ignore an adolescent's suicidal threats or self-injurious behavior; nor should they completely ignore them.

The dialectical balance that needs to be maintained here is responding appropriately to real danger, while not overresponding to all such behavior so that danger is increased.

In yet another case, a family behavior analysis revealed parental consequences that were problematic because the parents were repeatedly nonattentive or punitive in response to *appropriate* behavior, contributing to the learning history of their 18-year-old daughter. For example, the daughter had told them that her older sister, who apparently had antisocial tendencies, had physically attacked her; she even showed them the bruises, trying to elicit their help and protection. They had dismissed her, blaming her for "starting trouble" and stating that the older sister "had enough problems."[1] Her efforts to communicate distress to them were eventually extinguished by this and similar episodes of invalidation, and by the time they entered therapy, she had withdrawn from them. The behavioral analysis revealed the daughter's feelings of hopelessness about her parents as sources of support, as well as mistrust of their motives. Present sources of distress, then, would not only affect her in their own right but also cause secondary emotions of intense hurt and anger, because she could not talk to her parents. Instead, she resorted to regularly piercing her arms and eyebrows with safety pins to regulate emotion, and to getting validation from a drug-addicted but supportive boyfriend. During the solution analysis portion of the session, the therapist worked to increase the parents' understanding of their daughter's mistrust, withdrawal, and distress. He also encouraged them to pay more attention to their daughter and take her seriously. He worked with the daughter as well, coaching her to use distress tolerance skills.

The Family Crisis Plan

Developing a family crisis plan during a family session can help prevent future episodes of self-destructive or maladaptive behavior. For example, the initial part of a crisis plan for Jessica's family might go as follows: The next time Jessica's father saw that Jessica was becoming increasingly angry, he could first try to coach her to use distress tolerance skills. If the father himself was still unfamiliar with these skills, he might call the skills trainer for guidance on how to coach his daughter. Or he might strongly urge Jessica to page her own therapist directly for coaching. A crisis plan should also include several other options—including, in this case, taking Jessica to the emergency room if none of the other strategies worked. It is often helpful to have someone in the family write down the crisis plan and have everyone read, sign, and be familiar with it. The crisis plan often brings distressed families an immense sense of relief, because it provides them with a clear course of action during a chaotic and frightening time.

PHONE CONSULTATION WITH FAMILY MEMBERS

When involving family members in treatment, we have found it helpful to provide them with phone coaching as an additional mode of treatment. In phone coaching with an adolescent's family member, it is crucial to assign the role of phone coach to someone *other than* the adolescent's primary therapist—to avoid the problem of dual roles, the threat to therapeutic trust, and the potential violation of confidentiality. The skills trainer or coleader (if this person is not also the primary therapist) is an excellent choice for this role, since this person knows the fam-

---

[1]Note that because of this adolescent's age (she was not a minor), combined with the fact that the sibling's physical aggression was apparently confined to an isolated incident and was not ongoing, the therapist did not report the parents for neglect.

ily members yet does not hold a "privileged" relationship with the adolescent. In situations in which the primary therapist is also the skills trainer, and there is not a second skills trainer, we suggest caution in using the primary therapist as parental phone coach. In such a case, both the adolescent and parents must be oriented to the situation. In order to preserve trust with the adolescent, ground rules must be set. These ground rules ought to include the following: (1) The adolescent will be informed when parents have called; (2) if an adolescent and a parent call at approximately the same time, or regarding the same situation, the adolescent's call will take precedence; and (3) no details about the adolescent's treatment will be disclosed during a phone call with a parent. Whenever possible, however, we strongly advise having a separate therapist available for family member skills coaching. The dual role is rife with possibilities for feelings of betrayal on the adolescent's part.

We suggest that the purposes of phone consultation with family members should be *in vivo* skills coaching (including coaching through crisis situations) and, if needed, relationship repair with the skills trainer. Relationship repair, in which the phone contact can be initiated by either a parent or the skills trainer, is important so that family members (much like teens in treatment), do not ruminate until the next session about perceived slights, misunderstandings, or other difficulties in the therapeutic relationship. For example, in one group skills training session, a parent felt put on the spot by the skills trainer when asked to use skills to address a conflict with her son. The skills trainer could see her distress and followed up with a phone call to repair the relationship, which the mother very much appreciated. Note that phone contact for the purpose of reporting good news is not recommended with parents, although it is used with adolescents (since with parents there is not the same need to break the pairing of increased telephone contact with suicidal crisis).

HANDLING SUICIDAL CRISES

Involvement of Family Members in Suicidal Crises

When an adolescent is in a suicidal crisis, the therapist must consider the family, as well as the primary client. In addition to having rights concerning the adolescent as a minor child, parents sometimes provide the major context in which the adolescent's crisis behaviors occur. At the very least, parents are brought in so that their child's disorder can be explained to them and so they can work on minimizing any invalidation. Beyond this, parents can be helpful by providing additional sets of eyes and ears to monitor the client during times of crisis. They can also help alter the eliciting and maintaining events surrounding the crisis. If parents are part of the problem related to the crisis situation or are interfering with therapy, family sessions can be helpful in addressing these problems. If parents are generally helpful, they can be brought in to find ways to maximize their helpfulness in a particular crisis situation.

Santisteban et al. (2003) discuss general DBT family therapy strategies that lend themselves well to crisis situations, including identifying family interaction patterns that tend to create barriers to the effective use of skills; preparing the adolescent for family sessions, particularly by inoculating the adolescent against the family interactions that typically trigger emotion dysregulation; educating the parents about the adolescent's vulnerability to emotion and behavior dysregulation; helping parents to empathize, nonjudgmentally, with the emotional pain driving the adolescent's extreme behaviors; preparing parents to expect "ups and downs," so that they can stay more consistently connected; reducing invalidating and increase validating communications; increasing the size of the adolescent's support network; and modifying family interactions to reinforce adaptive and not reinforce maladaptive behaviors. Based on suggestions of Santisteban et al. (2003), standard DBT strategies, and our clinical experience with including families in treatment, Table 9.2 highlights useful crisis intervention targets with families.

Santisteban et al. (2003) also recommends steps for the therapist to take regarding family work within an inpatient setting when the adolescent has been hospitalized for suicidal behavior. These include holding meetings with the adolescent and family members within the setting; scheduling family sessions prior to discharge, both to address the transition to home and to plan for increased monitoring and safety; and reframing the hospitalization crisis as a step in the treatment process and as a potential springboard toward more adaptive functioning.

In general, the first family members to involve during a crisis are those directly involved in the adolescent's treatment (i.e., through skills training and as-needed family sessions). These family members already share a focus on the adolescent's treatment outcome, and are typically already versed in the nature of the teen's disorder and the DBT approach. They also usually already have some relationship with the primary therapist. However, at times other family members might be brought in. First, if the setting is one in which parents are not routine participants in treatment, they might nevertheless be brought in when a crisis situation develops. Second, if family members are participating in treatment, but a family member who has not been participating is playing a major role in the crisis, this member might be brought in. Third, if the therapist determines that a person not routinely involved with the client's therapy might be particularly helpful in supporting the adolescent during the crisis, this person might be brought in. In addition to parents and stepparents, who are typically the primary

TABLE 9.2. Targets of Intervention for Family Sessions in Crisis Situations

- Prepare the adolescent for family interactions.
  - Identify goals of the family meeting.
  - Consider possible familial sources of the adolescent's emotion dysregulation.
  - Rehearse effective skill use, including ways to handle the adolescent's emotion dysregulation in the family session.
  - Anticipate difficulties and troubleshoot.
- Increase parental understanding of the adolescent's emotional vulnerability.
  - Provide psychoeducation regarding emotion dysregulation.
  - Help parents to increase their empathy for the adolescent's pain while decreasing judgmental reactions.
- Address the parents' emotional dysregulation.
  - Anticipate despair, anxiety, and other strong emotional reactions from parents.
  - Validate parents' distress and concerns.
  - Cheerlead parents' ability to get through the crisis.
- Improve communication between the adolescent and family members.
  - Increase validating and decrease invalidating communication.
  - Decrease negativity in family interactions.
  - Increase use of behavioral skills.
- Modify contingencies in the familial environment.
  - Increase parental responsiveness during noncrisis periods.
  - Increase reinforcement of adaptive and decrease reinforcement of maladaptive behaviors.
- Take steps to keep the adolescent safe.
  - Provide psychoeducation to parents regarding risk assessment.
  - Increase parental monitoring of the adolescent.
  - Devise a detailed plan to keep the adolescent safe.
  - Anticipate crisis recurrence and stay in touch.

people involved in adolescents' treatment, we have on occasion held conjoint sessions with grandparents, godparents, boyfriends/girlfriends, and siblings.

Getting the Family Members Involved with the Crisis Plan

Engaging family members in a crisis plan generally involves a combination of soothing, validating, cheerleading, and providing psychoeducation to the parents. In addition, the therapist can apply the standard DBT crisis strategies and treatment-planning considerations, as outlined below.

Soothing and Validating

In most crisis situations, the therapist can expect the parents to be alarmed and emotionally dysregulated themselves. They may be eager to help or take charge, but may have little idea what they might do. The therapist must remember to take time to focus on the parents' needs and reactions as well as the client's, since the parents will be the major components of the environment to which the adolescent in crisis is exposed. Not only does the therapist want to avoid having the parents' responses exacerbate the crisis, but the parents will be needed to cooperate with a crisis plan. At the very least, the therapist may rely on the parents to bring the adolescent in to his or her next appointment and not interfere in the adolescent's attendance at this time. If time and circumstances permit it, the therapist should assess the parents' concerns and beliefs regarding the crisis situation. The therapist should validate the parents' emotional reactions and their perceptions of how difficult the situation is, while reinforcing any statements or actions on the parents' part that will be helpful in dealing with the crisis.

Cheerleading

Providing cheerleading to parents in such situations is important as well. For example, parents may feel overwhelmed and hopeless. Statements indicating a belief in the parents' ability to get through this crisis, handle it (with the therapist's help), and do what is needed can greatly encourage emotionally depleted parents.

Psychoeducation

A major step in securing the parents' involvement in the crisis plan will involve psychoeducation. Although the focus of the psychoeducation will be particular to the circumstances, it often concerns such topics as biosocial theory, emotion dysregulation, principles of learning, and validation. In addition, the therapist can educate the parents to apply many of the standard DBT crisis strategies (Linehan, 1993a). For example, parents can pay attention to their teen's affect rather than to the content of a situation. This can be important to teach parents, since parents may see the adolescent's affect as a prototypical expression of adolescent moodiness or overreactivity and thus may not take the response seriously. Parents can also explore the current (not past) problem; focus on problem solving; focus on affect tolerance; get commitment to a plan of action; assess suicide potential (parents may need the therapist to provide questions for them to ask their teen, such as whether the teen intends to commit suicide and has the means to do so, whether the teen feels able to refrain from self-harm, or whether the teen needs to page the therapist; Table 8.5, which lists signs of imminent risk, may be helpful here); and anticipate a recurrence of the crisis response and therefore closely monitor their child. These strategies are further expanded upon below, and we provide an example of a therapist's incorporating these steps into a family session.

Standard DBT Crisis Strategies and Treatment-Planning Considerations

The first DBT crisis strategy (Linehan, 1993a) concerns *paying attention to affect rather than content*. For example, if a highly distressed client says, "My parents grounded me again, and I want to die!", the therapist would pay attention to the suicidal thoughts and the related emotions rather than the issue of grounding. A crisis is not the time to focus on historical factors, but rather to *explore the current problem* by trying to identify key precipitants of the current crisis. Not only should the adolescent not focus on distal events, but parents should be dissuaded from bringing up historical factors as well. In staying present-focused, the therapist can guide the teen and family through *problem solving* to address some of the precipitating factors or to *tolerate the affect* generated by the precipitants. Note that the therapist might have to work with family members to tolerate the intense affect experienced during times of crisis, so as not to exacerbate the situation by reacting with panic or criticism. Once problem solving has occurred, key precipitants have been identified, and strategies to tolerate painful affect have been selected, the therapist must *obtain commitment to a plan of action*. This plan of action must include a series of steps that will enable all parties to get through the crisis situation by coping with or tolerating it, without engaging in self-harm or doing something to make the situation worse. It should also include troubleshooting—that is, anticipating where the plan is likely to go wrong, and planning what to do then. As discussed further below, with adolescents, family members will often be involved in this plan. *Assessing suicide potential* (including finding out about intent and access to lethal means, and considering the client's history) will be important in developing the plan of action. Imminent risk factors (see Table 8.5) should be considered in determining the potential for suicide. Finally, the therapist needs to *anticipate a recurrence of the crisis response*, and therefore to remain in contact with the client—and, ideally, involve the parents in monitoring the adolescent as well.

In addition to these crisis strategies, standard DBT includes treatment-planning considerations for suicidal behaviors (Linehan, 1993a). These considerations vary, depending on whether the suicidal behavior is respondent or operant in nature (see Table 8.6). If functional assessment indicates that the suicidal behavior is respondent, or primarily elicited by antecedents, the therapist works to change the nature of these eliciting events, teach skills for preventing such events, or teach skills for coping with the events. If assessment indicates that the suicidal behavior appears to be operant, or primarily controlled by consequences, the therapist responds by not reinforcing and by pulling improved behavior from the client before intervening. Note that the therapist often involves family members in these treatment-planning considerations as well.

An example of applying these crisis strategies and treatment-planning considerations involved an 18-year-old client in her third month of an unplanned pregnancy, whose parents had called to ask whether they could come in for a family session because of a crisis situation in which the adolescent was stating that she wanted to die, following a family argument about living arrangements. She was notably tearful and agitated. *Paying attention to her affect*, the therapist assessed her suicidal ideation, intention, and plans. The client then began a verbal tirade, attacking her father for years of past difficulties in their relationship. Rather than encourage the adolescent to continue this venting, the therapist redirected the conversation to *focus on the current suicidal crisis* and the events that led up to it. In response to the therapist's direct questions, the client stated that she wanted to kill herself, and that she would do it with the full bottle of Tylenol and bottle of antidepressant medication she had at home in her bathroom. In addition, she had ingested large amounts of pills twice before with ambivalent intention to die; these episodes had led to hospitalization.

The main precipitant of the current suicidal intent was that her father had told her she could no longer live in the family apartment, and wanted her to move out by the end of the week. Yet she was pregnant, and she perceived that she had no place to go and could not support herself or ultimately care for her baby without help. Thus she felt abandoned and unloved, and wanted to be dead. Her parents explained that their limits had been pushed one too many times, with the last incident leading to their extreme decision to ask her to move out. The night before, when the parents were not home, their daughter and her boyfriend had engaged in a loud argument in which he was cursing and threatening her while pounding on the windows and walls—all in the presence of the two younger siblings. The boyfriend finally stormed out. When the parents returned, the siblings told them of the incident, leading the father to confront his daughter angrily and demand that she move out. They were concerned about her well-being and her future, but were also concerned that she provided a negative role model for their other daughters. They had been allowing her to live with them because they wanted to keep a close watch on her and were afraid of pushing her to become suicidal, as she had in the past. However, this argument with her boyfriend proved a "last straw" for them. They felt that she had now gone beyond making a poor decision for herself and being a negative influence on her siblings, to actually traumatizing them and posing a danger to them. From her perspective, they were abandoning her in her time of greatest need, proving their greater allegiance to her younger siblings—and she felt panicked that she would end up homeless or in a shelter with her baby. She could envision only killing herself as a means to escape her predicament and emotional distress. As the parents and their daughter were recanting the events, the daughter intermittently became tearful and enraged. Thus the therapist worked with her in session to *tolerate her current affect* by use of mindfulness skills.

Exploring the current problem then allowed the therapist to work on formulating and summarizing the problem situation—a crucial step before problem solving. The therapist decided to focus on the precipitating factors of the suicidality; because the suicidal behavior appeared to be largely respondent in nature, she believed that addressing these factors could mitigate the client's distress and desperation. The therapist thus began by urging parents and teen to express themselves more effectively, using DEAR MAN and GIVE skills with a particular focus on validating each other's positions. To begin problem solving, the therapist referred them to the dialectical dilemma of *fostering dependence versus forcing autonomy* (see Chapter 5), which they had learned about in skills training during the Walking the Middle Path module (see Chapter 10). The therapist asked the family members how they thought this applied to them, and the parents immediately saw that they had flipped from one extreme position to another. For some time, they had been fostering dependence on their daughter's part by making allowances for her many maladaptive decisions and irresponsible behaviors, without demands for more responsible, adult behavior. When the consequences of this continued to mount, they reached their limit and rapidly switched to the other extreme of forcing autonomy by asking her to move out, even in her pregnant and unemployed state. Problem solving then naturally focused on finding a dialectical synthesis—a middle ground between these polarized positions. The corresponding treatment targets (see Chapter 5) of *increasing individuation while decreasing excessive dependence*, plus *increasing effective reliance on others while decreasing autonomy*, served as a guide for the therapist to help the family reach a middle path. The parents were reluctant to change their position of forcing their daughter out because of the self-destructive course they felt she was on, as well as the matter of the younger siblings' well-being. The father stated that his limits, which could not be compromised, were ensuring the safety of his younger daughters and respecting his position that the boyfriend was no longer allowed in the house. Thus the therapist helped devise a plan that satisfied their concerns.

In a suicidal crisis involving family members, the therapist faces the challenge of enlisting the parents' help in modifying their stance on the one hand, and not reinforcing suicidal behavior on the other. In this case, the therapist believed that the client's suicidal behavior also had an operant component, as her parents had inadvertently reinforced her suicidal behavior in the past. The therapist thus turned to the teen and said, "So you don't want to move out? We need to think of a way to talk to your parents about this where we take their concerns (which are realistic) into account, but where you also can get some of what you are asking for." The burden was then on the adolescent to replace her suicidal communication with validation of and negotiation with her parents (this was an example of pulling improved behavior from the client), with the assistance of the therapist's coaching. Also, the therapist did not encourage the parents to let her "off the hook" completely, by dropping all of their demands in response to her suicidal communication, but rather to clarify and assert their revised "middle path" demands. To clarify the contingencies operating, the therapist would then point out that the parents responded with reason and flexibility to the adolescent's effective (i.e., nonthreatening) communication regarding the matter of conflict (thus reinforcing a reduction in suicidal communication).

The problem-solving process led to the following: The parents agreed to let the client stay temporarily in the family apartment and to provide her with partial financial support, if certain conditions were met. She would have to take a series of steps to demonstrate her commitment to becoming more autonomous, more of a contributing member of the household, and more of a role model to her siblings. These steps would include demonstrating a concerted effort to find and keep at least a part-time job, contributing to the household with income and increased responsibility for household tasks, getting appropriate health care during her pregnancy, and (most important) keeping arguments with her boyfriend out of the house. At the same time, they asked that she look into alternative living arrangements. If these conditions were not met in a month, they would not ask her to leave immediately but would give her a warning, and she would have an additional month either to meet the conditions or to move out. However, if the conditions were met, she could remain home indefinitely, with the understanding that when the baby was born, new issues would arise and would have to be negotiated. They were also willing to consult with her on finding a job and on finding other living arrangements (this was an example of the consultation-to-the-patient strategy, which helped with the treatment target of increasing effective reliance on others; see Chapters 3 and 5), rather than expecting her to accomplish these steps without help. This plan satisfied the parents, in that they felt that their daughter would either remain home under tolerable circumstances for all members, or would move out but with ample time to plan for a feasible living situation. The plan also appeased the client, because she was better able to understand her parents' position while being relieved that they were flexible and willing to give her a chance to prove herself—which she claimed that she was motivated to do.

In addition to this broader plan, the therapist wanted to *obtain commitment to a plan of action* to address the adolescent's immediate suicidal risk. Upon reassessment of the client's suicidality, she reported no longer intending to kill herself (for now) and having more hope. It is important for therapists to err on the side of being conservative and to *anticipate a recurrence of the crisis response*. In this case, where family relations were likely to remain strained and where overdosing was a response that had been reinforcing for the adolescent in the past (numbing her immediate pain, arousing her parents' sympathy and support, and relieving her of certain responsibilities), suicidal behavior seemed a likely problem-solving mechanism for this teen. Thus the therapist obtained the client's *commitment to go home and dispose of the Tylenol* under her mother's watch, and to allow her mother to keep the antidepressants locked up and administer her daily dose. In addition, she agreed to practice self-soothing and mindfulness to help her tolerate her affect if her distress should intensify, and to page the therapist prior to any self-harm behavior if suicidal urges increased. If the therapist could not be reached immediately, she agreed either to call her best friend or to skillfully approach her mother to try to enlist her support. As part of anticipating a recurrence, it can be helpful to remain in contact to monitor the teen following a crisis session. The therapist thus made a plan to check in with the adolescent by phone later that evening and the next day, and to see the family in 1 week for a follow-up session. The parents also agreed to lend additional "eyes and ears" in observing their daughter, and to prompt her to call the therapist if they observed a marked decline in her mood or behavior.

Handling Suicidal Threats to Parents

Some teens' communications of suicidality are stated as threats (e.g., "If you don't let me go to see Johnny, I'm gonna swallow these pills right now!"). In response to such threats, parents have often understandably given in to the teen's demands repeatedly, fearful of the consequences. In such a case, the therapist will need to teach the parents not to reinforce the suicidal behavior, but to withhold reinforcement to work toward extinguishing it. This is difficult, especially because of "behavioral bursts" that occur (i.e., withholding reinforcement often results in an increase in behavior before a decrease begins). But a parent can be taught to use some of the very same strategies that the therapist uses in handling suicidal communications. These include dialectical strategies such as extending—in which the most extreme part of the teen's message (the suicidal threat) is addressed, rather than the request embedded in the communication (see Chapter 3). For example, in the example of an adolescent threatening to swallow pills if she is not allowed to go see her boyfriend, she desires to see her boyfriend and wants that part of the communication attended to by the parent. In extending, the parent would attend to the more extreme part of the communication, ignoring the wish to see the boyfriend. So the parent might respond with "Oh, really? You're planning to take those pills? Do we need to get you to the emergency room? I'll call an ambulance." This attention to the "wrong" part of the statement typically results in a deescalation of the extreme communication ("No, you don't have to call an ambulance! I'm not going to take them! But you've got to let me go see Johnny!")

Relatedly, there should be a matter-of-fact determination of risk by a parent, in which warmth is not increased but the parent ascertains whether there is danger. Can the adolescent commit to keep him- or herself alive? Can he or she commit to staying in contact with the parent, calling the parent or therapist before engaging in any self-harm behavior? Will the teen agree to dispose of pills or other lethal means? Does the parent's troubleshooting indicate that the crisis plan will be followed even if the teen's mood changes? If not, some form of closer monitoring might have to be considered. Overall, the parent must do what has to be done to keep the adolescent alive while not caving in to such threats. The parents must be reminded that temptations to "give in" in response to suicidal communications in the short run are likely to escalate suicidal behavior in the long run. Despite the fact that contact with parents during a crisis will typically occur during family sessions, some of this teaching can take place with the adolescent out of the room, if necessary. If the therapist feels a critical need to speak alone with the parents, he or she should first orient and get agreement from the adolescent: "I think at this point I can best help your parents be helpful to you if I talk to them alone for a few minutes. Are you OK with that?" A brief explanation and request to the adolescent convey respect and are likely to be met with an affirmative response. However, it may be best to avoid meeting with parents alone, to minimize risk of damaging the adolescent's trust.

The parents and therapist face tough decisions following suicidal behavior, because the goal of keeping the client alive in the short term (and thereby intervening in a more active fashion) might appear to conflict with the goal of avoiding intensive, reinforcing attention that increases suicidal behavior in the long term (Santisteban et al., 2003) or avoiding iatrogenic treatment programs that may be administered in some inpatient settings (e.g., being coddled by staff). That is why a parent should always try to determine actual medical risk and intervene as appropriate, while resisting the urge to increase soothing and warmth or respond to the adolescent's suicide-linked threats.

On the other hand, parents may have little idea how to determine whether a child's talk of suicide poses a real risk. Teaching family members suicidal risk factors (Table 8.5), as well as teaching them how to listen and suggesting some follow-up questions to ask their child, can be invaluable. For example, one adolescent broke down crying in front of her mother, stating that she did not want to "be here anymore." Her mother, anxious to find out what was going on, responded by forcefully saying, "Something must have happened! Come on, tell me what happened!" These words made the adolescent feel that she was being accused of something; they also missed the point that in her mind, no one thing had occurred, but there was an overwhelming accumulation of rejections and failures. The adolescent simply shut down, and the exchange became one more event confirming for her that she had no one she could rely on. In an ensuing family session, the therapist worked on helping the mother to see how she could have been more helpful in maintaining her daughter's communication and finding out her actual intent. The therapist provided suggestions of more helpful responses, some of which were volunteered by her daughter. For example, her daughter wished to convey how despondent she was and wanted a sign that her mother understood her pain. The daughter stated that an initial response such as "I'm sorry to see you are in so much pain. I'm here if you want to talk," would have made her feel that her mother cared, and she would have engaged in a conversation with her. In fact, that was the outcome the teen had been wishing for. The therapist pointed out that the mother could have then asked more about the suicidal reference and gotten a sense of whether any further steps had to be taken (e.g., obtaining commitment to a plan of action, contacting the therapist, etc.). Note that the therapist must also work with the family members to ensure that their validation and attentiveness are not primarily contingent upon suicidal communications; thus an overarching treatment goal with parents is to increase their ability to validate their teen in general. Moreover, the therapist emphasized in this case that the parent might have used mindfulness and distress tolerance skills to manage her own anxiety about her daughter's expression of suicidal thoughts.

When Parents' Interpretations of a Crisis Don't Match the Adolescent's

There may be times when parents' interpretations of a crisis situation do not match the adolescent's interpretations. One scenario is that the adolescent presents in crisis, but the parents minimize or negate the importance of the situation or the severity of the adolescent's risk. This tendency can be akin to normalizing pathological behavior, as discussed in Chapter 5, and can also be part of a pattern of pervasive invalidation of the adolescent (see the discussion of the biosocial theory, Chapter 3). An example of this was an adolescent who was intensely distressed; reported suicidal ideation, clear intent, and a specific plan; would not agree to a plan to keep herself alive; and was asking to be hospitalized. Her parents brought her to the session, but asked to speak to the therapist alone for a few minutes. With the client's assent, the therapist granted them these few minutes. They spoke of preparing the therapist for their daughter's "dramatic behavior" and urged the therapist not to "get sucked into it." They stated that she only wanted to be hospitalized because she missed her previous therapist, to whom she was very attached and who worked on the inpatient unit. Thus, according to the parents, the teen was inventing these symptoms because she knew "exactly how to manipulate the system" to get what she wanted. Upon assessment, the adolescent indeed expressed a wish to be hospitalized; however, she also expressed what appeared to be genuine distress, which was intensified by her perception that her parents did not take her seriously.

When a therapist encounters a disagreement between an adolescent and family members about whether something is a crisis situation or not, it is useful to remember the DBT assumption that there is no one absolute truth (see Chapter 10 for DBT assumptions). It is helpful to try to listen to both the adolescent's and the parents' perspectives, and at least to understand why both parties see things the way they do. The therapist should also consider the "both–and" possibility that both parties might hold a significant piece of the truth. For example, in the example above, it was true *both* that the adolescent missed her old therapist and wanted to see her, *and* that she was feeling as if she wanted to die. The therapist helped the parents to see that both positions could be true. The parents' position made sense; even if the adolescent was honest in her denial of seeing her old therapist as her primary motive, the expectation of seeing the therapist might have nevertheless been driving her suicidal ideation and misery, since learning takes place out of awareness. However, their stance did not validate her genuine distress. As the teen's suicidality seemed to have a large operant component, the need was to avoid reinforcing it; the solution thus would be either to hospitalize her in a different hospital, to hospitalize her in the same hospital but ensure that the old therapist would not be assigned to her, or (if possible) to develop a plan to monitor her and keep her alive as an outpatient. Note that while mental health professionals are typically trained to use hospitalization for suicidality, this choice does not necessarily best serve a suicidal client. In fact, although an inpatient stay may keep an individual alive in the short run, there is no evidence that it helps to keep one alive in the long run. Moreover, hospitalization may have iatrogenic effects, as it tends to reinforce behaviors not helpful to the client while doing little to facilitate the client's coping with difficulties faced in the context of life outside the hospital.

In general, when searching for a dialectical synthesis between extreme perspectives, the therapist can investigate whether there is something about the way the adolescent has communicated pain that has led family members to discrepant interpretations (e.g., not asking for help when needed, asking inconsistently, appearing periodically helpless, etc.). Behavioral rehearsal with the adolescent, followed by a family session in which the teen skillfully communicates his or her experience, often helps dramatically (see Table 9.3, below). The therapist should also consider whether the discrepant view of the crisis is part of a pattern of pervasive invalidation of the adolescent. If so, stressing validation of the adolescent may help bring them together.

Another possible scenario is that parents will perceive a crisis when the adolescent does not. For example, an adolescent may appear moody, withdrawn, and uncommunicative, or may be spending excessive amounts of time with friends, and a parent may believe that a crisis situation is occurring (e.g., suicidality, a drug problem, etc.); yet the adolescent reports a lack of any particular distress or subjective change in mood or thoughts. This can also happen when a parent perceives that an environmental crisis is occurring (e.g., parental divorce) and that the adolescent must be having an extreme reaction to it. This can be akin to pathologizing normal adolescent behavior (Chapter 5) and can also be a form of invalidation, if parents reject their children's input and do not take their statements at face value. This concern can be understandable, particularly when parents have had the experience of suicidal crises in the past and are now hypervigilant and fear missing key warning signs. But assumptions about crises can pose difficulties if the parents put excessive pressure on their child to "admit" what is going on or to behave differently, pressure the therapist to intervene in some way, or insist that the adolescent meet with the therapist (or enter therapy initially) to discuss the "problem."

A helpful response to this scenario can be to enhance the adolescent's empathy for the parent, in terms of both why the parent might remain concerned and how worried the parent must feel, given these concerns. The therapist can then work with the adolescent to communicate skillfully what is valid and invalid about the parent's perceptions. For example, one mother noticed that her daughter had become moody and was spending excessive amounts of time with her friends ("I don't know where they go. I have no idea what she's doing out until 2 A.M., and she won't tell me. How do I know she's not doing drugs, or having sex, or getting into some kind of trouble?"). Meanwhile, her daughter insisted that there was "nothing wrong" and they were just "hanging out"; the more she denied problems, the more her mother challenged her. In this case, the teen was doing very well in school, was engaged in many extracurricular activities, and (according to her reports in individual sessions) was not suicidal or engaging in risk behaviors. Based on their history together, her individual therapist trusted the client's self-report. She was, however, extremely anxious about leaving for college the following fall and felt guilty about leaving her single mom home alone. To address what the client experienced as her mother's "constant questioning" and distrust of her, the therapist devoted individual session time to figuring out how to "get Mom off her back." The therapist helped the client to see her mother's perspective; given the client's history of suicidal behavior and some ongoing family stressors, it was natural for a mother to worry about her daughter's long absences, particularly when she was uncommunicative about anything specific she did during those times. The client resented her mother for not allowing her privacy, and so resented sharing details of her times with her friends. Yet once she understood the basis of her mother's concerns, she was responsive to the therapist's next question: "Now how can we get her to trust and believe you?" The client then realized that by filling in her mother to a greater extent about how she spent her time with her friends, and by admitting the primary stressors on her mind (i.e., those concerning leaving for college), her mother would feel reassured, would be able to make sense of her daughter's behavior, and would be less apt to "nag" her. In addition, the therapist worked with the mother on observing her own limits regarding her daughter's late nights out. By limiting her daughter's late nights to weekends, and requesting a phone call if she were to be out past midnight, her mother felt more comfortable allowing her daughter this independent time without questioning her.

When Parents' Interpretations of a Crisis Don't Match the Therapist's

At times a therapist will find that the family members involved in a client's treatment do not hold the same view of a crisis situation as the therapist. They may think that it is either more or less serious than the therapist considers it—or, even if all adults hold a similar view of a crisis, they may hold differing views of how to handle it. This may pose a great challenge to the therapist, particularly if it results in the family members' not cooperating with what the therapist sees as essential recommendations. For example, parents may want to hospitalize their child immediately because of behavioral changes they observe, despite the therapist's belief that the situation can be handled on an outpatient basis with perhaps increased contact. Or they may, in a well-meaning way, be engaging in actions that reinforce suicidal behaviors. For example, one set of parents allowed their daughter to escape from all aversive demands the moment she expressed suicidal thinking (e.g., doing homework, attending school, meeting household responsibilities). For this client, suicidal behavior became so effectively operant that it became deeply ingrained, and minicrises occurred regularly. For these parents, treatment involved pointing out the pattern and working to change the contingencies. For example, the therapist taught the parents the dialectical strategy of extending, as described earlier, so they began to respond by seriously inquiring about the suicidality their daughter expressed instead of responding to the desire to escape from a responsibility. As predicted, she then began to deescalate her communications of distress. In addition, the strategy of contingency clarification was used with the adolescent to point out this pattern to her and actually get her to begin work on reducing suicidal communications.

Conversely, parents may not see a need for any special protocol or procedures, and may adopt a "watch and wait" attitude. For example, one of our adolescent clients was voicing strong suicidal intent and evidencing emerging delusional thinking in the beginning of treatment. The client's parents were convinced that hospitalization would *cause* a deterioration in functioning because of psychotropic medications (their daughter had had bad experiences with these medications in the past) and exposure to psychotic clients. The mother was actually in the medical field and held strong views based on her knowledge and experience—yet they were discrepant from the therapist's view that hospitalization should be considered immediately. In this case, it was important that the therapist assess further to determine exactly what the parents' concerns and the client's past negative experiences with psychotropic medications and exposure to other clients were. Their concerns were validated, and the therapist discussed with them the compromise of communicating with the pharmacotherapist to try different medications this time. The parents were also concerned that exposure to psychotic clients would make their daughter "sicker." Here a dialectical synthesis was sought: The therapist reassured (i.e., educated) the parents that psychotic disorders were not contagious, but validated the truth in their position—that the experience of inpatient hospitalization and forging connections with other inpatients could indeed influence their daughter's identity, as least in the short run, as a "mental patient." However, the experience of delusional thinking outside of the hospital setting would also be likely to make her feel like a "mental patient," and would perhaps even be prolonged by the lack of inpatient treatment. Since the parents felt taken seriously by the therapist, they were able to engage in a continued discussion and explore options. As the parents remained reluctant to consider hospitalization, the therapist discussed alternatives with them and warned of possible consequences associated with such alternatives. For example, the therapist warned that the risk of monitoring the teen closely at home might result in a deterioration of functioning and ultimately hospitalization anyway (which could possibly be even longer, because it would begin at a more advanced point in her psychotic episode). In this case, the therapist and parents agreed to a compromise of keeping the adolescent out of the hospital for the next 24–48 hours, but going immediately for a consultation with a pharmacotherapist for possible outpatient pharmacotherapy. The plan, developed with the adolescent and the parents in the room, included moment-to-moment details on how they would monitor her and keep her from harming herself, including overnight. With the adolescent's commitment that she would not engage in suicidal behaviors and the parents' agreement to the plan, the therapist let them go without insisting on hospitalization. In this case, the adolescent was on a new medication 48 hours later, and the adolescent and her parents remained compliant with their monitoring plan. The delusional thinking soon remitted; the parents agreed at this point to take their daughter to an emergency room if delusional thinking reemerged.

One of the most challenging aspects of conducting DBT with adolescents is encountering such a lack of shared perspective with a client's family members, a lack of parental cooperation, or (even worse) outright perceived parental sabotage of treatment goals or strategies. During a crisis situation, the ramifications of such mismatches can become even more serious. Just as in working with adolescents toward problem solving, the therapist may need to employ orientation, didactic, and commitment strategies with parents in responding to a crisis. There is no a priori reason to assume that parents will know just how to read an adolescent's signals or how to respond. Thus the therapist may need to spend ample time not only on psychoeducation, but also on commitment strategies to try to understand what will interfere with the parents' collaboration with the crisis plan (e.g., withholding certain reinforcers), as well as to shape them toward doing so.

On the other hand, unlike working with adults (where the therapist usually plays the sole expert role), working with minors necessitates considering the parents as expert consultants on their children. Although the parents may not have training as mental health professionals, and are not serving in such a capacity with their child, they certainly have expertise regarding their child and the child's history and patterns. The therapist must thus remember not to adopt an arrogant position of "expert" with regard to his or her knowledge of the client, and instead to consider the parents' perspective respectfully. This input from other observers in the client's natural environment (i.e., family members) may provide invaluable information on how the client comes across to others, communicates distress ineffectively, and so on. Thus, even if the therapist does not see eye to eye with parents regarding the assessment of the situation, the therapist should pay attention to any opportunities to learn more about the client. Table 9.3 summarizes strategies for handling mismatches in perceptions of crisis situations.

Referring or Reporting?

In the example above regarding the adolescent with emerging delusional thinking, a careful balance of assessment, validation, taking the parents' concerns seriously, orientation, psychoeducation, and flexibility on the therapist's part was needed to stay engaged in a productive dialogue with these parents and come up with a plan that was satisfactory to all. If the parents had not been amenable to adhering to the specific crisis plan, or in some other way could not

TABLE 9.3. Strategies for Handling Mismatches in Perceptions of Crises

When parents' and adolescent's perceptions of a crisis do not match
- Increase empathy and perspective taking.
  Aim: To achieve dialectical synthesis.
- Enhance accurate communication; employ behavioral rehearsal.
  Aim: To help adolescent increase accurate communication of distress.
  Aim: To help parents increase accurate communication of concern.

When parents' and therapists perceptions of a crisis do not match
- Assess further; consider input from parents seriously; empathize with their viewpoint.
- Consider parents to be additional experts on their children.
  Aim: To achieve dialectical synthesis.
- Explain therapist perspective; provide rationale; employ psychoeducation (e.g., regarding disorder, treatment, learning theory); employ commitment strategies.
  Aim: To gain commitment to crisis plan.

When synthesis cannot be achieved and therapist still differs from parents
- Provide a range of options when possible (i.e., alternative strategies or treatments).
- Consult team when possible.
  Aim: To maintain alliance while still providing optimal care.

If pursuing other options is not possible or there is still no agreement
- Refer parents and teen to another provider.
  Aim: To provide parents with a satisfactory option while therapist maintains values or works within areas of competence.
- Report for medical neglect.[a]
  Aim: To ensure adequate treatment for adolescent.

---

[a]This option should be considered only after other options have been exhausted and a second opinion has been sought, typically from the team.

reach an agreement with the therapist, the next step would have been for the therapist to refer them to a provider who could help them as they wanted. However, if parents insist on an intervention (or on a lack of any intervention or monitoring) that the therapist believes is absolutely a dangerous approach, given the adolescent's presentation, the therapist may be left with no option but to report them to a child protection agency for medical neglect. Reporting for such neglect depends on state laws, and providers should be familiar with these. This is a serious step that should only be considered when it is believed that a client's life is in jeopardy; when all other options have been exhausted; and after consultation with one's team, individual supervisor, or other trusted colleagues.

Using the DBT Therapist Consultation Team

Finally, these issues are appropriate for bringing to the DBT consultation team, particularly to help the therapist remain reasonably balanced and empathic toward parents as well as the adolescent client. The therapist must remember that a number of factors may be operating from the parents' vantage points that could make them either less or more likely to perceive a crisis. These include the difficulties of having an often emotionally and behaviorally dysregulated child; the pain and anxiety parents experience at believing that their child is in danger or at risk; their prior experiences of either missing real danger signs or jumping to conclusions for no reason; and the potential shame, self-blame, and fear of appearing incompetent or inadequate as parents merely because of having a child in treatment.

HANDLING ISSUES OF CONFIDENTIALITY

Confidentiality can be broken when a therapist believes that a minor client is at serious risk. Defining what level of risk is serious enough to break confidentiality, however, may not always be clear in work with adolescents and their parents. Certainly, if a therapist determines that there is a high and imminent threat of suicide, the choice to notify others (typically the adolescent's parents) is straightforward. However, does an increase in suicidal ideation with no clear plan merit breaking confidentiality? How about increased ideation and access to lethal methods, but a denial of intent? What about the case of NSIB (e.g., self-cutting with no intent to die)? Is NSIB, no matter how minor, indicative of posing a danger to oneself when we know that individuals who engage in such behaviors are more likely to complete suicide eventually (e.g., Cooper et al., 2005)? What about other risk behaviors that have lethal potential, such as unprotected sex or drunk driving?

These are complex decisions, and must be weighed against the fact that if confidentiality is ensured, the adolescent is likely to have a higher level of disclosure to the therapist. We thus suggest a number of guidelines, which are summarized in Table 9.4. First, it is critical to explain to the adolescent and parents the limits of confidentiality (i.e., if the therapist suspects or learns that the client is at imminent risk of committing suicide or homicide, or learns of ongoing child abuse or neglect) from the outset of treatment, to avoid later feelings of betrayal. In addition, the clinician must discuss how he or she will handle confidentiality regarding sensitive issues (e.g., NSIB, risky sexual behavior, drug use). Although the therapist can stress that he or she will make a serious effort to keep sensitive material private, the therapist must emphasize that this cannot be guaranteed, because sustained intense risk behaviors or a serious escalation of behavior that puts the minor client at risk of suicide or indicates the therapy is not helping will need to be discussed with the parents (Santisteban et al., 2003). The therapist can further explain that withholding such information from parents would not only be ir-

TABLE 9.4. Guidelines for Breaking Confidentiality

From treatment outset
- Explain limits of confidentiality.
- Discuss how therapist will handle confidentiality regarding sensitive issues (e.g., NSIB, risky sexual behavior).

Under these conditions, therapist does not need to break confidentiality
- Legal standards for breaking confidentiality are not met (therapist must know state laws).
- Therapist believes that disclosure would be likely to result in exacerbation of the crisis or place adolescent in danger.

Under these conditions, therapist might choose to break confidentiality
- Even when no clear-cut case for breaking confidentiality exists (i.e., no imminent danger to self or others), therapist may elect to encourage disclosure of crisis state to a parent or other family member if:
  - Such a disclosure would be likely to do more good than harm.
  - Therapist believes that parent's knowledge of situation would result in needed support for the adolescent.
  - Therapist believes that lack of disclosure would significantly interfere with client's ability to get through the crisis.
  - Therapist believes that lack of disclosure is seriously undermining family work or is somehow maintaining crisis situation.
  - Therapist believes that holding a particular secret regarding the adolescent's welfare is too great a violation of family trust.
  - Therapist sees parent as critical in monitoring and aiding the adolescent through crisis, even if therapist coaching is needed to assist the parent in being helpful.
- Therapist may initiate contact with family members directly if he or she determines that short-term gain in reporting crisis is worth potential cost of adolescent's (1) trust and (2) learning to communicate difficulties and seek help appropriately.

Under these conditions therapist does need to break confidentiality
- Behavior reaches threshold of legal mandate (i.e., suspicion) to report abuse or neglect.
- Behaviors escalate significantly.
- Behaviors are maintained at significant level of risk, so that:
  - Minor client is in danger.
  - Treatment does not appear to be helping.
  - Minor client is threatening to harm a particular person.

How to handle breaking confidentiality when adolescent agrees
- Engage adolescent actively in process.
- Inform adolescent about therapist's plans.
- Allow adolescent to voice concerns.
- Plan with adolescent how, when, and to whom the disclosure will take place.
- Use behavioral rehearsal to plan disclosure.

How to handle breaking confidentiality when adolescent does not agree
- Engage adolescent actively in process.
- Inform adolescent about therapist's plans.
- Explain rationale; communicate directly about intentions.
- Allow adolescent to voice concerns.
- Be sure to understand the adolescent's perspective (can conduct behavioral analysis of unwillingness to disclose if becomes therapy-interfering behavior).
- Discuss pros and cons of disclosing.
- Discuss potential consequences of *not* disclosing.
- Plan with adolescent how, when, and to whom the disclosure will take place.
- Use behavioral rehearsal to plan disclosure.
- Stress intention to work to ensure that family interaction around crisis remains adaptive.
- Consider alternatives (e.g., temporarily delaying disclosure to parents; disclosing to a selected and trusted family member).
- Employ commitment strategies (e.g., devil's advocate, shaping).
- Convey support and respect for adolescent's position.

responsible, but also undermine the protective function critical to parents' roles. Having said this, however, the therapist indicates willingness to make the adolescent's privacy a priority, and works hard both to rehearse with the adolescent how to disclose the issue him- or herself in the following session and to ensure that the family's interaction around the material remains adaptive, if sensitive material needs to be discussed (Santisteban et al., 2003). Rather than warning a parent about an adolescent's high-risk situation over the phone following a session with the adolescent, we might use session time to plan how and what the adolescent will communicate regarding the issue of concern, or use a family session to communicate this information (provided that essential time is not lost in doing so). In the interest of the safety of our minor adolescent clients, we err on the side of a lower threshold for determining what level of threat merits breaking confidentiality—especially in the early stages of treatment as we are getting to know the clients). But in the interest of maintaining a therapeutic alliance with each client, treating each client with respect, and following the principle of consulting to the client on handling the environment rather than consulting to the environment (see Chapter 3), we prefer to encourage clients to communicate to their caregivers about the issue of concern directly.

For example, one client cut herself regularly with razors and other objects, mostly in places on her body where the marks would be hidden from public view. The adolescent had kept these acts hidden from her mother and preferred to keep them that way. Behavioral analysis revealed that the client believed her mother's reaction to these acts would be overbearing and highly burdensome to her, and that avoiding such reactions by hiding the self-injurious behavior reduced the anxiety associated with it. Thus hiding the behavior was negatively reinforcing, in that it reduced anxiety about an aversive consequence. As part of a contingency management strategy, the therapist brought up the idea of revealing the self-cutting to her mother. As there was no immediate escalation of these behaviors or development of any suicidal intention or plan, it was determined that the therapist and client could take the time to discuss her views about revealing these behaviors to her mother, to coach her in doing so once she agreed, and to plan a family session where the client would share the information.

Some DBT therapists choose to address the issue of self-cutting with parents at the outset of treatment. The following example depicts a common exchange:

PARENT: I am worried that my daughter's cutting will get worse, she won't tell me, and I won't see it—and now, in the name of confidentiality, you won't tell me either.

THERAPIST: I understand your concern. I want you to know that your daughter has agreed to track her self-harm on a diary card that we will review together each week (and, as an aside, you know that the diary card is a private document that I would ask you not to view). Thus I am going to be keeping careful track of her self-harm. Given that this behavior is frequent (and typically not life-threatening), I believe it would not help Jessica or my therapeutic alliance with her if I contacted you each time she cut herself, or even if I encouraged her to tell you herself each time she did it. So I will say this: If I feel that her cutting is escalating either in frequency or in medical dangerousness, I will break confidentiality. Otherwise, this behavior will be something that we will work on together, and I will not be contacting you each time she engages in it. Does that seem reasonable?

Occasionally the therapist will decide that it would not be helpful at the present time to urge the adolescent to reveal a crisis situation to family members. This would be the case when the therapist believes that such a revelation would be likely to result in an exacerbation of the crisis or would actually place the adolescent in danger (e.g., realistic risk of getting severely physically disciplined by a parent, following an admission of pregnancy).

CONCLUSION

Including family members in therapy with adolescents adds a complex dimension to the treatment; yet this addition has the potential to be strongly supportive of the treatment, and highly beneficial to teens and parents alike. In addition, although any crisis situation with clients by definition poses a challenge to the therapist, crises that arise in work with adolescents and their family members pose special challenges. In this chapter we have attempted to describe various strategies for working with family members, and to capture those aspects of handling crises that we face most commonly in intervening with our adolescent population.

CHAPTER 10

Skills Training with Adolescents

As discussed in Chapter 4 and throughout this book, we strongly recommend that parents, guardians, or other caregivers be included in skills training sessions for adolescents. Although several skills training formats (depending on the setting) are reviewed in Chapter 4, we recommend that the multifamily skills training group format be used whenever possible. Throughout this chapter, we discuss our experience with running multifamily skills groups. But readers should also keep in mind the other possible formats for conducting skills training with adolescents.

WHO SHOULD CONDUCT SKILLS TRAINING?

If skills training is to be conducted in a group format, we recommend that two coleaders serve as skills trainers. Having two leaders is beneficial because it provides extra help, an extra pair of hands to help manage the group, and an extra pair of eyes to observe group members (for emotion dysregulation, signs of distraction, etc.). Some settings with limited resources might not be able to support two skills trainers in a group; in such settings, the skills trainer might attempt to recruit a trainee (e.g., an intern, resident, etc.) as coleader. When it is simply not possible to have two skills trainers in a group, the skills trainer should certainly make ample use of the therapist consultation meeting to share observations about clients and address any difficulties. When skills training is conducted with an individual family, a single skills trainer is sufficient.

Although the skills trainers are naturally a part of the DBT team, it can be helpful for them *not* to serve also as primary therapists to group members. Reasons for this include the benefit of having additional team members become familiar with each client, which enhances the team approach. It also allows clients to consult one therapist (primary therapist or skills trainer) regarding problems with the other, as opposed to having no one to consult with for coaching if the same person is serving both functions. Also, as mentioned in Chapter 9, skills trainers can provide phone consultation to family members in the group, provided that they are not also the primary therapists of the adolescents in this group.

Yet it is not always desirable to have separate primary therapists and skills trainers. For staff training purposes, for example, many clinicians value the chance to learn both roles, and it is often not feasible simply to run a group that does not contain therapists' individual clients. Some therapists gain a better understanding of their clients from viewing them in both individual therapy and skills training, and some settings simply do not have the staff resources to have separate therapists in each role. This situation can be workable as well, especially if there is a coleader available who can serve as phone coach to a client's parents.

WHO PARTICIPATES IN MULTIFAMILY SKILLS GROUPS?

Who are the participating family members, and how do we decide whom to include? Typically, this question gets answered easily; we first look for the availability of at least one parent, and there is often a "main" parent who brings an adolescent in from the outset of treatment. This parent is often either the sole custodial parent, or, when there are two parents in the home, the parent with whom the teen has the closer relationship. This parent often participates in the intake and orientation process. At times, however, we have taken the opposite approach by choosing to invite the parent with whom the teen has greater problems, in order to (1) have that parent learn the skills concurrently and (2) provide an opportunity for this dyad to have some additional therapeutic time together. Another common scenario is that an adolescent brings in both parents (either two biological parents or a biological parent and a stepparent). When a custodial parent is not available or appropriate, a clinician may have to decide whom to include among more than one possible family member. Criteria to consider include willingness, availability, and relationship to the adolescent client. The person should ideally reside with the adolescent. When this is not possible, the person should at least play an integral role in the adolescent's life. For example, some adolescents have brought fathers with whom they did not reside but whom they saw regularly. When one considers the purposes of family members' participation, including treating the environment directly as well as providing models and coaches, then obviously a family member should constitute a significant part of the adolescent's environment and should have enough contact with the teen to help with skill generalization.

We advise making every possible effort to engage parents in the group, especially those who initially refuse to join. An individual therapist can speak to a parent in person and over the phone to encourage the parent to attend, keeping the DBT commitment strategies in mind. Also, the therapist can coach the adolescent to skillfully invite his or her parent to join the group. The therapist can also offer to write letters to employers when necessary. Based on our clinical experience, we emphasize to parents that their children are likely to have a better outcome if they participate. For distressed parents, this becomes an easy sell. In some cases, however, no matter how skillful a therapist is, a parent may refuse to attend for a variety of reasons. Generally, we then attempt to identify the next closest relative to attend. In some cases, however, adolescents are left to come by themselves. Typically, these teens are "adopted" by other families in the group and receive ample validation and reinforcement from group members.

When family members participate in a group, we recommend limiting the number of clients, since parental involvement makes the group about twice as large. Depending on the number of parents participating, 5–6 adolescents per group tends to be ideal, for an average total of 10–15 group members when family members are included. With a larger size, the leaders risk not having enough time to review homework (4–5 minutes per member). In addition, the leaders are likely to have more difficulty keeping all members engaged in a larger group. A limitation of a smaller group is the periodic absence from the regular rotation of "senior members" helping to orient new members. Typically, those who have been there for one or more modules help engage new members by telling them why they should participate and how the program has been helpful to them.

WHOM TO CONSIDER EXCLUDING FROM MULTIFAMILY SKILLS GROUPS

We recommend a policy of requiring the same family member(s) to attend each time, and to make the same attendance commitment as the adolescent. Rotating family members based on who might be available that week would undermine the purposes of directly modifying the invalidating environment and providing a coach to the adolescent, since no relative would have the opportunity to learn the skills, practice, and receive feedback in any meaningful way. Furthermore, such intermittent attendance would certainly prove disruptive to group cohesion. Relatedly, we feel adolescents should not involve friends as the identified persons to accompany them, for two primary reasons: (1) Someone who lives in a teen's home is preferred to learn the skills and be able to provide group coaching as needed; and (2) including friends in the group unbalances the adolescent–adult ratio and risks fostering an atmosphere of play instead of work. Lastly, the presence of a boyfriend or girlfriend might also prove disruptive, given the volatility of many adolescent relationships. Thus we discourage practitioners from permitting romantic partners to serve in this capacity as well. The one exception we have made has been for a married teenager to invite his or her spouse.

Conditions under which we recommend excluding family members include the following: (1) A parent's work schedule or other obligations make it impossible for him or her to attend; (2) there is estrangement between the parent and the adolescent; (3) there is such an intense degree of parent–adolescent conflict that their being in a group together would be likely to result in explosive or otherwise therapy-destroying behavior; (4) there is an ongoing abusive situation, and the adolescent is looking to maintain distance and safety; or (5) a parent has a serious unmanaged mental disorder. In these cases, the adolescent can identify another relative or someone in a caregiver role to attend the group. We also exclude parents who are non-English speaking even if one of the group leaders speaks the parental language, as it would be disruptive for the leader to repeat everything said in a second language. In such a case, we invite the teen to attend the group alone. If the individual therapist happens to speak the language of the parents (e.g., Spanish), several of the individual sessions can be divided in half to include collateral family visits. In this context, the non-English-speaking parents can be exposed to a modified (albeit limited) skills training course, tailored to the specific needs of the teen and parents. If the parents cannot attend for some reason, we still attempt to get them involved through granting them at least some exposure to skills handouts and their application through family sessions. Ideally, if a skills trainer speaks the language of the parents, and other families speaking this language join the program, a multifamily skills group could be conducted in the families' native language.

OPEN GROUP VERSUS CLOSED GROUP

There are advantages and disadvantages to both open and closed groups, but we recommend keeping a group open whenever this is feasible. A closed group is one that is formed and stays together for an agreed-upon period of time. The primary advantage of this type of group is that the members get to know each other better, trust each other more, and therefore are likely to reveal more material in the group. The disadvantage is that once the clients feel comfortable with one another, it becomes more difficult to keep the focus on behavioral skills training and more likely for the group to drift into process issues. Hence, since the multifamily skills training group is skills-oriented, this serves as one reason to keep the group open (i.e., to add new families at the start of each new module).

A second reason to keep the group open is that these adolescents need practice adapting to changes in their environment. Adolescents diagnosed with BPD or borderline features, like their adult counterparts, have enormous difficulty dealing with change. Thus an open group allows for exposure to controlled but continual change in a therapeutic context.

A third reason to keep the group open is that it creates a "seniority system" within the group. By allowing new members into the group at each module start and having others graduate, the DBT program creates a culture in which senior members help orient junior members to DBT. Having senior members in the same group with new initiates has several advantages: (1) the seniors help build commitment and model "sticking it out" with newer members who might otherwise drop out of treatment; (2) the senior group members also model skillful behavior as well as give constructive feedback to the more junior members, especially at the monthly graduation ceremony; and (3) the junior members can see that there is an end in sight—that many people who commit themselves to DBT do improve and ultimately graduate.

SKILLS TRAINING CONTENT AND SCHEDULE

Skills training with adolescents in multifamily groups can follow the same didactic behavioral format as outlined in Linehan's (1993b) *Skills Training Manual for Treating Borderline Personality Disorder*. Standard DBT for adults covers four sets of skills, taught as independent modules; as noted in earlier chapters and discussed in detail later, we have added a fifth set of skills for adolescents and families. Each module employs didactic presentation of skills, role plays and other experiential components, and review of homework exercises. The nature of the skills group blends a classroom environment with a group therapy environment. The classroom aspects stem from the fact that group members are given handouts, notebooks, and paper for writing notes, and each session follows a curriculum. Each week, members are given additional handouts that are three-hole-punched and go into their loose-leaf binders, which are organized by major skill areas (e.g., core mindfulness, distress tolerance, etc.). Skills trainers teach skills (sometimes writing on a whiteboard), assign homework weekly, and provide constructive feedback. However, the group therapy aspects stem from the often personal content of material discussed as teaching examples or in homework review (e.g., using skills to assert oneself with a boyfriend or girlfriend, coping with memories of trauma), and from the supportive and validating climate that develops between group members.

The four skills modules in standard DBT are Core Mindfulness Skills, Interpersonal Effectiveness Skills, Emotion Regulation Skills, and Distress Tolerance Skills. Since *mindfulness skills* are central to the treatment, they are referred to as "core" skills. Drawn largely from Zen practice but also compatible with most Eastern meditation practices and Western contemplative practices, "the skills are psychological and behavioral versions of meditation skills" (Linehan, 1993a, p, 144). They involve learning to observe, describe, and participate—that is, respectively, to notice or attend to events, emotions, and behavioral responses; then to be able to describe these events in words; and to enter completely into this experience without self-consciousness. Additional mindfulness skills involve how one observes, describes, and participates. They include being nonjudgmental, being one-mindful (i.e., doing only one thing in the moment), and being effective (i.e., keeping an eye on one's goals in a situation and doing what is needed to achieve them, rather than focusing on being "right").

Interpersonal effectiveness skills involve strategies for asking what one wants or needs, saying no, coping with conflict and maintaining relationships, and maintaining self-respect. The Interpersonal Effectiveness module also includes components such as identifying beliefs that interfere with interpersonal effectiveness, and factors to consider when deciding whether to and how strongly to assert oneself.

Emotion regulation skills aim to help clients regulate painful affective states. The Emotion Regulation module includes didactic material on the functions of emotions, identifying and labeling emotions, reducing emotional vulnerability through self care and building a sense of mastery, increasing positive emotional events, increasing mindfulness to the current emotion (i.e., nonjudgmental observation and description of one's emotional experience in the moment), and changing the behavioral–expressive component of an emotion by acting opposite to the action urge associated with the emotion.

Finally, distress tolerance skills teach clients strategies to *survive* painful emotions or situations without *succumbing* to them, or without engaging in maladaptive problem-solving behavior that makes the situation worse (Linehan, 1993a). The Distress Tolerance module contains two sets of skills: crisis survival skills and acceptance skills. The crisis survival skills include strategies to distract, self-soothe, improve the moment (through strategies such as using imagery, making meaning, and self-encouragement), and consider the pros and cons of tolerating the distress (i.e., coping) versus not tolerating the distress (i.e., acting impulsively or otherwise maladaptively). Acceptance skills teach clients radical acceptance of situations as they are ("acceptance" does not imply approval of a situation), turning the mind toward acceptance, and the notion of willingness (i.e., doing what is needed; deep, accepting participation in the processes of life) versus willfulness (i.e., not doing what is needed; resisting the processes of life; cutting off one's nose to spite one's face).

Table 10.1 lists the specific skills within each standard DBT module, together with the schedule for their rotation. Virtually all of the skills handouts are accompanied by homework sheets that skills trainers distribute in group for practice during the week. In skills groups and in this book, many of the skills are referred to by acronyms (e.g., DEAR MAN); these serve as mnemonic devices for clients. Table 10.2 offers a key to decoding these acronyms. For adolescents and family members, we have developed a fifth module: Walking the Middle Path Skills (Miller, Rathus, & Linehan, 1999, adapted from Linehan, 1993b).

Some programs may consider shortening the length of treatment with adolescents; this may enhance adolescents' willingness to commit to, and the likelihood of their completing, treatment. Compared to adult clients with BPD, some adolescent clients may not yet have severely entrenched behavior patterns and could be served as well by a shorter treatment course. The schedule for the 16-week version of adolescent outpatient skills group at Montefiore consists of four rotating modules (Interpersonal Effectiveness, Emotion Regulation, Distress Tolerance, and Walking the Middle Path), with the fifth, Core Mindfulness, repeated before the beginning of each of the other modules. Table 10.3 shows this schedule. Table 10.4 outlines a sample schedule for the rotation of skills training topics with adolescents in a shortened 16-week treatment format. Yet the original randomized controlled trials studying the efficacy of DBT were conducted within a 1-year time frame for Stage 1 of treatment, and included a proportion of older adolescent participants. Since then, other lengths of treatment have been investigated, including 6-month outpatient treatments and shorter-term treatments in outpatient and inpatient settings (Miller, Rathus, et al., in press). For example, 2 weeks of mindfulness skills can be interspersed with skills modules that run for 6 weeks each, as in standard DBT. On acute inpatient units, skills might be taught in independent daily skills groups, or in rotating topic-based modules lasting 1 week at a time. Note that until further data are available, the more conservative approach is to follow a format supported by data from the randomized controlled studies of DBT.

TABLE 10.1. Standard DBT Skills and Rotation Schedules

Two weeks (repeated at each module start)

Orientation (Week 1 only)
 What is DBT?
 Goals of skills training (DBT problem areas)
 DBT assumptions
 Biosocial theory
 Guidelines for skills group
Core Mindfulness
 Three states of mind
 "What" skills
 "How" skills

Six weeks: Distress Tolerance

 Crisis survival skills
  • Distract with ACCEPTS
  • Self-soothe
  • Improve the moment
  • Pros and cons
 Guidelines for accepting reality
 Observing-your-breath exercises
 Half-smiling exercises
 Awareness exercises
 Turning the mind/radical acceptance
 Willfulness versus willingness

Six weeks: Interpersonal Effectiveness

 Situations for interpersonal effectiveness
 Goals of interpersonal effectiveness
 Factors reducing interpersonal effectiveness
 Myths about interpersonal effectiveness
 Cheerleading statements for interpersonal effectiveness
 Options for intensity of asking or saying no, and factors to consider in deciding
 Suggestions for interpersonal effectiveness practice
 Getting what you want (DEAR MAN)
 Keeping the relationship (GIVE)
 Keeping self-respect (FAST)

Six weeks: Emotion Regulation

 Goals of emotion regulation training
 Myths about emotions
 Model for describing emotions
 Ways to describe emotions
 What good are emotions?
 Reducing vulnerability to negative emotions (PLEASE MASTER)
 Steps for increasing positive emotions
 Letting go of emotional suffering: Mindfulness of the current emotion
 Changing emotions by acting opposite to the current emotion

With an ongoing, open skills group, a family can enter treatment at the start of any module. When possible, it is best to have at least two adolescents join a group at the same time, so that each adolescent can feel part of a "cohort." This may foster better compliance. Although families can begin with different modules, depending on the point at which they enter, they will have all been exposed to the same sets of skills by the time they complete the five modules.

TABLE 10.2. Key for Skills Acronyms

Distress Tolerance

Distract with ACCEPTS
    (Activities, Contributing, Comparisons, opposite Emotions, Pushing away, other Thoughts, other
      Sensations)
Self-soothe with five senses
    (hearing, vision, smell, taste, touch)
IMPROVE the moment
    (Imagery, Meaning, Prayer, Relaxing actions, One thing in the moment, brief Vacation, self-
      Encouragement)

Interpersonal Effectiveness

Getting what you want (DEAR MAN)
    (Describe, Express, Assert, Reinforce, stay Mindful, Appear confident, Negotiate)
Keeping the relationship (GIVE)
    (be Gentle, act Interested, Validate, use an Easy manner)
Keeping self-respect (FAST)
    (be Fair, no Apologies, Stick to values, be Truthful)

Emotion Regulation

Reducing vulnerability to negative emotions (PLEASE MASTER)
    (PhysicaL illness, balance Eating, avoid mood-Altering drugs, balance Sleep, get Exercise; build
      MASTERy)

Note. See Linehan (1993b) for detailed descriptions of each skill.

INITIAL MULTIFAMILY GROUP SESSION:
ORIENTATION AND TECHNIQUE

As in standard DBT, whenever a new skills module is started and new families begin the group, we recommend conducting an orientation specific to the DBT skills group. This generally occurs during the first half of the first 2-hour session that introduces a new skills module. In other words, it should take between 45 minutes and 1 hour, but may vary depending on the setting and length of the skills training session. We recommend that leaders cover the following in the orientation session: (1) introducing group members and skills trainers, (2) reviewing

TABLE 10.3. Sample Schedule for Rotating Skills Group Modules

Four-week module: Distress Tolerance

    One week: Orientation and core mindfulness skills
    Three weeks: Distress tolerance skills

Four-week module: Emotion Regulation

    One week: Orientation and core mindfulness skills
    Three weeks: Emotion regulation skills

Four-week module: Interpersonal Effectiveness

    One week: Orientation and core mindfulness skills
    Three weeks: Interpersonal effectiveness skills

Four-week module: Walking the Middle Path

    One week: Orientation and core mindfulness skills
    Three weeks: Walking the middle path skills

TABLE 10.4. DBT Skills for Adolescents and Family Members: 16-Week Format

One week (repeated at each module start)	*Three Weeks: Interpersonal Effectiveness*
Orientation	Goals and what interferes
What is DBT?	Worry thoughts and cheerleading statements
DBT problem areas	DEAR MAN
DBT assumptions	GIVE
Biosocial theory	FAST
Guidelines for skills group	
DBT agreement	*Three weeks: Emotion Regulation*
Core Mindfulness	Goals and what good are emotions?
Three states of mind	Why bother regulating emotions?
"What" skills	Model of emotions
"How" skills	PLEASE MASTER
	Increasing positive emotions
Three weeks: Distress Tolerance	Acting opposite
Goals and why bother?	The "wave" skill (being mindful of emotions)
Crisis survival skills	
Distract with ACCEPTS	*Three weeks: Walking the Middle Path*
Self-soothe	Dialectics/dialectical dilemmas
Pros and cons	Validation
Turning the mind/radical acceptance	Behaviorism
Willfulness versus willingness	

the limits of confidentiality, (3) providing a rationale for why these adolescents were chosen for this special program, (4) orienting members to the skills training goals, (5) reviewing DBT biosocial theory (or other relevant theoretical approach), (6) reviewing DBT assumptions, (7) orienting members to group rules, and (8) asking members to sign an agreement. A discussion of how to carry out these steps follows below. The group then normally takes a break, followed by the second half of the session. As in standard DBT, the second hour of the orientation session then follows the same format as all other sessions, covering the rationale, description, discussion, and practice of a new skill. Table 10.5 outlines a format for the initial session, as well as the three subsequent sessions of each module.

Introducing Group Members and Skills Trainers

When skills training takes place in a group format, skills trainers can model an introduction and then ask each member to introduce him- or herself. Some skills trainers ask for only names; others ask for more information, such as a brief statement of an interest or hobby. Or, if the skills trainers wish to wait until after treatment goals are explained, introductions can include names and a brief statement about which treatment goals apply to each adolescent member. In multifamily skills training groups, it is helpful if parents are asked to introduce themselves in the same way, such as by stating which treatment goals they feel they themselves can benefit from (as discussed below). Sometimes leaders use ice-breaking exercises in an initial group skills training session. These might include having the first person state his or her name, having the second person repeat that name and then state his or her own name, having the third repeat the first two names and then state his or her own, and so on. Or members can break into dyads (family members should be separated for this exercise), exchange information for 2 minutes (name, interests, etc.), and then introduce each other to the group.

Note that some adolescents enter the group with extreme social anxiety and may find introductions difficult. With such teens, skills trainers can accept little in the first session and

TABLE 10.5. Sample Multifamily Skills Group Session Format

Week 1 of each skills module (initial orientation session)

50–60 minutes:
   Introduce all group members and skills trainers
   Review limits of confidentiality
   Present rationale for why these adolescents were chosen for this program
   Present group treatment goals
   Orient members to DBT biosocial theory and DBT assumptions
   Orient members to group rules and format
   Ask adolescents and family members to sign contract

10 minutes: Break (snack, etc.)

50–60 minutes:
   Present didactic material on new core mindfulness skills
   Assign homework exercise
   Wind-down exercise

Weeks 2, 3, 4 of each skills module

50–60 minutes:
   Mindfulness exercise
   Announcements and overview of session content
   Homework practice review

10 minutes: Break (snack, etc.)

50–60 minutes:
   Present didactic material on new skills
   Assign homework exercise
   Wind-down exercise

---

shape participation with positive feedback, or can choose an introduction method that minimizes performance anxiety (e.g., just asking for names on the first day, or asking a shy teen to introduce a partner rather than him- or herself). Teens tend to feel less self-conscious about reporting on someone else than about describing themselves.

Reviewing Limits of Confidentiality

After the introductions, group leaders should review confidentiality issues, including the limits of confidentiality. For example, in New York State, we tell our group members about the state's three exceptions to confidentiality: suicidal ideation that includes plan or intent, homicidal ideation that includes plan or intent, or a suspicion of abuse or neglect.

   Handling confidentiality may at times present a challenge. Because of discussions in the weekly therapist consultation meetings, group leaders know more about clients than they may have revealed in group sessions, and possibly more than their parents know. This can become even more complicated when a group leader is also the primary therapist. Confidentiality issues pertaining to parents' roles, group leaders, and so on are discussed initially during orientation (see Chapters 7 and 9), and basic guidelines for confidentiality are followed.

Presenting Rationale for the Skills Program and Group Treatment Goals

Skills trainers explain that group members were chosen for this program because DBT is a treatment for a specific set of problems. This can then be linked with the rationale for the skills program and the program goals. Skills orientation proceeds here much as it does in pre-treatment: The adolescents' specific problems are linked to the five areas of dysregulation (confusion about oneself, impulsivity, emotion dysregulation, interpersonal problems, and adolescent–family dilemmas). Early in the initial group session, participants can be referred to a handout outlining the five common problem areas addressed in DBT for adolescents. (See the "Goals of Skills Training" handout in Linehan, 1993b, p. 107.) These core problem areas are discussed in Chapters 3 and 4.

Therapists can ask adolescents to identify for the group which areas are most problematic for them and to offer one or two behavioral examples. For example, frequent physical fights and persistent boyfriend or girlfriend problems would be classified as impulsivity and inter-personal problems, respectively. We advise starting with the more senior members, so that they can model how to describe these problem areas. In our experience, some of these senior members will happily report the reduction or remission of some of the problem areas since the beginning of skills training. The problem areas are then linked with treatment goals—the behaviors to increase.

We recommend that after reviewing the areas of dysregulation with all of the adoles-cents, the skills trainers then ask the family members to reveal which (if any) of the problem areas either relate to them presently or did so in the past when they were teenagers. Often parents experienced similar sorts of difficulties when they were adolescents, and sometimes experience them presently as well. These disclosures are typically enlightening for the adoles-cents, who often have not known of the parents' teenage problems or have not heard the par-ents admit a current set of problems. Inviting parents to participate in this fashion fosters a sense of camaraderie among all ages.

Reviewing DBT Biosocial Theory

The next step is to present the biosocial theory of BPD (see Chapter 3). The discussion can be handled similarly to the way it is presented in pretreatment orientation (see Chapter 7). The group can be asked: How is it that this group of adolescents has such a similar constellation of problems? As in pretreatment orientation of families, the discussion of the invalidating environ-ment needs to be sensitively handled. We find it helpful to frame the invalidating environment as particular behaviors or ways of communicating, rather than as characteristics of family mem-bers; it is also useful to point out potential external sources of invalidation (see Chapter 3).

To reduce the parents' guilt or defensiveness, the skills trainers can ask whether the par-ents experienced any invalidation in their own childhood homes. In fact, many of these par-ents have reported to us that invalidation was the *only* type of communication they experi-enced. Skills trainers need to make the point here that it makes perfect sense that they are inadvertently invalidating their own children, since a validating environment was never mod-eled for them while they themselves were growing up.

Another way to prevent parents from feeling blamed is to emphasize the transactional na-ture of the biosocial theory. For example, sometimes a parent and child may have different temperaments, as in the case of a hyperactive toddler with a quiet, mellow mother. That is, emotion dysregulation in a child tends to pull for invalidation by a parent. We have found that often parents actually report feeling *validated* by this discussion. The trainers can point out that the style of downplaying emotional experiencing (e.g., "Come on, stop crying; it's not that bad") may have a neutral or even beneficial impact on a different type of child—one who is not emotionally vulnerable. Some parents report having felt inadequate for years because they were unable to soothe their children and always felt that they were doing or saying the wrong thing. It now begins to make sense.

Orienting Members to DBT Assumptions

Obtaining agreement on DBT's basic assumptions is an essential part of orienting multifamily skills training groups. Although these assumptions by definition cannot be proved, they can be particularly influential in treating suicidal adolescents with their families. In fact, we announce to the multifamily group members that buying into these assumptions will promote nonjudgmental interactions, which will in turn facilitate therapy. If family members are not participating in treatment, then adolescents should nevertheless be oriented to these treatment assumptions, either at pretreatment or in an adolescent skills training group. We present these assumptions on a written handout.

Presenting the assumptions to adolescent–parent groups differs in two ways from their presentation in standard DBT. First, we apply most of the assumptions to family members as well as to the adolescents, in the belief that they are applicable and will help to motivate and support family members. Second, the discussion that ensues is not limited to adolescents' talking about their own experiences; family members inevitably join in and comment on their children's experiences. This often sparks a lively debate on the various points within families. Note also that several of the assumptions differ slightly from those in standard DBT. Group leaders must be prepared to note and respond to polarized positions regarding these assumptions.

The first three assumptions can be used to highlight the core dialectic in the treatment— acceptance and change. This simultaneously helps move everyone toward a synthesis by validating both the adolescents' and parents' perspectives. These first three assumptions are as follows:

1. *People are doing the best they can.*
2. *People want to improve.*
3. *People need to do better, try harder, and be more motivated to change.*

The third assumption appears to contradict the first one. However, even if all group members are doing the best they can and want to do better, this does not mean that their efforts and motivation are up to the task. Skills trainers can explain that the first and third assumptions, which seemingly are opposites, can be true at the same time and form the core dialectic in DBT: balancing acceptance of what group members are doing in the moment with change, which is necessary to become more motivated and function better. Skills trainers can elaborate that for numerous reasons, including past learning and certain skills deficits, adolescents and family members (and skills trainers) are doing the best they can at this point in time. However, they still need to learn new skills and do better, try harder, and become more motivated to change. This discussion is often enlightening for adolescents and families alike.

To reinforce this point further, the skills trainers can engage the parent who appears the most frustrated with his or her child's behavior by asking something like the following:

THERAPIST: Mrs. Ruiz, please read Assumption 1. (*After she reads*) Do you think that Vanessa is doing the best she can?

MRS. RUIZ: Absolutely not. She is doing this on purpose, just to get me angry and. . . .

THERAPIST: Mrs. Ruiz, do you think Vanessa wants to be in this room at 6:00 P.M. every Monday night?

MRS. RUIZ: Well, no. Who knows what she wants? She never tells me anything.

THERAPIST: If Vanessa could control her behavior well enough not to require 3 hours of therapy per week and could hang out with her friends instead, do you think she would do so?

MRS. RUIZ: I guess so (*tentatively*).

THERAPIST: In other words, if Vanessa could do better, she would do better . . . but for whatever reasons, she is not currently capable of doing that and therefore must be doing the best she can, just as we believe you are doing the best you can to manage the relationship with your daughter. This is Assumption 1. And since you are both here, we believe you want to improve. This is Assumption 2. But, by the same token, Mrs. Ruiz, you and Vanessa have ongoing conflicts. So you both need to figure out how to do better, try harder, and be more motivated to change. This is Assumption 3. These three assumptions together create a dialectic. Both sides can be true: accepting yourself and other family members as doing the best they can in the moment, while also acknowledging that everyone needs and wants to do better, try harder, and be more motivated to change.

At this point, an adolescent whose parent has refused to attend the group may state that his or her parent is not doing the best he or she can, because the parent is not even making the effort to participate. What stance should be taken on family members who are not supporting the adolescent in treatment? We believe it is still useful to hold to the position that even these individuals are doing the best they can at the present time, given their own situation and capabilities. But group leaders can also validate that it can be hard to see it that way sometimes, and it can still be painful when a loved one's "best" does not feel satisfying.

This may be the first time an adolescent has gotten the validation inherent in the transactional model of BPD. In other words, it is not just that the teen is lazy, emotional, or the like; the teen is doing the best he or she can and wants to improve, and the parent as well as the teen must do better, try harder, and be more motivated to change. Once these three important assumptions have been discussed and accepted, the trainers can move on to the others.

4. *People may not have caused all of their problems, but they have to solve them anyway.* Adolescents sometimes balk at this assumption, saying, "That's not fair." We have found the following example useful:

"I am walking along the Hudson River carrying my laptop computer and wearing my jacket and tie, and someone accidentally or purposely pushes me into the water. Did I want to be swimming in the less than purified Hudson River water, fully dressed, with my laptop? No. Is it my fault that I am presently in the water? No. But the fact that I did not put myself in the water does not mean that I do not have to swim to get out."

Adolescents sometimes cannot solve their problems on their own to the degree that adults can. For example, unpaid medical bills, a family move to an undesirable residence, and a lack of transportation are all examples of problems that may be beyond adolescents' capacity to solve. Parents or other authority figures (e.g., teachers, guidance counselors, other care providers) may be the only ones who can alter certain situations. The group leaders should acknowledge that this may be the case at times. In fact, this is why DBT with adolescents balances consultation to the client with environmental intervention (see Chapters 3 and 4); therapists at times may have to act on their clients' behalf with family members or others. However, by presenting the idea that individuals need to solve their own problems, therapists are encouraging an active problem-solving approach and openness to learning new skills.

5. *The lives of group members are painful as they are currently being lived.* This assumption is reworded slightly from standard DBT, in which clients' lives are described as "unbearable" as currently lived. This assumption was intended to validate the experience of suicidal clients. Although clients' family members' lives are certainly painful, given the circumstance of having suicidal children, we did not want to equate the children's and parents' emotions (by labeling both "unbearable") and thereby risk invalidating the adolescents and mislabeling the experience of the family members. However, the term "painful" is still intended to validate the difficulty experienced by both teen clients and their families. It also helps to increase parents' empathy by targeting their misattributions of their adolescents' maladaptive behaviors as a mere lack of motivation. When considering this assumption, parents become more likely to see problematic behaviors as related to painful emotions than to stubbornness, manipulativeness, vindictiveness, or laziness. Similarly, adolescents can come to see their parents' problematic behaviors as in part stemming from painful emotions rather than only negative qualities.

6. *Group members must learn new behaviors in all important situations in their lives.* Suicidal adolescents commonly engage in mood-dependent behaviors. As a result, they must learn how to manage these emotions and resulting behaviors differently. Maladaptive responses to painful emotions may often occur at home, at school, at work, with friends, or with family members. Periods of stress offer opportunities to learn new ways of coping. However, this does not mean that clients are on their own. Therapists stay in close contact, actively coaching with skills, cheerleading, and helping with problem solving. Similarly, it is assumed that parents of suicidal teens need to learn new behaviors to cope more effectively with their lives, and in particular, with their adolescents.

7. *There is no absolute truth.* This assumption takes on special significance when family members are present in group, because it can be described immediately in terms of the parents' versus the adolescents' perspectives. Skills trainers explain that no one is the sole proprietor of the truth. Both parents and children have valid points to make, and at any given time, a grain of truth can be found in either position. We search for a synthesis between opposite points of view. After reviewing the assumptions for the third time in group, one authoritarian father reported that since beginning the group, he had been carefully monitoring his tendency to assume his "absolute truth" stance with his daughter. He reported that trying to abide by this assumption helped to reduce some of their conflicts.

8. *It is more effective to take things in a well-meaning way than to assume the worst.* We developed this assumption specifically for adolescents and their family members, after seeing that they regularly manifested a hostile attributional bias in their interactions with one another, leading to attacks and escalations. Adolescents often manifest extreme interpersonal sensitivity and are thus highly reactive to any perceived criticism, deprivation, rejection, or other slights from the people in their lives. Parents, influenced by repeated displays of anger or other negative communications, may overinterpret their children's behaviors as intentional or malicious. Thus skills trainers encourage both adolescents and parents to consider neutral or benign interpretations for each other's behaviors, rather than automatically making the worst assumptions. For example, a teenager may accuse a parent of checking up on him or her, while the parent's questions may simply reflect an interest in the adolescent's day. Or a parent may believe that a child is shutting him or her out, while the adolescent's pleas of "Leave me alone; I don't want to talk about it now" may reflect an attempt to avoid exploding when the teen feels unable to calm down immediately.

Note that at times it is correct to assume the worst about another's intentions, and this must be acknowledged. In fact, some individuals with BPD or borderline features err on the side of being overly trusting, which can lead to its own set of problems. However, in this population, we commonly see the hostile attributional bias operating within families and provoking unnecessarily conflictual exchanges. We thus emphasize that particularly with family members, it is more effective (and thus worth the risk) to assume benign intentions. Such an assumption is likely to increase communication while reducing anger and conflict escalation.

9. *Clients and their family members cannot fail in DBT.* The inclusion of family members in this assumption is the only change from its standard DBT version. We believe that if clients drop out of treatment or fail to get better, the therapy, the therapists, or both have failed. If the therapy was applied according to protocol, and clients still do not improve, then the failure is attributable to the therapy itself. This contrasts with the assumption of many therapists that when clients drop out or fail to improve, it can be attributed to a deficit in motivation on the clients' part. Even if this is true, the job of therapy is to enhance motivation sufficiently for the clients to progress.

Orienting Members to Group Rules

After discussion of the DBT assumptions, skills trainers review the rules of the multifamily skills training group. Most of these derive from standard DBT; we have made only slight modifications. These ruled are listed on a handout, and we review them in group. The rules are as follows:

1. *Each adolescent must be in ongoing individual therapy.*
2. *Group members are not to come to sessions under the influence of drugs or alcohol.*
3. *Information obtained during sessions (including the names of other group members) must remain confidential.*
4. *Group members who miss four skills training sessions (and/or four individual sessions, for adolescents) may not remain in treatment.* They can reapply for skills training one skills module after their cohort has completed treatment. We feel that if four sessions are missed, this it reflects a lack of commitment, and the client or family member has also not received sufficient content for the treatment to be fruitful. Thus it is deemed a disservice to allow them to remain in treatment. Furthermore, applying a consequence to missed sessions should serve to enhance attendance. Reapplication one module after their cohort has completed treatment is the chosen time period, so that those clients or family members who drop out near the end still experience a natural consequence and have to wait at least one skills module before reentering. It would seem inconsequential if one could drop out during the next to last week and resume 1 week later.

At times, a family member will miss his or her fourth group session when an adolescent has not. In such situations, we warn the adolescent after the second and third miss by the family member that the family member will be terminated from the group, but the teen can remain. Our own team has disagreed about the decision to exclude a family member after the fourth miss, even though he or she is not the identified client. The argument goes, "Isn't it better to have a family member attend even some of the group sessions than none at all?" Our belief after much discussion is that family members, especially parents, should be held to the same standard as the adolescents. If we do not expect this much from the parents, then what message might we be sending to the teenagers?

5. *Group members who come more than 15 minutes late will be allowed in the group but will be considered absent.* We developed this rule to discourage lateness to the group. We decided to have significant lateness count as an absence but not to exclude latecomers from attending the group, since it would be counterproductive to block adaptive behaviors (i.e., mak-

ing it to group to learn skills, even when arriving late). We did not want to punish members' efforts to attend. Furthermore, not being allowed in group when lateness occurred for benign reasons (e.g., delays on public transportation) seemed punitive and demoralizing. Counting lateness as an absence, in contrast, simply holds group members accountable for trying even harder to make it on time in the future, and helps to convey the point that they are missing significant content when they arrive late.

6. *Clients are not allowed to discuss past suicidal behaviors with other clients outside of sessions.* Hearing about other adolescents' cutting or overdosing behaviors may elicit self-harm urges in teen clients. There is a documented contagion effect of suicidality, particularly among adolescents (e.g., Velting & Gould, 1997). In addition, group members' reactions to suicidal behaviors may include sympathy, interest, and concern, all of which may reinforce these behaviors. Thus clients are instructed to discuss these behaviors with their individual therapists instead.

7. *Clients who call one another for help when feeling suicidal must be willing to accept help from the person they call.* It is not acceptable for a client to call someone and say, "I am going to kill myself," and then refuse to let the person help him or her. This rule helps to teach group members how to reach out for and accept help when needed, while not putting other group members in positions of frustration and helplessness.

8. *Clients may not form sexual relationships with one another while they are in DBT.* If such a relationship were to become unstable or dissolve, one or both partners might feel uncomfortable about attending group. For similar reasons, we have not allowed clients to have their boyfriends or girlfriends serve as the accompanying "family members."

9. *Group members may not act in a mean or disrespectful manner toward other group members.* This last rule is especially important to spell out for an adolescent population. Compared to their adult counterparts, we have found adolescents more prone to disrespectful behaviors in group, such as rolling their eyes, giggling, or impulsively interrupting with jokes or sarcastic comments. Sometimes these may be directed at teens' own family members rather than at peers. In any case, when we present the handout of group rules, we elicit from group members examples of disrespectful behaviors; they are usually proficient at providing such examples. We then ask them how these would be likely to make others feel, and again, they are adept at generating responses. We find that when we ask them to generate the examples and consequences, they take on the role of arguing for the rule and are thus likely to become more committed to it; this is similar to the devil's advocate commitment strategy (Chapter 7). At times, however, they will of course need to be reminded of this and the other rules.

Handling Consequences When a Parent Is Responsible for an Adolescent's Breaking DBT Rules

At times a teen will miss sessions because of the participating family member. This may happen when the adolescent is dependent on the parent for transportation and the parent intentionally or unintentionally creates a scheduling conflict (e.g., scheduling a doctor's appointment during session time). Although it is unfortunate for an adolescent to be penalized for a parent's lack of commitment to the treatment, it is important to be consistent in applying the policy regarding missed sessions or other issues. If it is clear that a parent is interfering with or hindering the adolescent's attending, the trainer can use a combination of coaching the adolescent in interpersonal effectiveness skills to stress the importance of making it to treatment and coaching in problem solving regarding other solutions (e.g., an alternate means of transportation). For example, one adolescent whose mother had erratic work hours arranged on several occasions to get rides to group with the members of another family who lived nearby.

Asking Members to Sign an Agreement

Having been oriented to the DBT rules, assumptions, biosocial theory, and treatment goals, adolescents and family members are asked to sign an agreement stating their willingness to commit to the DBT program. As originally developed, DBT did not include a policy of asking clients to sign an agreement; only a spoken commitment was elicited. However, we believe that a written agreement increases the commitment levels of adolescent clients. First, social psychology research informs us that making both a written and a spoken commitment is more likely to result in behavioral follow-through. Second, behavior therapy has precedents for using written contracts to effect behavior change in a variety of problem areas. Third, the very act of signing an agreement conveys to adolescents a seriousness about treatment and an adult-like responsibility for it, which from the outset differentiate their role in therapy from the more passive and youth-like role they may be accustomed to playing in school or with other care providers. Finally, although teens and parents are only asked to make oral commitments in individual therapy, we find that the written agreement in group acknowledges the enormous commitment required for attending a 2-hour group plus doing homework. If a teen chooses to sign an agreement, the skills trainers cosign, and then the client is asked to have the individual therapist cosign as well. Parents are asked to sign their own agreements, which are placed in the front of their skills notebooks; skills trainers cosign their agreements as well. Figure 10.1 presents a sample adolescent–family member DBT agreement.

SKILLS TRAINING SESSION STRUCTURE

Usually skills training sessions are divided into two parts with a break in the middle. In standard outpatient DBT (Linehan et al., 1991), skills training sessions were conducted in a group format and were 2½ hours long. For adolescents, we typically run multifamily skills training groups for 2 hours. This decision was based on two major factors: (1) the somewhat shorter attention span of a younger population, and (2) the scheduling needs of families and adolescents (i.e., balancing therapy with parents' work schedules and kids' school homework demands). When skills training is conducted with a single family, it is often shorter (1–1½ hours). Although the skills trainer covers the same material, homework review, discussion, and practice of new skills take less time with only one family. In some programs, skills training is divided into two shorter sessions over different days of the week—one for teaching new skills, and one for homework review and practice This schedule works especially well with a "captive audience," such as an inpatient or juvenile justice population.

First Half of Skills Session:
Mindfulness Skill Practice, Homework Practice Review

The first half of each skills training session follows a similar format regardless of setting, and regardless of whether the second half takes place directly following it or on a different day. The session generally begins with a several-minute practice of specific mindfulness skills (see Appendix A). With teens, we recommend starting out briefly (usually 1–2 minute), and gradually working up to longer exercises. After asking for a handful of group members to volunteer to share their observations from the mindfulness exercise, skills trainers then relate what the content will be for the rest of that group session. The skills covered are determined by the treatment manual, as skills are taught in sequence within a given module. (Skills trainers plan ahead of time how the skills are to be covered, including, ideally, what exercises will be used

DBT Agreement

I am familiar with the theory, assumptions, and format of dialectical behavior therapy (DBT).

I agree to participate in the full DBT program.

I will come to group on time, with my materials and homework. If I don't do my homework, I agree to do a behavioral analysis.

(For teens) I am fully aware of the attendance policy, which is that if I miss more than four individual sessions and/or four skills training group sessions, I will have dropped out of DBT.

(For family members) I am fully aware of the attendance policy, which is that if I miss more than four skills training group sessions, I will have dropped out of DBT.

_____   _____
(Your signature)   (Date)

_____   _____
(Skills trainer's signature)   (Date)

_____   _____
(Skills trainer's signature)   (Date)

_____   _____
(Individual therapist's signature)   (Date)

FIGURE 10.1. *Sample DBT agreement for adolescents and family members*

and what homework will be assigned.) Also at this time, skills trainers make any announce-ments that are relevant.

Then homework review begins. If group size allows, we recommend asking all group members (adolescents and family members alike) to review their homework practice aloud, allowing several minutes each. Although it is preferable to review homework with each mem-ber each week, if a skills group is overly large the trainers can ask only a proportion of mem-bers to go over their homework, and be sure to ask the other group members to do so in the following session. Another possibility is to break into two smaller groups for homework re-view, with one skills trainer meeting with each smaller group. Group members can then re-convene in a larger group for the second half. Homework review offers a chance to ascertain whether clients have correctly learned the skills, to review concepts in which clients need ex-tra help, and to reinforce clients for making the effort to practice.

Session Break

Purposes of the Break

Following the first 50–60 minutes of each skills training session, the group generally takes a 10-minute break. We have found this break important for several reasons. First, it is a practical ne-cessity to allow participants to use the restrooms or make phone calls. Second, this time allows for informal conversation that inevitably strengthens the alliances among participants and be-tween participants and coleaders. For example, parents sometimes "compare notes" as to how they are coping with their adolescents' behaviors. Adolescents often discuss activities occurring at school, boyfriend- or girlfriend-related issues, and weekend plans. Third, the break serves as a periodic opportunity for the skills trainers to check on members who came in late or appear emo-tionally dysregulated, or to give specific feedback to someone about his or her behavior. For ex-ample, one adolescent who had arrived late for several weeks, and appeared disengaged during the first hour of group, seemed to come alive during the break while socializing with his peers. The leader asked to speak with him for a moment outside of the group room and explained:

> "José, when you express yourself and talk with your peers during the break, you are very en-gaging and likeable. I've been wondering why you've been coming in late and not partici-pating in the group during the last few weeks." [José shrugged his shoulders.] "Well, maybe you can think about it and discuss it with me or your individual therapist. All I can tell you is this—you're a good guy who is well liked by the group, but I think you would get more out of this group if you participated by paying attention and speaking up a bit. The question is, can you try to push yourself harder to get here on time? Also, how about if you can try to say one thing during the second half of the group today? Anything at all, OK?"

José nodded and said, "OK, I'll try." This type of brief interaction often has a positive effect.

A fourth reason to take a break is that participants require reinforcement for attending the group. For adolescents, we recommend that this take the form of receiving snack foods, such as crackers, potato chips, cookies, and juice or soda. In fact, it has often been noted that food appears to be a strong motivator for youth.

The Great Snack Break Debate

Our staff of adolescent DBT therapists has engaged in a debate over the years about the snack break. Should the snacks be used merely as reinforcers? If so, we should bring a variety of junk foods to the group, such as chips, cookies, and soda, and hope that these snacks will help lure clients back to group next week. Or should the snacks consist of healthy foods that exemplify healthy choices? The Emotion Regulation module's PLEASE MASTER skills specifically refer to balanced (and healthy) eating as a means of reducing vulnerability to negative emotions. Thus it also makes sense to have food that does not increase vulnerability to negative emotions or contribute to unhealthy dietary habits.

Despite several years of teaching PLEASE MASTER skills and being struck by the adolescents' and their families' limited understanding of food and its impact on emotions, we were reluctant to withhold the junk foods during our snack break. Our rationalization was "What good is it to have healthy food if they do not show up?" However, we have gained confidence about our ability to treat teens and families and have them return; it's apparent that the treatment itself engages them, not just the snacks! Thus the DBT therapists have achieved a dialectical synthesis, based on conversations with our adolescent clients. Most of the teens preferred to have some junk food snacks while also being exposed to healthier snacks, such as fruit and fruit juices, seltzer, crackers or pretzels, and low-fat cookies. As a result, many teens who have worked with us to date have reduced their junk food intake while increasing their healthy snack intake (e.g., fresh fruit).

Second Half of Skills Session: Teaching New Skills

Following the break, new skills are taught in the second half of every group session, including sessions that begin with the orientation described above. Orienting is a skills trainer's primary means of selling new behaviors as worth learning and DBT procedures as likely to work. Before teaching each new skill, the trainers should provide an overall rationale for why this particular skill or set of skills might be useful. The important point to make here, and to repeat as often as needed, is that learning new skills requires practice, practice, and more practice. Equally important, the trainers should emphasize that practice has to occur in situations where the skills are needed. The skills teaching format begins with a rationale for each new skill and follows the presentation structure described by Linehan (1993b). Thus it is not reviewed in detail here, although we do offer some helpful exercises and tips for teaching adolescents (see below). By the end of the session, homework is assigned for practicing the new skills that have just been taught. This homework is then reviewed in the first half of the next week's session. The session typically ends with a wind-down exercise, typically an observation.

Group Wind-Down

At the end of each session, after assigning the practice exercises for the upcoming week, the skills trainers then devote about 3 minutes to a process-observing wind-down (see Linehan, 1993b, p. 21). Skills trainers ring the mindfulness bell and ask participants, in no particular order, to nonjudgmentally describe an observation about anything that is relevant to that day's group experience. Moreover, participants are instructed not to respond to anyone else's descriptions. The primary skills trainer goes last, often adding a final observation of concern about any member who did not attend that day's group session. Although it is initially challenging to apply their skills in this format, the adolescents typically enjoy the opportunity to share one nonjudgmental observation about themselves, the group, or other members. This exercise again strengthens their mindfulness "muscles" while helping to bring a quiet, thoughtful closure to each session.

Note that over time, skills trainers shape these responses to be sure that they are consistent with nonjudgmental observing and describing, giving feedback in response to any comment that is not. For example, if a client says, "I feel like I did a terrible job today," the skills trainer might say, "Shelly, did you hear how that observation sounded *a bit* judgmental? Can you try it again, observing and describing without the judgment?" Shelly then might say, "I was quiet and had a lot on my mind today, so I didn't get as much out of group as I usually do," and the skills trainer might respond with "OK—that time it was more descriptive with less judgment!" In general, between modeling of comments by skills trainers and shaping of group members' comments, clients learn quickly and make closing observations that demonstrate nonjudgmental observing and describing.

CLINICAL TIPS FOR TEACHING DBT SKILLS TO ADOLESCENTS

Although our format and teaching points for adolescent skills training reflect standard DBT (see Linehan, 1993b), we have found that teaching in as lively and experiential a way possible engages adolescents most effectively. In addition, while keeping the content the same, we have made minor to moderate revisions on most skills handouts—using more "teen-friendly" words and language, using larger type and varied fonts along with some graphics, and putting less text on a page. We have found that these revised handouts seem to engage adolescents better, while seeming less daunting to teens with lower reading levels. We have also shortened the skills training content, both to fit within a shorter treatment length and to allow room for our new module, Walking the Middle Path. If clinicians are conducting skills training within a shorter time frame, it is possible to cover fewer skills. However, one must keep in mind that altering the skills handouts can be risky, as it strays slightly from the empirically supported treatment package and could possibly alter the meaning or emphasis of the skills. Reducing the number of skills covered is risky as well, until empirical research demonstrates which skills are essential and linked to treatment outcome. If trainers choose to revise the handouts in this manner, it is important for them to maintain the original meanings and follow the teaching points in the skills training manual (Linehan, 1993b) corresponding to each handout when they are teaching the skills in group. Figures 10.2a–10.2d are samples of DBT skills handouts adapted for adolescents in the Montefiore program. Table 10.4, presented earlier, provides a model of a shortened skills training format. In what follows, we provide several examples of lively, experiential exercises that work well for teens in the four standard DBT skills modules. We then describe the new fifth skills module, Walking the Middle Path.

Core Mindfulness Skills

The Core Mindfulness Skills module is always the first module taught to new members. We employ many of the same exercises as those used with adults (Linehan, 1993b). But we also use others that involve humor and silliness and are more interactive. Appendix A describes a number of mindfulness exercises we use with adolescents; these kinds of exercises can break the ice and help strengthen adolescents' commitment to the group. The "snap, crackle, and pop" exercise, for example, involves everyone getting up and standing in a circle, pointing to others with arms in specified positions that correspond, in sequence, to the words "snap," "crackle," and "pop." Getting mixed up with the arm movements is inevitable and leaves almost everyone laughing and energized. It emphasizes participation without judgment and focusing on one thing in the moment. Skills trainers make the teaching points while everyone is feeling more engaged and relaxed by the exercise. As a rule, skills trainers should tie each exercise to at least one specific mindfulness skill (observing, describing, etc.). They should also

Mindfulness
Three Steps to Achieve Wise Mind: "What" Skills

OBSERVE

- Just notice the experience in the present moment.
- *Wordless watching:* Watch your thoughts and feelings come and go, as if they are on a conveyor belt.
- Don't push away your thoughts and feelings. Just let them happen, even when they are painful.
- Observe both inside and outside yourself.

DESCRIBE

- *Wordful watching:* Label what you observed with words.
- Put words on the experience—for example, "I feel sad," or "My heart is pounding."
- Describe only what you observe (without interpretations).

PARTICIPATE

- Try not to worry about tomorrow or focus on yesterday. Throw yourself into the present moment fully (e.g., dancing, cleaning, taking a test, feeling sad in the moment).
- Fully experience your feelings without being self-conscious.
- Listen to your WISE MIND to help you choose to participate (a) in your discomfort; (b) in an alternate activity to escape/avoid distress; or (c) in order to experience life fully.
- Remember to use your "HOW" SKILLS while participating.

FIGURE 10.2a. *Example of an adapted skills handout for adolescents.*

Emotion Regulation

Taking Charge of Your Emotions: Why Bother?

Taking charge of your emotions is important because:

> Suicidal and depressed adolescents often have intense emotions, such as anger, frustration, depression, or anxiety.

> Difficulties in controlling these emotions often lead to suicidal and other self-destructive behaviors.

> Suicidal and other self-destructive actions are often behavioral solutions to intensely painful emotions.

FIGURE 10.2b. *Example of an adapted skills handout for adolescents.*

Distress Tolerance

Crisis Survival Skills: Distracting

A good way to remember these skills is the phrase "Wise Mind ACCEPTS."

Distract with...

Activities — *Do something.* Call, e-mail, text-message, or visit a friend. Watch a favorite movie or TV show. Play sports. Play video games. Write in a journal. Clean your room.

Contributing — *Contribute (do something nice) for someone.* Help a friend or sibling with homework. Surprise someone with a card, flower, or hug. Consider volunteer work. Send a thoughtful instant message.

Comparisons — *Make comparisons that will help you feel better.* Compare yourself to those less fortunate. Compare how you are feeling now to a time when you felt different. Consider those who are coping in the same way as, or less well than, you are.

Emotions — *Create different emotions.* Watch a funny TV show. Rent a scary movie. Listen to music. Read comics. Get active when you are sad. Slow down when you are wound up.

Pushing away — *Push the painful situation out of your mind temporarily.* Leave the situation mentally by moving your attention and thoughts away. Build an imaginary wall between you and the situation. Block the situation from your mind. Remind yourself that you aren't thinking about that situation. Put the pain and situation in a box, on a shelf, or in a drawer, and leave it there.

Thoughts — *Replace your thoughts.* Read. Do word puzzles. Count to 10. Notice the colors in a poster. Repeat the words to a song in your mind. Go to "reasonable mind" and stay there for a while.

Sensations — *Intensify other sensations.* Hold or chew ice. Listen to loud music. Wear a rubber band on your wrist. Take a hot or cold shower. Squeeze a ball or toy. Run fast.

FIGURE 10.2c. *Example of an adapted skills handout for adolescents.*

Interpersonal Effectiveness
How to Get Someone to Do What You Want

A good way to remember these skills is the term "DEAR MAN."

<u>D</u>escribe   <u>M</u>indful
<u>E</u>xpress   <u>A</u>ppear Confident
<u>A</u>ssert   <u>N</u>egotiate
<u>R</u>einforce

<u>D</u>escribe	Describe the situation. Stick to the facts.
<u>E</u>xpress	Express your feelings by using "I" statements ("I feel . . . ," "I would like . . ."). Do not assume that the other person knows how you feel. Stay away from "You should . . . "
<u>A</u>ssert	Ask for what you want or say "no" clearly. Remember, the other person cannot read your mind.
<u>R</u>einforce	Reward (reinforce) the person ahead of time by explaining the positive effects of getting what you want. Also, reward him or her afterward.
(Stay) <u>M</u>indful	Keep your focus on what you want, avoiding distractions. Come back to your assertion over and over. Ignore attacks; keep making your point.
<u>A</u>ppear Confident	Make (and maintain) eye contact. Use a confident tone of voice—do not whisper, mumble, or give up and say "whatever."
<u>N</u>egotiate:	Be willing to "give to get." Ask for the other person's input. Offer alternative solutions to the problem. Know when to "agree to disagree" and walk away.

FIGURE 10.2d. *Example of an adapted skills handout for adolescents.*

leave time for at least some sharing of experiences by group members afterward, so a teaching point can be made.

Another adolescent program (DeRosa et al., 2006) uses a "states of mind" charades game. Participants volunteer to act out one of the states of mind (i.e., emotion mind, reasonable mind, and wise mind). They can use both verbal and nonverbal communication to portray the mind state, and members must guess which state they are depicting. Leaders can act out states of mind too, if no one volunteers at first. Group members are then asked how they recognized the state of mind (by facial cues, body language, voice tone and content, etc.). This exercise helps familiarize adolescents with the states of mind and with the role that facial expressions, body language, and other cues play in communicating emotions—again, while they laugh and have fun. For adolescents, this playful and active component of group exercises helps engage them, helps differentiate skills training from most of their classroom experiences, and makes the attending the group more reinforcing for them. It also creates shared laughter between adolescents and their parents, which can be refreshing after the periods of strain and stress that have typically preceded their entry into treatment.

We have been asked whether using games or other active mindfulness exercises risks causing strong shame reactions in adolescents who lose a game or otherwise "make fools out of themselves." This possibility can be minimized by making most of the exercises noncompetitive, by having leaders participate themselves, and by being strict about maintaining an atmosphere of respect among group members—which means no teasing, whispering, rolling eyes, or similar behaviors (see the discussion of group rules above). Occasionally however, shame may occur, and a group leader who notices it can handle it by asking *all* group members to practice being nonjudgmental or by speaking to the client either during break or after group. If it comes up in individual therapy, the primary therapist should address it with the adolescent. If it becomes a problem for a group member, leaders can use less interactive exercises for a while. Yet we have found that the benefits of such exercises outweigh the risks, because of the engagement with the learning process they create for the vast majority of group members.

When possible, we also try to tie mindfulness exercises into the content of other modules. For example, when teaching distress tolerance, we may begin by playing a piece of classical music and asking participants to listen mindfully (i.e., to concentrate on one aspect of mindfulness, such as observing and describing, listening without judgment, focusing on only one thing in the moment, or fully participating in the experience). Then later that session, we may tie this exercise in with the notion of self-soothing with music. Or, when teaching interpersonal effectiveness skills, we sometimes use a mindful communication exercise. We break group members up into pairs and have one member speak about his or her day for a minute or so, while the other "listens" while acting clearly distracted. We then stop them and have them resume, this time with the listener attending "one-mindfully" (emphasizing the mindfulness skill of focusing on only one thing in the moment). When time allows, the partners can then switch speaker and listener roles. We then ask the speakers of the dyads to comment on what it felt like to have an attentive versus a nonattentive listener. This exercise always elicits a powerful response. It not only helps demonstrate mindful listening, but also creates empathy for family members, as participants (adolescents and adults alike) realize that they may rarely give them full attention.

Distress Tolerance Skills

When teaching distress tolerance, we find it helpful to spend group time on applications of these skills. With self-soothing, for example, we have had group leaders bring in a variety of self-soothing "tools" for the various senses. These have included beautiful pictures and art books (vision); soft, pleasant music (hearing); scented candles and potpourri (smell); soft pillows, velvet or silky fabrics, and plush stuffed animals (touch); and herbal teas, chocolates, and other treats (taste, smell). To conduct group practice, we set up all objects on a table during break, before group members enter. We also try to turn off fluorescent lights and use lamps to make the lighting softer. We ask group members to come in and select items to soothe some or all of the senses, and go back to their seats with them. We briefly orient them to the idea of using these objects to soothe themselves through the various senses. We then play the music and have group members begin self-soothing by looking mindfully at the pictures, sipping their tea, stroking their stuffed animals, and so on. We do this for several minutes, and then ask members to describe the experience, including how they felt before and after. We find that adolescents *love* this exercise. Although they may be self-conscious at first, they tend to throw themselves into it fully and, while enjoying themselves, to take the business of self-soothing quite seriously. We then introduce the self-soothing handout and begin making the teaching points. Because the group members have just experienced the self-soothing firsthand, they learn the concepts immediately.

We have had similar success with group practice of the skill of distracting. We bring in various distracting items, such as upbeat music, video clips of funny or uplifting scenes from movies or popular TV shows, crossword puzzle books, popular magazines, decks of cards, and even manicure kits. We have helped group members access sad or distressing feelings by asking them to recall and imagine a recent time they felt sad. Then we ask them to participate fully in one of the offered activities for 5 or 10 minutes (e.g., we will show a funny movie scene or have them select a distracting activity to participate in). Afterward, we ask participants to comment on whether they were able to take their minds off the distressing content. The experience of actively distracting themselves in session, rather than simply reading about it on a handout, has proven helpful in getting teens to believe in the skill and use it outside of the group. Note that these group practices can be done when skills training is being conducted with only one client or family as well.

As an alternative to inducing sadness, members can just observe their current moods and thoughts, and notice whether a distracting exercise succeeds in distracting them from these. This actually works quite well, as many members come in feeling stressed, sad, anxious, or otherwise distressed anyway. If the leaders attempt to provoke mild distress in group and a group member gets very upset, this is best handled by having one leader check in with the group member, spend a few minutes outside the group discussing the reaction if needed, talk with the member after group, or perhaps follow up with a phone call to check in and provide coaching about ways to feel better. Checking in with this member the following week is also advised, and the primary therapist can address the issue in individual therapy as well. Other group members might need to be reassured too, if they feel upset that a group exercise has proven disturbing to a fellow member. It is helpful to remember that group members get upset from time to time in group for various reasons—ranging from reactions to another group member's contribution, to upsetting comments made by their family members, to their own thoughts.

Interpersonal Effectiveness Skills

For teaching interpersonal effectiveness skills, we always employ role plays in group, either between two adolescents or between an adolescent and a parent (the teen's own or someone else's). In first teaching an interpersonal effectiveness skill such as DEAR MAN, we sometimes present a hypothetical conflict that will allow them to see the application of the skills. This conflict might concern a hypothetical parent–adolescent dyad, two adolescents, a skills trainer and another party, or even the two skills trainers. Whereas group members typically become engaged by conflicts that might relate to them, they really seem to enjoy beginning with a conflict involving skills trainers. For example, we have presented hypothetical conflicts between a skills trainer and an outside party such as an auto mechanic (e.g., over when the trainer's car will be ready) or a neighbor (e.g., over the noise level of the neighbor's music), or between the group coleaders (e.g., over who is responsible for picking up the snacks before group that day). Note that hypothetical conflicts involving the skills trainers are best kept relatively benign and not deeply personal. Adolescents can then be asked to coach the skills trainers on how to handle the situation skillfully, or for volunteers to play both sides. Perhaps because of their generally strong curiosity about their therapists, and perhaps because of the validation they experience from seeing that therapists are fallible beings, adolescents nearly always become highly engaged by such exercises and perform impressively skillfully. This allows them to see how the skills can be used in a more neutral way before they apply it to something more emotionally laden for them. Adolescents truly participate in these exercises—often hamming it up and loving to be tough opponents in a role-played conflict—and they can be disarmingly skillful! One particularly helpful thing we have found is to ask an adolescent to play the role of a parent and a parent to play the role of an adolescent. This helps with skill acquisition, while also increasing perspective taking and empathy.

Emotion Regulation Skills

As in the other modules, we make the teaching of emotion regulation skills as experiential as possible. For example, to teach the model of emotions (the diagram of emotions and their connections to behaviors, thoughts, urges, aftereffects, etc.), we typically present a hypothetical prompting event that group members can relate to, such as being yelled at by a teacher after making a mistake in class. We then take them through the cycle of emotions, writing the diagram on the board and asking them to fill in thoughts, body changes, urges, actions, emotion labels, and so forth. We find that the group members become heavily invested in this exercise, often shouting out a variety of appropriate responses. When the diagram is completely filled in, we then discuss the complexity of emotions with them, noting all the different things that are going on when emotions get triggered. We then ask for a volunteer to provide a real-life example, and we complete the diagram a second time, again engaging the group members with questions about how they might feel or react.

Another example is our use of a group exercise we call "the wave" (called "mindfulness to the current emotion" in standard DBT). Rather than simply reviewing the handout, we have actively practiced this skill in group. We have sometimes used music or movie clips, both designed to provoke reactions (moods, body sensations, etc.). We find that these are very powerful stimuli for evoking emotions in adolescents. We then ask members to listen or watch nonjudgmentally, and to direct their attention to their inner experience in response to the clip. We then ask for observations on this, and then repeat it with a very different piece of music or movie clip. Group members are readily engaged by this activity; they eagerly share their nonjudgmental observations and descriptions of their emotions as they come and go, along with accompanying thoughts, body sensations, actions, and urges.

Similarly, with the emotion regulation skill of "acting opposite to the current emotion," we have begun by having the group coleaders act out a brief angry interpersonal exchange that begins to escalate. We then ask the group to identify the emotions, action urges, and behaviors. We ask them to describe what the opposite action would be, and then "replay" the incident—either by having the group members coach the skills trainers in opposite action, or by asking for group member volunteers to role-play the opposite-action version.

Walking the Middle Path

Walking the Middle Path, our new skills training module developed for adolescents and family members, is described below.

WALKING THE MIDDLE PATH: A NEW SKILLS TRAINING MODULE

Walking the Middle Path is a new skills training module developed specifically for adolescents and families. This module helps clients to balance change-oriented skills with acceptance-oriented skills. The name of this module grew out of the dialectical dilemmas apparent among our adolescents and their families. We believe that this title captures the essence of DBT and is certainly relevant to the other four skills modules. The module was developed to focus on issues that regularly required more attention in adolescent and family skills groups, and in the overall therapy: the notion of dialectics in general, followed by specific examples of balancing validation (i.e., acceptance) with problem solving (i.e., change), and balancing extreme behavior patterns as discussed in Chapter 5.

The format is similar to that of the other modules, in that we use handouts and homework sheets, present the material didactically, and ask for examples from group members. However, more than the other modules, the content of this material is aimed at parent–adolescent interactions, and even at parenting styles in their own right. The module is thus especially relevant for inclusion when parents participate in the skills training. We find that parents are highly engaged by this material; however, the module can be useful even for skills training without parents or other adults present. Adolescents can discuss their experiences with parents regarding "middle path" skills, as well as applying some of the skills to themselves. Table 10.6 outlines the content of the Walking the Middle Path module. The complete module is provided in Appendices B (lecture notes/discussion points) and C (handouts). The present section overviews the three main skill areas in the module: dialectics, validation, and behavioral principles.

Dialectics

General Content

The dialectics segment teaches an alternative world view that fosters a capacity to consider opposing perspectives and to work toward achieving a synthesis (i.e., "walking the middle path"). These concepts are applied to group members' own polarities in thinking, feeling, and behavior, as well as to managing opposing stances that cause tension in interactions with others. The dialectical dilemmas grew out of themes of behavioral extremes repeatedly described by families (Rathus & Miller, 2000). Although the three dialectical dilemmas presented in Linehan's (1993a) original text continue to inform case conceptualization and treatment with suicidal adolescents who have BPD or borderline features, the behavioral patterns in this skills segment characterize familial interactions in particular, especially those between parents and teens.

Parent–Adolescent Dialectical Dilemmas

As explicated in Chapter 5, the parents of suicidal adolescents, the adolescents themselves, and even the treating therapists commonly vacillate and become polarized along three dimensions: (1) excessive leniency versus authoritarian control; (2) normalizing pathological behav-

TABLE 10.6. Walking the Middle Path Module: Content Outline

Dialectics

Parent–adolescent dialectical dilemmas
    Excessive leniency versus authoritarian control
    Normalizing pathological behaviors versus pathologizing normal behaviors
    Forcing autonomy versus fostering dependence

Balancing validation and change

Validation
    Why validate?
    Steps to validate self and other

Behavioral principles
    Positive reinforcement
    Negative reinforcement
    Self-reinforcement
    Extinction
    Effective and ineffective punishment
    Shaping

iors versus pathologizing normative behaviors; and (3) forcing autonomy versus fostering dependence. In our adolescent–parent handouts, we have simplified the terms for each of these dilemmas as follows: (1) being too loose versus too strict; (2) making light of problematic behavior versus making too much of typical adolescent behavior; and (3) pushing away versus holding on too tight. Again, consistent with the theme of this module, we teach adolescents and their family members that balancing the extremes are important skills. While these dialectical dilemmas and their corresponding skills are often first highlighted in group sessions, they can also be addressed in depth in individual and family sessions. Additionally, these dilemmas may be found between two parents, between a therapist and teen, or within the very same teen.

The two skills areas that follow, validation and behaviorism segments, highlight the two sides of the treatment's core dialectic: acceptance and change.

Validation: Working on Acceptance

The validation portion of this module teaches acceptance of one's own and others' experiences. Swann et al.'s (1992) self-verification theory suggests that challenges to one's self-constructs increase emotion dysregulation. This in turn interferes with cognitive processing and impedes new learning. One can extrapolate from Swann et al.'s self-verification data to the constructs of self- and other-validation. That is, self-validation is likely to enhance emotion regulation and processing of new information; validation of others is likely to maintain interpersonal connectedness while helping to deescalate conflicts. Data from marital interaction research lend support to the importance of validation in improving affective and verbal aspects of communication (e.g., Weiss & Tolman, 1990). Reinforcing this notion with youth is the fact that over 70% of suicidal adolescents report some form of "interpersonal conflict" as the precipitating event for their suicidal behavior (Miller & Glinski, 2000).

Skills trainers orient participants to this topic by alluding to the validation component of the GIVE skills taught in the Interpersonal Effectiveness module, and discussing the pull individuals sometimes feel to be either overly validating or overly change-focused. We find extended teaching of validation particularly important in working with adolescents and their family members. Although we considered keeping the extension of the validation topic within the Interpersonal Effectiveness module, we decided to include it in the Walking the Middle Path module, because it provides the dialectical balance with the change-focused behavioral strategies that are also included in the latter module. Thus, although we teach validation in Interpersonal Effectiveness, we highlight it and teach it in more depth in Walking the Middle Path.

Behaviorism: Working on Change

The change-oriented behaviorism segment of the new module teaches individuals how to increase adaptive behaviors while decreasing maladaptive behaviors in themselves and others. Specific learning principles taught include positive reinforcement, negative reinforcement, shaping, extinction, and punishment. After years of conducting DBT with teens and family members, it became apparent that many participants were lacking basic knowledge in this area. For example, numerous behavioral analyses with suicidal multiproblem adolescents revealed the inadvertent positive reinforcement of suicidal behaviors by unsuspecting family members and boyfriends/girlfriends (see Chapter 8). At the same time, family members and teens often missed opportunities to reinforce adaptive behaviors in each other and themselves, and inadvertently punished or extinguished preferred behaviors.

SPECIFIC GROUP STRATEGIES FOR HANDLING TYPICAL CONCERNS

Issues inevitably arise in skills groups with adolescents and family members, such as motivation, homework compliance, therapy-interfering behaviors, and others. Here we discuss specific group strategies to handle these concerns.

Increasing Motivation

Group leaders can use various strategies in group to increase members' motivation to participate actively in skills training (i.e., to answer questions, share observations, review homework, or role-play a skill). One common method is to try positive reinforcement and shaping principles when a client makes a "just-noticeable improvement" along his or her behavioral chain. For example, one reticent client, who previously had not participated, received a "Good man, thanks" comment from the skills trainer after volunteering to read an excerpt from the skills handout. Another client received a high-five from the coleader after doing her homework for the first time in a month. Since both clients subsequently increased the frequency of these adaptive behaviors, we can assume that the skills trainers' responses were positively reinforcing, thereby increasing the clients' motivation.

However, for some clients, such positive reinforcement may not work in increasing participation. For such clients, skills trainers can try other strategies—such as directly asking them to review their homework or participate in an exercise, or asking the clients about their reticence during session break. Depending on the client, it may not be a good idea to conduct a brief behavioral analysis and problem-solve in group, as one would for problems with homework compliance (see below). This is because there may be factors interfering with motivation that a client does not feel comfortable discussing in front of other group members or his or her own parents (e.g., experiencing severe social anxiety, being emotionally dysregulated in group, feeling hurt by a skills trainer's comment, or feeling punished for efforts to participate by the perceived mocking reactions of other group members). Thus the client's apparent lack of motivation should be shared in the team meeting, so that the primary therapist can be informed; the primary therapist can then address this as a therapy-interfering behavior and conduct a behavioral analysis and solution analysis in the individual session. Note that some teens will always be less active participants than others; even shy or quiet members can learn the skills capably and do not necessarily need to be shaped toward more active involvement. Skills trainers need only attend to what appears therapy-interfering, such as an apparent lack of motivation that interferes with an individual's skill acquisition or hurts the morale of the group.

Increasing Homework Compliance

Motivating Adolescents to Complete Homework

The concept of homework for many adolescents, particularly depressed and suicidal ones, is an aversive one. We choose to use the term "take-home practice exercises" in lieu of "homework" as much as possible, to reduce this negative connotation (others have similarly substituted terms for homework as well, such as using the term "worksheet" for skills practice forms and "journaling" for filling out the diary card). Obviously, however, using different terminology by itself will not appease all adolescents. Using metaphors helps to emphasize the importance of practicing, such as a track star's practicing with short runs weekly for months in order to build up to running a marathon, or the now-retired basketball player Mugsy Bogues's working on his dribbling and shooting skills to compensate for his short stature and proving all of his critics wrong. Ultimately, the most effective way to elicit compliance with homework is to employ the behavioral principles of shaping, positive reinforcement, and use of slightly aversive consequences (e.g., disappointment or withholding attention). Problem solving following a mini-behavioral analysis can be used as well.

Shaping behavior begins in the first group by reinforcing all target-relevant behaviors with praise (provided that praise is a reinforcer for a given adolescent). Thus, when an oppositional and defiant teen shows any sign of interest in a skill (e.g., raising his or her hand to ask an appropriate question or to give an answer), the coleaders reward that client with plenty of attention by smiling, making eye contact, and offering praise. If a client fails to bring in the homework, a group leader can show a bit of disappointment and then ask, "What happened?" Then the skills trainer conducts a brief behavioral analysis to help identify the problem and develop solutions to prevent it from recurring, while withholding more positive attention. This is important, as a number of factors can contribute to noncompletion of homework, ranging from motivational or emotional factors interfering to forgetting or not understanding the assignment. We have been shaped by our clients to take an extra minute or so to explain the take-home practice exercise carefully and clearly, including exactly the form we expect to see it in (filled-out worksheet vs. oral report, etc.). We then often ask a group member to repeat the assignment aloud, to be sure it has been understood as we intended. We find that making this extra effort to orient group members to the homework results in better compliance.

If a client fails to bring in the homework the following week, the therapist questions the client again in a deliberate, firm manner. However, the therapist never judges, demeans, or criticizes the client. In fact, the skills trainers give that client as little attention as possible (unless it is deemed that avoidance of attention is reinforcing), and await some just noticeable improvement to reinforce. For example, one client failed to do her homework for 3 consecutive weeks, reporting that she failed to think about it at all after leaving the group each week. By the third week, the client reported having thought about the assignment and almost practiced her skill until she became dysregulated and unable to follow through completely. The client received considerable reinforcement from the coleader, which helped promote the completion of homework for the next week. In other words, reinforcement for merely thinking about doing her homework proved fruitful eventually in shaping the client to complete it. As an aside, the skills trainers consistently alert each client's individual therapist when the client fails to do his or her homework. It is incumbent upon the individual therapist to address all therapy-interfering behaviors, including noncompliance with homework, especially when the group skills trainers' behavioral interventions are not effecting change.

When several members of the group fail to complete the homework, the coleaders consult openly with one another in front of the group and discuss how it is that they, the coleaders did an ineffective job of either teaching the skill itself or orienting the group to the practice exercise for that week. Thus the skills trainers, and not the group members, take responsibility when a pattern of noncompliance occurs within the group.

What reinforcers for completing homework work well for adolescents? There are both immediate and delayed reinforcers for homework completion. Immediate social reinforcement from peers, parents, and group leaders can be a strong motivator. For instance, skills trainers can allow the first volunteer with completed homework to lead the homework review as a reinforcer (however, leaders must be confident that this would actually be reinforcing for the particular group member!). Delayed reinforcers include the natural reinforcers of becoming more skillful in life and making overall greater progress in treatment. Some groups even have concrete reward policies in place, such as awarding some type of small prize (e.g., key chain, movie pass) to individuals who complete homework for four weeks in a row, or giving a collective prize (e.g., pizza party during break) to groups whose members complete all homework for 4 weeks in a row. Some groups have such policies regarding attendance as well.

Motivating Family Members to Complete Homework

Once the family members have disclosed their own behavioral problems and skills deficits during the group orientation (i.e., the first week of every module), the coleaders use the family members' own words to reinforce the need to practice the skills themselves. Two of the DBT assumptions reviewed during this orientation are that all group members (including skills trainers) are doing the best they can, *and* that everyone needs to do better, try harder, and be more motivated to change. These tenets help adolescent and adult group members alike accept the need to practice new behavioral skills in order to help themselves and their family members. In addition, the same principles of shaping, reinforcement, mildly aversive consequences, and problem solving described above apply to family members as well as teens.

Handling Clients' Expression of Dissatisfaction with Their Individual Therapists in Group

At times, adolescents will voice dissatisfaction with their primary therapists in the skills training group. A skills trainer does not dismiss such a client's feelings, nor does he or she condone back-stabbing and judgmental statements. Rather, the trainer helps the client to observe and describe the difficulty quickly and nonjudgmentally, and then provides brief coaching on what skills the client might use directly with the individual therapist (consultation-to-the-client strategies). Ideally, the skills trainer can link this coaching to the present subject matter of skills training, such as use of DEAR MAN skills, acting opposite (e.g., approaching rather than avoiding a feared situation), or radical acceptance. The skills trainer might find it appropriate to validate the client's feelings, but to state that things are not likely to change if the client fails to discuss what bothers him or her directly with the individual therapist. After addressing this problem, the skills trainer should immediately move on to the next issue. If the problem is interfering with the skills training agenda, the skills trainer can offer to consult with the client briefly about it during break or after session.

Handling Therapy-Interfering Teen Behaviors in Group

It is common for teens to engage in therapy-interfering behaviors in group, such as cross-talking, doodling, giggling, interrupting, moving around the room, and passing notes or objects to other group members. However, decreasing therapy-interfering behaviors is a lower-order target in group skills training than in individual therapy. In skills groups, increasing behavioral skills is a higher-order target. The purpose of this shift in ranking is to help maintain the agenda of skills training and not get sidetracked by the numerous potential therapy-interfering behaviors of emotionally dysregulated teens. Thus such behaviors, if mild, are at first ignored in group, with attention and praise selectively applied the moment an adolescent shows signs of reengaging with the group. Skills trainers regularly employ contingency management strategies in order to change the motivation of the client in each context as well. If a problem behavior is more than a passing phenomenon, group leaders can speak to the adolescent about it during a break and also alert the individual therapist, so that it may be addressed in individual sessions. If the problematic behavior occurs for an extended period of time, to the point of seriously distracting leaders or other members, the leaders will address it directly in session, modeling interpersonal effectiveness skills in bringing it up and requesting change.

Addressing Therapy-Interfering Behaviors of Family Members

Therapy-interfering behaviors of family members in group (such as cross-talking) are handled in the same way as those of adolescents. That is, the skills trainers ignore these at first but reinforce other, compliant behaviors; if a problem behavior persists, they speak to the family member during break or use interpersonal effectiveness skills to address the problem in group. Since family members do not receive individual sessions in which a behavioral analysis could take place, the skills trainers must rely on one of these other methods to address the problem. A therapy-interfering behavior occurring outside of group skills training (e.g., arriving late to a family session) might be addressed through a "microanalysis" of the problem (e.g., 2 minutes), with an attempt to come up with one solution and obtain a commitment to try it. If such a behavior is a more substantial problem, it may be addressed as part of a planned family therapy session.

Handling the Dropping Out of a Family Member When the Adolescent Remains

At times, an adolescent's family member will drop out of therapy, either of his or her own accord or because of violating the rule of no more than four missed sessions. When this occurs, the adolescent often feels anger, disappointment, or shame. These feelings may be directed at the parent (for not caring enough, not trying hard enough, or not following the rules) or at the DBT program (for enforcing the rules). This is a useful scenario to bring to the therapist consultation team for discussion. In this case, the primary therapist will need to check in with the adolescent regarding the impact of the family member's dropping out, its impact on the relationships with the skills trainers, the impact on motivation to continue treatment, and how the teen would like to handle it in group skills training (although it should be addressed only briefly, there will need to be some acknowledgment of the parent's dropping out, and the skills trainers and the adolescent might collaboratively decide who makes this statement and how it is worded to the group). In any case, the adolescent's continued efforts are acknowledged and praised by the primary therapist and skills trainers. Furthermore, in the few cases we have seen in which this happened, the client received a great deal of support from other group members. Note that when family members drop out of skills training, they may still be given the chance to participate to some degree through attending scheduled family sessions.

GOODBYE RITUAL AND GRADUATION CEREMONY

In an open group, at the end of the final week of each skills module, some group members will have completed the rotation. In a closed group, members complete the group at the end of the contracted skills training period. In either case, leaders have the option of providing some type of goodbye ritual or ceremony to mark the completion of skills training (see also Chapter 11). We recommend conducting some type of ritual, despite the time it takes away from open groups. The time is worth the reinforcement it provides for those completing skills training, as well as the motivation it provides the remaining members.

In our outpatient open group, participants and skills trainers engage in a goodbye ritual (typically lasting 30 minutes) whenever people complete the skills rotation. The ritual begins with each group member's and each skills trainer's offering specific feedback to the graduates about the work they have accomplished, as well as what potential pitfalls to anticipate upon graduation. Following this go-around, each graduate proceeds to say goodbye to each remaining member, as well as to each peer and family member who is also graduating. These goodbyes are opportunities for adolescents, family members, and therapists alike to share their honest feelings and to provide constructive feedback. The exchanges are typically taken quite seriously; the comments are thoughtful and poignant. It is important that the parents receive the same goodbyes and acknowledgments of accomplishment as the teens do after completing the program. The ritual ends with a graduation ceremony, in which graduating clients and their family members are each awarded a diploma for successful completion of the DBT program.

During these goodbyes, if continuing treatment is available, the skills trainers might remind the graduates of the opportunity for them to enhance their gains and remain connected to the program in some way by entering the next phase of treatment. For example, standard DBT is typically followed by a treatment addressing Stage 2 targets such as unresolved trauma. Standard DBT and some adapted programs have also incorporated other continuation phases, such as graduate groups or advanced groups. The graduating adolescents have usually already discussed these options with their individual therapists. But the reminder during their graduation from skills training is helpful in reinforcing their commitment to continuing to work in therapy; participating in the next phase of treatment is likely to help maintain and even increase their gains. This point is supported by research data with depressed adolescents, which suggest that a continuation phase of therapy enhances the likelihood of maintaining the therapeutic effects of a short-term treatment (Brent, Kolko, Birmaher, Baugher, & Bridge, 1999b; Birmaher et al., 2000).

HANDLING GRADUATION IN A SHORT-TERM TREATMENT FORMAT

Teens are considered to be in Stage 1 of DBT as long as they evidence significant behavioral instability. In most settings, regardless of the agreed-upon time frame of therapy (e.g., 16 weeks, 6 months, 1 year), adolescents are kept in standard DBT until they are out of Stage 1.

There are two main possibilities for how this might occur (see also Chapters 4 and 11). First, if a client's behaviors remain severe (e.g., continued suicidal behaviors or other severe, out-of-control behaviors), the client should repeat the first phase of therapy, addressing Stage 1 targets. In this circumstance it is critical to maintain therapy with a primary therapist who can monitor and intervene in the case of suicidal and other crisis or out-of-control behaviors. Second, a continuation of the first phase of DBT in a more intensive format may be needed at times. For example, we had one teen who continued carrying out life-threatening behaviors routinely, and in several weeks it became apparent that her suicidal urges were not responding to the treatment and that she was unable to make a commitment to reduce self-harm behaviors. In this case, we added family sessions focused on developing a plan of action and a suicide-monitoring plan, and we increased phone monitoring with the primary therapist. Depending on the situation, other modalities offering more intensive treatment might be considered. For example, DBT day treatment might be fitting for a teen with severe, out-of-control behaviors who is not attending school, as it would address the targets of safety and behavioral control while providing a structure.

If at the conclusion of the agreed-upon time frame of therapy, the client's behaviors have shown improvement and are no longer considered Stage 1 targets (i.e., the client is no longer evidencing suicidal and other severe behaviors), the client can be invited to continue in the next phase of treatment offered in the setting. (Note that some clients might need a break between phases.) Standard DBT follows the Stage 1 work of addressing severe behavioral dyscontrol with the Stage 2 work of emotionally processing past trauma, grief, and loss. Stage 2 DBT primarily addresses PTSD, using an exposure therapy format. Some programs offer other continuation options, either in addition to or in place of standard Stage 2 DBT. A common continuation phase is one of a number of versions of a "graduate group." Note that if PTSD work is indicated, and if Stage 2 DBT is not available in one's setting (because of a shortage of resources or of therapists trained in exposure therapy), we would recommend either problem solving to be able to offer this mode of treatment, or referring the client to a therapist who can provide exposure therapy. This might occur either in lieu of another type of continuation phase, or as an adjunct to it.

Assuming that exposure therapy can be made available to clients who need it, it can be beneficial to offer an optional graduate group as well. This group can follow numerous formats, but its goals generally include skill maintenance, generalization, and strengthening, along with opportunities for problem solving and peer support. These goals can be pursued either in a structured format with planned didactic presentations for each group meeting, or in a process-supportive format, where the group follows its own course but DBT skills are worked in whenever applicable. Note that to be in any type of DBT group, a client must have a primary therapist to take responsibility if the client should become highly suicidal. For a graduate group, this primary therapist could be the therapist conducting the exposure therapy, if this mode is occurring. When this mode is not occurring, the graduate group leader could serve as the primary therapist, in which case groups are best kept small. Yet another option is for a client to continue working with the primary individual therapist from the first phase of treatment. In this case, the frequency of visits might decrease, and the session targets and format might be altered to be appropriate to the client's current clinical presentation.

CHAPTER 11

Assessing Progress, Running a Graduate Group, and Terminating Treatment

This chapter first discusses various means of assessing progress in treatment, including what to do when the therapy seems stuck. (We also offer advice on handling the devastating experience of a completed adolescent suicide.) The chapter then goes on to discuss a continuation phase of treatment in the form of a graduate group. Finally, termination from DBT is covered, emphasizing the ending of various phases of treatment (i.e., transitions) as well as formal termination from treatment.

ASSESSING PROGRESS

There are several means of assessing progress in DBT; some of these involve clinical observation, and some involve formal assessment measures. Aside from the goal of assessing initial functioning and outcome for clinical and research purposes, using the formalized assessment procedures discussed in Chapter 6, a clinician is also interested in assessing progress over the course of a client's treatment. This interest relates to the well-being of the client, the formulation of the case, and the determination of whether the client is making sufficient progress on Stage 1 targets to enter the next stage and phase of DBT. The following discussion delineates methods of using clinical judgment to assess an adolescent's progress in DBT.

Clinical Observation

A teen client's primary therapist continually monitors the adolescent's progress through a number of means. These include observing changes in the diary card content, monitoring changes in therapy-interfering behavior, noting progress in individual session content, observing changes in family functioning, and obtaining feedback from the DBT consultation team. Skills trainers, pharmacotherapists, and primary therapists can all exchange relevant feedback at this meeting. The clinician thus can conceptualize the client's progress in terms of whether the client has addressed the targets of the particular treatment stage he or she is in.

Monitoring the Diary Card

As we've seen in earlier chapters, the diary card records a client's behaviors and identifies the items in the treatment hierarchy that need attention. The primary therapist uses the client's diary card to organize the agenda of individual sessions and to drive the treatment. Thus the therapist can place a great deal of emphasis on the diary card. The way in which the adolescent complies with the diary card task also provides important information on treatment progress. A client who has had difficulty with the card has made progress if over time he or she fills out the card more accurately or more thoughtfully, fills it out completely, does it every day or nearly every day (instead of during a session or at the last minute before a session), and remembers to bring it in each week. Completing the diary card consistently throughout treatment is a demanding task. Yet we find that most adolescents do ultimately comply with this component of treatment. However, completion of the diary card does not always go smoothly, and careful attention to this can be essential for making progress in therapy. For example, one of us had an adolescent client whose entire treatment revolved around her not doing her diary card. Conducting repeated behavioral analysis of this therapy-interfering behavior was valuable, because the factors controlling the behavior were the same as those influencing her inability to initiate or complete other important tasks in her life. Each week the therapist could make an easy transition from the card to other important tasks. Another adolescent client would not complete the diary cards, and after many months of behavioral analyses, it finally came out that she primarily did not want herself or her therapist to know how many drugs she was using. Therapy progressed when the therapist first had the client fill out the card but not bring it in; then fill it out, bring it in, but get it back before the therapist read it; and finally bring it in and give it to the therapist to read.

Learning to fill out the card accurately also indicates the client's progress. We have had adolescents who have minimized ratings on the diary card, either because they wished to downplay their problems or distress level, or because they had little insight into identifying and labeling their emotions. For instance, some troubled adolescents brought in diary cards reporting low urges to self-harm and only little emotional distress. In individual sessions, however, it became clear that the adolescents were indeed minimizing their own experiences. For such adolescents, we would consider it progress for their cards over time to reflect greater urges and indications of distress. Since this is often the case, clinicians should not be alarmed if after weeks in treatment clients who seem to have a minimizing response style appear worse on their diary cards.

For most adolescents, progress is reflected in the diary card by decreases in reported urges to commit suicide or NSIB, in actual suicide attempts or NSIB, in other impulsive target behaviors (i.e., quality-of-life-interfering behaviors recorded on the diary card, such as reductions in alcohol and drug use, unsafe sex, problems with housing, problems with school truancy, etc.), and in negative emotions. Such decreases reflect progress on Stage 1 treatment targets. An increase in ratings of positive emotions also indicates progress.

Monitoring Therapy-Interfering Behaviors

Examining a clients' therapy-interfering behaviors is another means of assessing progress. Some therapy-interfering behaviors will involve the diary card, such as not filling it out regularly or not bringing it in to session. Other behaviors will not be reflected on the diary card, but will be displayed in the interaction with the therapist (e.g., remaining mute during sessions, throwing things in the therapist's office, dissociating during sessions, refusing to leave the office at a session's end, calling excessively, or calling with suicide threats and then hanging up). Therapy-interfering behaviors may cover a wide range: trouble with the therapeutic alliance, inability to regulate anger or hostile behaviors in session, arriving late to session, not completing homework assignments, not participating in the skills training group, problems with motivation, and/or not calling the therapist prior to a suicide attempt or NSIB. Patterns of therapy-interfering behaviors typically reveal themselves early in treatment; progress occurs when such behaviors subside following behavior and solution analyses. For example, in the early part of treatment one teen was self-cutting continually, but was not calling the therapist ahead of time. She simply reported the self-injurious acts on her diary card to be analyzed in the next session. Behavior analysis revealed that her lack of calling to avert the acts was mainly influenced by two factors. The first was the client's lack of any strong commitment to work on reducing self-harm behaviors, as she found them too effective for emotion regulation. She was terrified of what her experience of misery would be if she did not cut herself. The second factor was a social phobia that included a fear of calling the therapist on the phone. For the first problem, the therapist returned to commitment strategies (linking present commitments to past commitments, examining the pros and cons of continuing to cope with distress through self-harming, etc.; see Chapter 7). The therapist and teen also used problem solving to arrive at specific distracting and self-soothing skills to replace the cutting. For the second problem, the therapist used exposure to reduce anxiety, by having the client go into the next office and telephone the therapist during session time several times in a row and initiate conversation. In addition, the therapist instructed the client to practice paging the therapist later that night (when she was presumably not in distress). Over several weeks, the client did increase her calling of the therapist prior to cutting herself. Although fully stopping her self-harm behaviors took additional time, her increases in timely calling of the therapist were considered a sure sign of progress.

Monitoring Individual Session Content

The therapist can also observe progress by noting positive changes in the content of individual sessions with the client. Among such changes are improved insight and participation in conducting the behavioral analyses. In the early sessions, the client is just learning the steps of behavioral analysis, and the therapist may do most of the work while the client passively answers questions. As time passes, however, the adolescent may come in to a session ready to report the point at which the chain started, his or her vulnerability factors, the key links on the chain, and even possible solutions. For example, one adolescent male who at first had little insight into his impulsive behaviors progressed to the point where he would come to a session having completed a mental behavioral analysis himself! His therapist would attempt to write out the links in a visual chain, and he would report them so fluently that the therapist could not keep up and had to ask him to slow down. When behavior analyses go more quickly and efficiently—both because the therapist is more familiar with the client's patterns, and because the client is developing greater insight—the therapy is progressing. Of course, if such changes are not accompanied by decreases in behaviors targeted for reduction (e.g., reduction in suicidal behaviors) or increases in behavioral skills, the therapist and client must slow down to see what important links have been missed or where solutions have been ineffective.

The therapist can also observe the client's improvement through the session content as the content changes to reflect a progression through the DBT Stage 1 treatment targets. Since the first phase of DBT for adolescents involves the primary Stage 1 aims (see Chapter 3) of increasing safety, stability, and behavioral control, these areas will ideally show improvement as treatment progresses toward Stage 2. Obviously, improvement will be evident with decreased ratings of suicidal or self-injurious thoughts, urges, and actions, or other signs of severe behavioral dyscontrol. Thus, whereas the early treatment sessions are likely to be dominated by behavior and solution analyses of life-threatening and therapy-interfering behaviors, progress is indicated by greater attention to analyzing quality-of-life-interfering behaviors and increasing behavioral skills. For example, one of our teenagers presented for treatment in a suicidal crisis. Her suicidal urges remained for several weeks and were the focus of many sessions. However, as treatment progressed, the therapist noted that the highest-priority targets of suicidal behaviors and urges were no longer occurring, and thus session time was increasingly devoted to topics such as the client's arguments with her parents and her efforts to secure an after-school job. In other words, as session content progresses along the hierarchy of targets, a client is moving closer to the overall aim of increased behavioral control. (Note that it is critical for the therapist to ensure that the session focus is changing in response to behavior change, and not changing even when behavior has not changed!) True progress on Stage 1 targets indicates that the adolescent is capable of moving into Stage 2 and phase 2 therapy.

Monitoring Family Functioning

DBT for adolescents directly targets the adolescents' environment by including family members in the treatment, and it teaches skills for improving family interactions, especially between adolescents and parents. Progress should certainly be evident in improved relations and functioning between adolescents and family members. Problematic family interactions themselves often serve as a stimulus for emotional and behavioral instability for adolescent clients (and parents), or exacerbate difficulties that an adolescent (or parent) is already experiencing. Progress can be noted in any number of ways around family functioning, depending upon the particular case. For example, improvement can be reflected in a decreased need for scheduling family sessions, an increased willingness to schedule family sessions, decreased reports of familial discord, improved communication and emotional regulation in the presence of family members, and increased or improved interaction with family members in the group setting.

For example, one adolescent girl entered the multifamily skills training group with both her mother and her stepfather. Whereas she had a fairly stable relationship with her mother, she had an acrimonious relationship with her stepfather—as indicated by sarcastic exchanges in group, her storming out of family sessions in tears, his critical remarks about her in both group and family sessions, and his inconsistent attendance in the group. According to the adolescent's and her mother's reports, the stepfather's and teen's behavior at home toward each other was highly conflictual, characterized by limited contact and frequent angry flare-ups when interaction was attempted by either party. By the end of treatment, though their interactions were far from perfect, these had improved substantially. Both parties had reduced the frequency of sarcastic exchanges and were attempting to be more interpersonally effective (expressing feelings and desires more directly and gently). The teen remained for a whole family session, even when things got heated. The stepfather was no longer making frequent critical comments and had increased the frequency of validating his stepdaughter. Although he still did not attend every scheduled family session because of stated work conflicts (much to his stepdaughter's dismay), he did attend most of them, and on their "graduation night" he shared observations about his stepdaughter that were glowing in his praise of her improvement and what she meant to him. (This also resulted in her tears, but with no urge to storm out of the room!) Clear improvement was mirrored in other aspects of this teen's functioning as well.

Note that in cases in which parents have themselves been engaging in highly maladaptive behaviors—such as abusing alcohol, behaving aggressively toward their children, having too severe or too liberal limits, reinforcing dysfunctional behaviors, or having in the past sexually abused their children—mending relations might be complicated or nearly impossible, or at a minimum might take additional family sessions to accomplish. Progress might be marked by an adolescent's beginning to confront a situation he or she had previously avoided (e.g., by assertively expressing the impact of the parents' behavior patterns), by a family's agreeing to attend an intensive and perhaps specialized family-focused treatment following Stage 1, or by a parent's admission of and willingness to begin addressing the problematic behaviors. Conversely, progress might be marked by an adolescent's work toward radically accepting the parent's behaviors (or even protectively distancing him- or herself from a dysfunctional situation), while focusing on adaptive steps toward self-care, such as building other sources of social support and taking steps to achieve long-term goals.

Obtaining Feedback from the Therapist Consultation Team

Problems with specific clients—such as therapists' difficulty in regulating their own emotions during sessions, difficulty in implementing treatment effectively, or difficulty in the therapeutic relationship—often dominate therapist consultation team discussions. Certain therapists may need more attention than others because of their clients' difficulties, and the team quickly learns which therapists need support regarding cases with which they are struggling. Additional signs of progress can be found in the team's lessening focus on a particular therapist. That is, when team attention shifts away from such a therapist, when his or her discussion takes less time, or when the therapist becomes more balanced and emotionally regulated in discussing problems in relation to the client or family, progress has probably occurred.

A note of caution, however, involves the fact that a shift away from discussing a problematic situation can indicate not improvement, but possibly avoidance or hopelessness on the part of the therapist or team. Thus, if team members notice the absence on the agenda of a therapist whose case has been the focus of much recent discussion, the team should check in with the therapist, follow up on the case, and clarify the reason for the lack of discussion (and reconsider placing the therapist on the agenda, if needed). It must be remembered that burnout—of therapist, of team, of group leaders, and/or of clinic staff— is a common scenario in work with suicidal multiproblem adolescents. Thus, if team discussion has drifted away from a therapist because of burnout and not because of improvement, the burnout must be addressed. The team can work with the therapist to assess the source of the burnout and attempt to alleviate it with such strategies as suggesting new approaches, identifying where the therapist has become unbalanced, enhancing empathy for the client, generating hope about the case, reviewing the biosocial theory, revisiting commitment strategies, or (in more extreme cases) suggesting that the therapist take a vacation from the therapy. In essence, the therapist's skills in treating the client must be enhanced, and improvements in a therapist's and a client's skills typically go together.

When the Therapy Gets "Stuck"

How does the therapist know whether the treatment is working or not working? Essentially, if over time a client is attending, complying with the various demands of treatment, participating actively in treatment, and making progress on identified target behaviors, then treatment is having its intended impact. However, some client–therapist dyads seem to get "stuck," and the therapy stops progressing or does not seem effective.

If progress is not occurring, the therapist's implementation of the treatment will need additional examination by the therapist consultation team (or through the therapist's individual supervision, if applicable). Some change in approach is likely to be warranted. Is there some lack of "buy-in" to the treatment on the therapist's part? Has the therapist been properly trained, or could he or she benefit from more training? The team (and, if relevant, the individual supervisor) must troubleshoot with the therapist to discover what is not working. The problem may lie in the application of behavior and solution analyses. For example, the thera-pist may not be devoting enough time to identifying factors that interfere with engaging in so-lutions and determining how to overcome them. Often the problem will lie in the therapist's losing balance in the treatment, such as placing too much emphasis on validation or on prob-lem solving; being too flexible or too rigid; or applying too great a degree of warm, nurturing communication or irreverent communication. Sometimes the problem will lie in the fact that the client has shaped the therapist into doing ineffective therapy, such as not adhering to the DBT session format (e.g., behavioral analysis of behavioral targets according to the target hi-erarchy). At times, the therapist will have lost the ability to remain nonjudgmental and empathic to the client; at other times, the therapist will have lost this ability with regard to cli-ents' family members. Working with adolescents requires DBT therapists to have an equal ca-pacity for validation, problem solving, and reestablishment of commitment with the teens' family members—especially when the teens are reliant on their family members to get them to and from the office.

With a highly suicidal client in particular, the therapist's own emotional responses to the threat of an impending suicide (e.g., fear or anger) may immobilize the therapist or lead to overly protective or punitive responses. It can take all of a team's combined skills to ferret out what the actual problem is. For example, a group leader in the University of Washington clinic reported weekly that clients were angry and hostile toward him. Several threatened to quit; suicide threats in group sessions were not uncommon; and the therapist was so miserable that he was getting burned out and wanted to quit himself. He had felt too ashamed to bring the topic up in team, and it was not until two group members quit that the topic was discussed by the team. The most frequent complaint from clients was that the therapist was dismissive and nonvalidating; the therapist reported that he was doing his best to validate. When the team members got the therapist to role-play with them how he responded to group clients, it was immediately apparent that he indeed did sound dismissive. Further investigation revealed that when he was attacked, the therapist got quite anxious—and when he was anxious, not only did his cognitive processing decrease, but his responses sounded dismissive instead of validating. In addition, his shame that his therapy was not as good as that of other team mem-bers was so great that he could not discuss the topic in team meetings without great difficulty. The treatment, organized by the team, was for the therapist to record his group sessions and then listen to them daily until both his shame and his anxiety went down. He was instructed to employ opposite action when discussing his group in team meetings: keeping his shoulders back, making his voice confident, and maintaining good eye contact, while telling the team all the details without apologies or self-judgmental statements. For several weeks, part of each team meeting was devoted to role-playing with the therapist situations that arose in his group. His homework assignments were to notice when his anxiety started increasing while he was leading his group, and to share with his group the advice he was receiving in team meetings. The conclusion of this was that his group members became allies with him in changing his behavior; his shame disappeared; and he became more skillful at managing his anxiety in his groups.

The therapist and team should consider also whether it is possible for the therapist to be missing signs of progress—assuming that treatment is not working, when in fact change is oc-curring. For example, consider the case mentioned earlier of the therapist's spending the whole therapy on the diary card. This client may have appeared "stuck," but her therapy-interfering behaviors were a microcosm of the controlling variables for most of her problem behaviors, and eventually change in these targets occurred.

Whatever the reason for therapy's getting off track, the therapist is advised to access his or her own "wise mind" to reflect on the situation, and to bring the situation to the therapist consultation team for discussion. The team's purpose is to "treat" the therapist; in making use of this critical component of DBT, the therapist can become reenergized and recommitted, and ideally will get unstuck.

Handling the Suicide of an Adolescent Client

When a therapist is working with a suicidal population, it is likely at some point that the therapist will experience a client's suicide. When that client is an adolescent, this experience can be especially devastating. Moreover, a therapist who has been working with the teen's family faces not only the loss of the client, but also the grief and despair of the parents. Responding to an adolescent suicide is thus a delicate and complicated matter.

When the individual therapist or other primary therapist learns of an adolescent client's suicide through someone other than a family member, the therapist should call the family promptly and should offer condolences, as kindly and empathically as possible. The therapist should also go to the funeral, demonstrating his or her connection to the client and family. In all family interactions, the therapist should monitor any tendency to blame either the family or him- or herself. Both of these are within the realm of normal reactions, but neither should be communicated to the family. The family may desire ongoing support and treatment from the same or from a different therapist. Regardless, the therapist should make ample use of the consultation team concerning the inevitable range of strong emotions that will occur, the potential impact on work with other clients, the decision regarding whether or not (and, if so, how) to proceed with the family, and ways to handle the incident with the skills training group.

In general, if the client who committed suicide is also in a skills training group, we recommend that the other adolescent members' primary therapists (ordinarily their individual therapists) call their clients prior to the next skills group meeting, inform them of the group member's suicide, and handle whatever interventions are needed for each client (e.g., validation, distress tolerance skills, etc.). Then group leaders should process the suicide in the next couple of group sessions. Allowing significant time to attend to the suicide in the skills group indicates sensitivity to group members' inevitably strong reactions, demonstrates the caring and concern of skills trainers, and allows both skills trainers and group members to process powerful emotions that would surely interfere with the normally scheduled skills training. Skills trainers can help facilitate the processing of the suicide in a number of ways: by answering questions, to the extent possible (which must be balanced with respecting the deceased client's confidentiality and the family's right to privacy); by allowing members to make comments and share their reactions; by normalizing the reactions shared; by eliciting skillful ways of coping with painful reactions; and/or by inviting members to share thoughts or memories of the deceased client. A particularly helpful process is to invite group members to plan a tribute session or memorial ceremony for the deceased client. The skills trainers might also want to encourage close contact with individual therapists, family members, or other supportive figures during this difficult time. Adolescents might experience an increase in suicidal ideation; family members in the group might need additional contact as well, because they feel grief for the other parents' loss and fear that their own children are at heightened risk. In group, it is important that after about two sessions, the skills trainers gently turn the focus back to the didactic curriculum. This acknowledges that clients in treatment still need to enhance their capabilities; it demonstrates continuity and consistency, which group members may experience as reassuring; and it models a balance between grieving and moving forward.

Formal Assessment Measures and Additional Objective Ratings

In any evidence-based treatment program, it is critical to include at least some evidence-based assessment instruments. What measures to include depend primarily on the focus of the treatment program or the goals of specific clients. In our Montefiore DBT program for adolescents, we assess progress through a series of formal measures; these include a number of standard measures that target suicidality, features of BPD, and related behavioral patterns. These measures and the time frames for administering them within our outpatient program are described in detail in Chapter 6. We will not describe them again here, except to mention that filling out measures at the end of treatment or treatment modules may, for adolescents, be reminiscent of school exams. They may feel they have to mark down the "right answer," and thus their responses may be especially subject to demand characteristics. It is thus important to orient them to these assessments by stressing that there are no right or wrong answers, and that their honest answers to the items are the best responses.

We also suggest using objective ratings of several relevant factors to determine improvement as a result of treatment. These include the number (and days) of psychiatric hospitalizations and emergency room visits during treatment; the number of suicide attempts during treatment, defined as self-injurious behaviors with the intent to die, and based on clients' self-reports during the course of treatment; the number of NSIB incidents, also based on self-reports during the course of treatment; and treatment completion, indicated as a dichotomous rating of "yes" or "no" based on whether clients complete the agreed-upon treatment program.

In sum, the suggested assessment battery we describe in Chapter 6 is intended to serve as a guideline to assemble an outcome battery in a particular treatment setting to help determine whether the adolescent clients have improved on standardized assessment tools.

A MODEL FOR AN ADOLESCENT GRADUATE GROUP

Since documented rates of relapse and recurrence among depressed adolescents are high, clinical researchers have recommended either booster or continuation treatment to address this problem (Birmaher et al., 2000). Thus, in work with suicidal adolescents, we recommend the use of a second group phase of treatment. It not only makes clinical sense to have a continuation phase in treating multiproblem suicidal adolescents, most of whom also have mood disorders; but it can also help them make the transition out of therapy. For example, our graduate group helps wean adolescents from first-phase group skills training by reducing the role of group leaders (i.e., greater use of peer coaching and problem solving, and of adolescents themselves as teachers of skills). This section reviews the rationale for a graduate group for adolescents, and describes the particular model employed at Montefiore Medical Center. This is one of many possible continuation-phase models. Also note that participation in a graduate group can occur concomitantly with standard DBT Stage 2 individual therapy focused on emotionally processing the past.

In an advanced skills or graduate skills group, the primary goals are (1) to prevent relapse by reinforcing the progress made in the previous skills training group; (2) to help clients generalize their behavioral skills; and (3) to help clients increase behaviors instrumental to a positive quality of life, while decreasing behaviors interfering with a positive quality of life. To achieve these primary goals, the group leaders encourage the adolescents to "consult" with, validate, and reinforce one another to manage their current life problems more effectively, with less emphasis on the leaders. Ideally, the clients will continue to rely on one another after the group ends, having become less reliant on the adult therapists. Group therapy is an especially powerful therapeutic tool with this age group, since peer relation-ships promote the development of social skills and identity formation (Brown, 1990). Posi-tive peer relations can also foster improved self-esteem, provide buffers from stress, and (in the case of academically successful peers) improve adolescents' view of school (cf., Berk, 2004; Eccles et al., 1993). Moreover, the transition from the first phase of treatment to the second-phase graduate group is characterized by placing increased responsibility on group members in terms of participating without parents, taking active teaching and consulting roles in group, and solving problems with peers. These changes mirror the adolescent de-velopmental trajectory toward separation, individuation, greater self-sufficiency, and greater importance of peers.

The Montefiore graduate group is an optional program continuation consisting of adoles-cent first-phase graduates and two therapists. We find that more than half of these graduates elect to participate in the graduate group. Individual therapy and the multifamily skills train-ing groups are discontinued at this point; less intensive contact is needed, since the eligible clients are no longer in a state of severe behavioral dyscontrol. On a case-by-case basis, how-ever, we will at times provide a more intensive second phase of treatment, with some contin-ued individual therapy and family sessions supplementing the graduate group.

The graduate group is less time- and therapist-intensive than first-phase group skills training. The graduate group consists of a 2-hour group session once per week for 16 weeks, with the opportunity to recontract for an additional 16 weeks if an adolescent is able to iden-tify clear treatment goals. Some teens recontract several times, resulting in their graduate group participation for more than 1 year. Telephone consultation is still used as needed in this modality, as are individual or family sessions led by one of the group therapists. The two ther-apists are expected to participate in the weekly DBT therapist consultation/supervision meet-ing for the same reasons described in Chapter 4. Table 11.1 summarizes the treatment modes used in this graduate group. Typically, four to five teens participate in the graduate group at one time; more than five teens in one group would potentially preclude some of the group members from getting enough attention paid to their respective problems.

Target Hierarchy for a Graduate Group

In the Montefiore program, we have developed a target hierarchy for adolescents participat-ing in the graduate group. In contrast to the first-phase skills training groups, where little at-tention is paid to in-session interpersonal process issues, the graduate group utilizes behav-iors that occur outside as well as within the group sessions as a means to change. Hence the

---

TABLE 11.1. Graduate Group Modes of Treatment

- Group therapy (weekly)
- Telephone consultation (as needed), with group therapist
- Individual and family sessions (as needed, and typically led by previous individual therapist, or someone other than graduate group leader)
- Therapist consultation meeting (weekly)
- Pharmacotherapy (as needed)

---

major targets address in-session behaviors that are inevitably linked to maladaptive behaviors outside of treatment.

The hierarchy of treatment targets for a graduate group is outlined in Table 11.2. Decreasing life-threatening behaviors is not included as a target here, because it is assumed that once clients are in a graduate group, life-threatening behaviors have been eliminated. (If such a behavior should recur with increasing frequency, the therapist should address it as a top priority, but should also seriously consider whether the client needs to be back in more intensive treatment addressing the standard Stage 1 targets.) It is also assumed that once clients are in a graduate group, therapy-interfering behaviors will be eliminated or nearly eliminated, but if they show up, they are addressed as a high priority. Decreasing therapy-interfering behaviors (e.g., not coming to group, coming late to sessions, not doing homework, not taking medications, verbally attacking or being disrespectful toward other clients or group leaders) therefore becomes the primary concern. Targeting these behaviors for elimination allows the therapists and other group members to address the second most important target, which is strengthening interpersonal effectiveness skills. Inevitably, conflicts and problems arise in group members' relationships; the group is seen as a microcosm of their lives in which to practice the use of these skills, while receiving constructive feedback from peers and staff. The third target is increasing behaviors that are instrumental to a positive quality of life, while decreasing behaviors that interfere with a positive quality of life. These behaviors include addressing the secondary treatment targets that affect life quality and derive from the behavioral patterns common among clients with BPD or borderline features, as identified by Linehan (1993a) and Rathus and Miller (2000) (see Chapter 5).

An example of addressing the secondary treatment targets involved Jennifer, a 17-year-old Asian female, who grew up in an extremely invalidating environment. Her father had left the family when she was 2, and when she attempted to reconnect with him at the age of 15, he stated that he did not want to be around her because she had so many problems. Her mother repeatedly invalidated her. The first phase of treatment helped reduce some of the day-to-day invalidation, with the help of the mother's participation in the multifamily skills training group and family sessions, but Jennifer was still prone to invalidate herself on a regular basis. Self-invalidation became an explicit target behavior addressed in the graduate group. Thus any time Jennifer invalidated herself, one of the group leaders or a peer would gently say, "That sounds like self-invalidation . . . can you describe how you feel without invalidating yourself?" In the beginning, this was difficult for Jennifer to hear and even more difficult to correct. However, as time went by, Jennifer became better able to catch herself in the act of self-invalidation and to restate her thoughts and feelings without self-invalidation and without prompting.

Another example of addressing secondary targets in the graduate group pertained to Latoya, a 14-year-old African American female. Latoya had a history of severe trauma and a long psychiatric history, including multiple hospitalizations, multiple suicide attempts, self-cutting, PTSD, depression, panic disorder with agoraphobia, drug and alcohol abuse (pres-

---

TABLE 11.2. Target Hierarchy for a Graduate Group

1. Decreasing therapy-interfering behaviors
2. Strengthening interpersonal effectiveness skills
3. Increasing behaviors instrumental to a positive quality of life, while decreasing behaviors interfering with a positive quality of life

---

ently in remission), and dissociation. She was a likeable young woman with a tragic past. Her active passivity in sessions was evidenced by her lack of response to obvious problem-solving situations. She would often present a problem, and when asked what she tried or could have tried to address the problem, she would passively reply, "I don't know." The group leaders experienced tremendous sympathy and empathy for her, which resulted in their becoming overly active in trying to solve her problems for her. It took several months before the coleaders recognized that they were inadvertently reinforcing her passivity by solving problems for her. While active passivity became one of her target behaviors (as discussed between therapists), the phrase used to describe this target behavior to her was "a need to increase active problem solving for yourself." She recognized her difficulty in actively solving her own problems. She was oriented to the treatment plan for her, which entailed the coleaders' and peers' "sitting on their hands" until Latoya produced at least one or two possible solutions to her own problems, before chiming in with other feedback.

Graduate Group Format and Procedures

Montefiore graduate group sessions follow the basic structure outlined in Table 11.3. The following discussion describes what happens within each segment of the session.

Mindfulness Practice Exercise

Each meeting starts with a 10-minute mindfulness practice exercise. A different adolescent or group therapist leads the exercise each week, based on a prearranged rotating schedule. Adolescents who lead these exercises reap several benefits. First, they have an opportunity to be creative in the development of their own mindfulness exercises. Second, they practice taking on the role of "leader," which can enhance their self-esteem and sense of mastery. Third, the more they teach, the more likely they are to employ their mindfulness skills on command in their lives outside the group.

Virtual Diary Card Review

Since they are no longer in the first phase of treatment, graduate group members are not required to complete or return diary cards, However, we believe that it is clinically imperative to continue to assess certain target problems and behaviors in the group each week. Therefore, a semistructured assessment is built into the group's agenda; we call this the "virtual diary card." In this way, therapists learn how each individual has been functioning over the past

---

TABLE 11.3. Format of Montefiore Graduate Group (2 Hours)

- *10 minutes:* Mindfulness practice exercise
- *20 minutes:* Check-in/virtual diary card review
- *15 minutes:* Skill review
- *5 minutes:* Snack break
- *70 minutes:* Consultation and problem solving
- *5 minutes:* Closing observation and commitment

7 days, what needs to be addressed during the group session, and what information will be documented in each client's progress note/medical record.

The virtual diary card review begins when one of the group leaders asks each group member to rate the following behaviors quickly on a scale of 0–5 (except as noted), based on the previous week: depression, anger, anxiety, self-harm thoughts, self-harm actions (yes–no), suicidal thoughts, and suicidal actions (yes–no). Each client is also asked to rate current self-harm thoughts/suicidal thoughts (i.e., today); to list any positive emotions and rate their intensity; to list which specific skills were used (referring to the diary card list) and give an example of applying one skill; to indicate compliance with pharmacotherapy (yes–no); and to review homework. The virtual diary card is tailored to the individual needs of the client, just as a standard diary card is. Hence some clients are asked to rate urges to use drugs/alcohol, and then to report the frequency and intensity of actual substance use behavior. Similarly, for clients with eating disorders, restriction, bingeing, and purging urges and behaviors are assessed. A group leader writes down their responses.

These ratings take approximately 5 minutes per person. If an adolescent endorses NSIB or suicidal action, or changes in ideation in either domain, time is spent discussing this later during that client's allotted consultation problem-solving portion of the session. Regardless of the adolescent's preference, the group leader will conduct a behavioral analysis of these target behaviors and will engage the adolescent and the other group members in the solution analysis. Chronic self-harm urges or suicidal ideation does not necessarily require the same intensity of analysis as NSIB or suicidal action, since many of our clients retain their thoughts about such actions long after the actions are extinguished. Clinical judgment determines whether a behavioral analysis is required. Senior group members are sometimes asked to help "conduct" the behavioral analysis of a peer by standing at the blackboard, asking questions, and writing down the responses. Ultimately, the individual client who engaged in the behavior is asked to conduct his or her own behavioral analysis in front of the group.

Some research suggests that a detailed discussion of self-injurious behavior in a group setting may serve as a form of contagion (Velting & Gould, 1997). The dilemma is that when a group becomes the primary modality of treatment, it also becomes the only context in which to discuss any target behaviors, including life-threatening behaviors. Our synthesis is that we ask clients not to provide any specific details about the self-harm itself. However, we do ask them to identify the vulnerability factors, the precipitant, the key links in the chain preceding the target behavior, and the consequences. Lavish reinforcement is provided to the identified client and peers who help identify effective solutions in the solution analysis. The skillful graduate group therapist has to be capable of conducting a behavioral analysis and engaging peers in the solution analysis, while not reinforcing pathological behavior or fostering contagion.

Skill Review

Each week, the group members are asked which skill they would like to review. The group therapists try to obtain a consensus and then ask which adolescent would be willing to lead the review. If no one volunteers, the group therapists either teach the skill themselves or ask one of the more senior members whether he or she would be willing to teach the skill standing at the blackboard. Often this adolescent agrees, with some mild encouragement and reassurance that the group therapists will provide help if necessary. Typically, the adolescent who requests the skill is asked to give a real-life example to bring the "lesson" to life.

For example, one adolescent named Shanti, a 15-year-old Hispanic female, asked for a review of the pros and cons skill. Michelle agreed to lead the discussion and went to the blackboard, where she gave the rationale for using pros and cons. She asked Shanti for an example in which she might need to use the skill. Shanti, who had recently been living in foster care, was now reunited with her biological mother. Although both parties many challenges faced during this reunification period, Shanti stated that a major stressor for her right now was her mother's "nagging behavior." The client stated that she was unaccustomed to having anyone "parenting" her; thus, while she understood that her mother was trying to do her job, it was "too much, too soon. . . . Did you do this? Did you do that? Can you do this? Can you do that?" The client continued to describe her efforts to tolerate her distress, since she did not want to hurt her mother's feelings, but recognized her urges to "tell Mom to back off" if her mother did not stop her "repeated requests" (newly described term without judgment). The group helped her review the pros and cons of tolerating her distress versus the pros and cons of not tolerating her distress. In addition, the group helped Shanti identify which of those pros and cons were short-term and which were long-term. Shanti was easily able to identify that it made sense to use her GIVE and DEAR MAN skills. Shanti role-played with a DBT group leader how she was going to validate both her mother's and her own perspectives, while also directly asking her mother to make one clear request of her at a time without repeating herself. Shanti received significant praise from the group, and Michelle, the adolescent who had led the "lesson," received a round of applause from her peers. Shanti's homework assignment for the upcoming week was to follow up with her mother using her DEAR MAN and GIVE skills.

Snack Break

The group takes a 10-minute snack break after the skill review.

Consultation and Problem Solving

The consultation and problem-solving stage of the group is the most important and the longest component of the group (70 minutes). A primary function of the graduate group is to provide consultation to adolescents regarding the management of their current life problems. To achieve this function, the group members must be able to employ their interpersonal effectiveness skills and provide heavy doses of validation and positive reinforcement to one another.

Group leaders divide this time by the number of members to determine how much time each member is allowed to receive consultation. Since a preferable number of teens per group is four or five, each member is typically allowed approximately 15 minutes to discuss his or her problems. Naturally, exceptions are made to the time limit. For example, when one girl discovered she was pregnant and wanted to make a decision regarding abortion, some of her peers willingly forfeited their time to lengthen the discussion. However, in some cases it is important to balance the clinical necessity of discussing certain issues further with the potential for inadvertently reinforcing certain maladaptive behaviors and inadvertently extinguishing adaptive behaviors by ignoring members not in crisis. Group leaders make an effort to reinforce adolescents' progress, positive life events, and effective use of behavioral skills by spending sufficient time discussing these "positive events" as well as the problematic ones.

Adolescents are reminded to frame their discussions in such a way as to encourage feedback. Moreover, those who provide feedback are encouraged to use and reference DBT skills whenever possible, both to reinforce the learning process and to ensure that clients are sharing the same language. Unfortunately, at first, many teenagers exhibit profound difficulty expressing validating comments and behavior. Given their histories of pervasive invalidation, adolescents tend either to remain quiet and expressionless or to bring the conversation back to their own experience without making the validating link by saying, "I know how you must feel. . . . I have been through something similar." Instead, they may inadvertently invalidate their peer by "stealing" the problem and not returning to the first adolescent's original problem. Group therapists must highlight this inadvertent maneuver and teach, via role plays, how to validate peers more effectively.

In one case, Beth, a 17-year-old white female, described her anxiety and anger toward her boyfriend for looking at and flirting with other girls in front of her. A male peer responded with bravado, "What's the big deal? Just 'cause you're looking at the menu doesn't mean you have to order." The group stopped in surprise, and another female exclaimed, "Peter, that's so messed up. You totally invalidated Beth. I think Beth has every reason to be upset. I'd be upset if my boyfriend was doing that!" Peter replied, "I didn't mean to invalidate her. . . . I was actually trying to validate her by saying this is what guys do these days and not to take it personally." The group leader asked Beth how she had experienced Peter's comment. Beth reported that it felt invalidating; however, Peter's explanation made her feel a little less hurt, since he was trying to help. The leader asked Peter whether he could retry validating Beth, using a slightly different approach, but he expressed uncertainty about what to do. When indicated, a brief didactic presentation may be employed. In this case, the group was referred to the validation skills, which include listening skills and specific validation techniques. The group reviewed key ingredients missing from Peter's effort to validate Beth. The leader then asked Peter to formulate another validating statement, given Beth's feelings. The group gave Peter feedback as he tweaked his statement further. Finally, Peter was instructed to say it to Beth directly, with appropriate tone and eye contact. Although such a statement often feels artificial since it has been constructed by the group, it is important for an adolescents to say it in as natural a way as possible, without avoiding it or stating it sarcastically.

In addition to validation and reinforcement, teens consult to one another in a variety of ways, such as how to solve certain current problems. Peers might suggest the use of new or different skills, suggest alternative ways of thinking about a situation, or help clients work toward radically accepting certain "unacceptable" events in their lives. When they are senior enough in skills application, teens can volunteer to serve informally as peer coaches outside of the group. The group phone list is regularly updated, and teens are permitted to call each other for coaching outside of sessions, under two conditions: (1) Distressed teens are required to call the group therapists after they speak with a peer if they require more coaching; and (2) teens are not permitted to discuss prior self-harm behaviors with one another outside of therapy sessions.

One teen reported in a group session that she had called another group member the night before to discuss a problem. The problem involved a conflict this 15-year-old girl was having with her mother about her poor school performance. She was feeling extremely invalidated by her mother's criticism that "You clearly aren't trying in school, and that if you cared at all about me, you'd try harder so that it wouldn't give me so much worry." The teen explained to her peer on the phone that she was actually trying as hard as she could, but that because of her depression, she had trouble concentrating and consequently was performing poorly at school. The distressed teen reported with appreciation to the group how the peer coach first validated her feelings, then encouraged the teen not to judge herself as her mother was doing. Rather, she helped the teen validate herself. Finally, the peer coach suggested that the teen remind her mother the next day that (1) the problem was not one of motivation, but rather one of her depression symptoms, which were presently interfering in her academic achievement; and (2) the teen too felt bad about her poor grades. The distressed teen expressed enormous gratitude in group to the peer coach for making herself available, for offering her validation, and for suggesting specific strategies for what to say to her mother the following day. The peer coach responded, "It's much easier when it's not your own mother. I don't get in emotion mind when it's your mother." The group leader reminded the peer coach that she had still offered support and helpful concrete advice to her peer, and suggested that the next appropriate response to give would be: "You're welcome . . . any time." She followed through with the recommendation, and the group proceeded.

Closing Observation and Commitment

The last activity of each graduate group session is a ritual called "closing observations and commitment." The group is given the following instructions: "Assume the mindfulness position, and after the sound of the bell, group members in any order may share one nonjudgmental observation about today's group. After that, please state what you commit to work on this week." One of the group leaders always goes last, and often includes as part of his or her closing observation a comment about any members not present and the wish for them to return next week.

The function of the closing observation is to help the clients (1) practice mindfulness skills, including observing, describing, not judging, and staying focused; (2) return to wise mind, since they may have been in emotion mind earlier in the group; and (3) practice self- and other-validation skills as well as reinforcement skills. The observations may range from "I am glad I came today . . . the group helped me feel better about myself," to "I observed that Susan worked hard today talking about her relationship problems with her mother," to "I am feeling very sad." Typically and fortunately, the closing observations help provide closure to an often emotionally intense group session.

The commitments often include individual assignments given during the group. Examples of commitments include "I am going to work on radically accepting the fact that my classmates are unable to handle the news that I am gay," "I am going to submit my college applications by the next group," and "I am going to commit to using my DEAR MAN skills with my friend who keeps wanting to discuss her self-cutting with me, since it really upsets me."

TERMINATING TREATMENT

Two factors determine when treatment should be terminated: a client's progress and the constraints of the treatment setting. In settings in which research protocols are being implemented, or in clinic or hospital settings with standardized treatment programs and strict time frames, the treatment structure determines the timing of an adolescent's treatment completion. However, even in such settings, exceptions must be made when severe behavioral instability persists. This may involve, for example, inviting the adolescent to repeat a portion of or an entire treatment program. At a minimum, clients entering therapy with high-priority Stage 1 target behaviors (i.e., with out-of-control behaviors that are life-threatening or severely compromise functioning) should ordinarily remain in treatment until adequate behavioral control is achieved. Once behavioral control is achieved, clients may terminate therapy altogether, take a break from therapy for some time period, or end one programmatic treatment and enter another program. When the latter is the case, the program transition may require terminating treatment with one or more therapists while still remaining in a coordinated DBT program. The exception to this rule of keeping clients in treatment throughout Stage 1 is when treatment is carried out as part of a research protocol where one of the outcomes is clients' functioning at the end of a specified time period. In these cases, particularly when suicidal behavior is not under control by the end of the protocol, it is essential that the program therapist organize a referral to continuing treatment.

In private practice settings, inpatient settings, or clinic or hospital settings with more flexible time frames, treatment length can be more of a general guideline than a policy. Generally, in these settings, an expected treatment length is negotiated at the start of treatment (e.g., 16 weeks, 24 weeks, 1 year); then, as the termination date approaches, therapy is reviewed to decide wither treatment should end at the agreed-upon time or a new agreement should be made. It is ordinarily important, however, to set specific time points for "go–no-go" reviews to prevent therapy from drifting or becoming a supportive relationship with little or no therapeutic change demanded or expected. Holding open rather than closed skills training groups facilitates the flexibility of a client's participation in treatment; the client can remain for additional modules in the skills training modality, rather than having to begin with a whole new cohort of clients.

In work with an adolescent, transitions in the client's life may result in termination's being determined by timing rather than clinical judgment. For example, once the school year ends, many adolescents may accept summer employment that interferes with the therapy schedule. They may also go away to summer camp, depart for their countries of origin, or leave for college. Still others will terminate abruptly because their parents decide to cease the therapy. When such abrupt terminations occur, the therapist can work to ease the transition in a number of ways. First, when such terminations are anticipated (e.g., leaving for college), planning in advance can occur, and referrals can be made if needed. Second, in some cases phone contact can be maintained for a specified period of time (and perhaps faded) to ease the transition away from therapy. Third, some adolescents and parents will at least be willing to arrange a termination session to handle issues of referrals, future plans, or the possibility of returning to the therapy at a future date.

How Are Termination and Phase Transitions Handled?

The handling of termination depends on the setting and the program structure. For inpatient, residential, institutional, or day treatment programs, termination is normally planned with arrangements made for follow-up care, typically in a less restrictive and time-intensive environment. In outpatient settings, termination may be delayed; instead, a transition may involve moving to a less structured phase of DBT (e.g., an exposure-focused treatment or some type of client graduate group), a different form of therapy, a gradual tapering process, or less frequent maintenance or "check-in" sessions.

If the treatment program is divided into phases, a transition takes place to the next phase, and termination is addressed at the end. Yet the end of the first phase is significant and marks a change in the format of the therapy. The intensive contact and format of individual therapy and the skills-acquisition-based multifamily skills group are often completed, and give way to a less time-intensive form of treatment (either individual therapy alone or a client graduate group). This phase shift makes for a "weaning" of sorts, with the adolescent taking a more active and independent role in his or her treatment. To determine whether the adolescent can move beyond the structured skills training, the primary therapist and the skills trainers should ensure that the adolescent demonstrates sufficient knowledge and practice of skills. This can be done by noting whether the client has shown understanding and application of skills in group, as well as whether the teen is putting those skills into practice by no longer being in Stage 1. In at least one setting we know of in Seattle, skills trainers require clients to pass a test to get into graduate groups; in this way, clients must demonstrate that they have learned the skills.

Making the Transition from the First Phase of Treatment

Individual Therapy

The first phase of treatment requires getting severe behaviors under control—suicidal behaviors and other severely maladaptive behaviors, such as not attending school, homelessness, severe substance abuse, or high-risk criminal behavior. In other words, clients must engage in normative behaviors. They must also be able to function in the skills training group. As completion of the agreed-upon length of the first phase of treatment nears, the individual therapist prepares the adolescent to complete this phase and move on to the next. Although the session format continues (i.e., review of diary card and behavioral analysis), the therapist will nevertheless allow some time for addressing the transition or termination. This involves feedback about progress, strengths, skills acquired, and areas that still need to be the focus of attention. This assumes, of course, that session time at this point is available for such discussion and not consumed by behavioral analyses of higher-order treatment targets. For many suicidal, emotionally dysregulated adolescents we see, the Stage 1 overarching targets of stability and behavioral control can be attained within 16 weeks (e.g., see Rathus & Miller, 2002). However, if these overarching targets remain (as they do in a subset of adolescents with more chronic and severe problems), the therapist should be discussing a continuation of addressing Stage 1 targets (which often corresponds to the first phase of treatment) with the client, rather than planning termination or a move to a second phase of treatment. Even when these target behaviors have substantially subsided, the therapist can point out areas that still need clinical attention. These areas should be actively addressed by the adolescent in a continuation phase of treatment, whether this involves individual therapy or some type of graduate group. In addition to feedback, the therapist anticipates with the adolescent potential areas that could cause setbacks or crises, and troubleshoots possible skillful responses. Often there is some exacerbation of old behaviors when termination nears. Stylistically, it is important that the therapist assess and validate the client's concerns about termination, while also engaging in problem solving and cheerleading.

When adolescents are engaged in a shorter-term outpatient treatment format, their therapists strongly encourages them to repeat a cycle of therapy when there is a need for continued work on Stage 1 targets. When clients have demonstrated control over the severe types of behavior targeted in Stage 1, they can move on to another phase of treatment. Typically, they are told about continuation phases available to them at the outset of treatment during orientation, but a therapist discusses continuation phases in more detail as a transition approaches, in terms of how they might benefit a particular adolescent. If clients have made substantial progress toward their Stage 1 goals (i.e., decreasing life-threatening behaviors and other severe forms of behavioral instability), they may wonder about the rationale for continuing in another form or mode of therapy. The therapist reiterates the rationales for the next phase of treatment, depending on what this phase is to consist of (e.g., to work on PTSD, to address problems in a less structured individual therapy format, to continue in a group setting to provide a forum for generalizing and strengthening the gains made, to prevent relapse, and/or to offer continued therapeutic contact should additional challenges arise). When a therapist believes that an adolescent has much to gain from continuing in treatment, orientation and commitment strategies can be applied at this point, as discussed in Chapter 7. However, many adolescents themselves desire additional treatment and are eager to continue in some format, especially when this involves continued contact with the program.

In preparing the adolescent for moving on to the next phase of treatment, the therapist might communicate a sentiment such as the following:

"I know it's going to take a little time to get to know and trust your new therapists [e.g., graduate group coleaders] and peers. Yet I expect you will learn to trust, like, respect, and get help from them. And, at the same time, I will always be your former therapist; hence, I would love to hear how your life proceeds—for example, when you graduate from high school, what college you choose to attend, and so forth. So if you feel like dropping me a note or postcard from time to time, send it to the clinic [or give it to the graduate group leaders and ask them to pass it along]."

Termination or Transition from the Multifamily Skills Training Group

Ideally, clients should continue skills training until they have mastered enough skills to be no longer engaging in life-threatening or therapist-interfering behaviors. When a multifamily skills group is being conducted in an open format with rotating entry points, some adolescents and their family members will graduate at the end of each module, as described in Chapter 10. During the last session of each module, the group leaders can conduct skills training according to the regular agenda for approximately three-quarters of the session, but devote the last quarter to acknowledging those who are graduating. This acknowledgment might involve presenting each graduating adolescent and family member with an attractive certificate of completion (e.g., rolled in ribbon like a diploma); encouraging each other group member (teen and parent) to make observations and provide feedback about the graduating group members' progress, as well as feelings about their leaving; and encouraging the graduates to offer feedback to each remaining group member (and leader). This type of exercise invariably proves emotional, moving, educational, and reinforcing of the good work clients have done. We are always impressed at the insights and perceptive observations about graduating clients offered by fellow group members. Perhaps most moving is the feedback the graduates provide to their own family members. Lastly, the group leaders might provide each teen or family with a small symbolic gift, to help them to remember or practice skills. For example, we have recently been giving departing members a CD called *The Wise Movement* (Behavioral Tech, 2004), a review of DBT skills put to music. Teens in particular respond well to such ceremonies and symbols of completion, similar to what occurs with school transitions.

Termination in the DBT Team

As individuals who are also taking responsibility for the treatment (since DBT is the treatment of a community of patients by a community of therapists), it is the responsibility of the team members to help each therapist both stay within the DBT treatment parameters on the one hand, and respond flexibly to new problems on the other hand. With respect to termination, the team has three major tasks. First, the team assists the therapist in determining when a client's treatment should be terminated. Although in a time-limited treatment program this may not be a major issue, it can become an important issue to think through when a client does not appear to be improving sufficiently, even though the end of the agreed-upon time for therapy is approaching. In our experience, both therapists and clients often want to extend therapy when an extension is not necessarily needed. This ordinarily occurs in cases where a therapist, a client, or both underestimate the client's abilities to cope and/or overestimate the problems the client is facing.

A second major role of the DBT team—somewhat the reverse of the first task—is to "remoralize" any therapist who is not only getting burned out with a particular client, but also starting to believe that the client simply isn't ready to change. In these cases, particularly with an adolescent who intermittently threatens to quit therapy prematurely, it is easy for the therapist to pull back and do little to reengage the client in the therapeutic process. In working with clients addicted to heroin in particular, therapists at our University of Washington program became very aware of their own frequent tendency to give up when the clients gave up. In such instances, it is essential that team members go into high gear to keep the therapists involved in the treatment.

A third task is to develop a process for handling therapists' termination from the DBT team. Leaving can be difficult because a tremendous sense of intimacy often develops, at least on long-running teams. There may also be a few instances when a therapist simply cannot or will not learn DBT sufficiently to put it into practice. Although this is rare, when it occurs it is similar to a treatment that does not lead to client improvement. Managing termination here is fraught with the same difficulties a therapist has in ending an unsuccessful therapy. For a person who wants to learn DBT but simply cannot "get it," the team may want to suggest additional coursework in areas of weakness. For example, a therapist on a University of Washington team was extremely motivated to learn DBT individual therapy. However, he had no background whatsoever in behavioral therapy or theory, and no amount of teaching on the team could overcome the deficit. The team finally asked him to audit several graduate courses in behavioral change. He did so, returned to the team, and became one of the best therapists on the team.

Termination from a Second Phase of Treatment

Termination from a second phase of treatment can vary for clients, depending on the modality of treatment they have been receiving, the progress they have made, and their plans for continuing some form of treatment. When individual therapy has continued, termination is considered when therapist and client agree that goals of a second phase of treatment have been accomplished, which often correspond to achieving DBT stage 2 and 3 targets. When some form of graduate group has been the modality, termination may come at the end of a full cycle of the group. However, a leader can also invite an adolescent who needs or desires continued group therapy to continue for another cycle. As noted earlier in this chapter, some graduate group members choose to recontract once, twice, and sometimes more before they officially graduate from the program. At that time, another graduation ceremony takes place.

In addition to the ritual described in Chapter 10 and above for clients moving on from the multifamily skills group, clients moving on from our graduate groups receive a more sophisticated diploma and a DBT tool kit. These kits contain items identified by the former individual therapist, former skills trainers, and current group leaders. For example, one adolescent female received distress tolerance tools (a "stress squeeze" ball and a small bottle of her favorite scented moisturizer) and mindfulness/emotion regulation tools (a journal for writing her thoughts and a pad for sketching, both of which the client considered pleasant activities). Therapists enjoy tailoring these DBT tool kits for each adolescent. Graduate groups typically become intense experiences for their members. The ending of this phase of treatment marks a substantial length of participation in the program, and clients often feel highly committed to the group and connected to one another.

In a sense, the entire concept of the graduate group prepares adolescents for termination. Adolescents have now mastered skills, and have typically made the transition from individual therapist intervention to a more peer-focused model in group. In the particular graduate group model used at Montefiore, adolescents must master skills to the point of teaching them to their peers, and follow a peer coaching model of treatment. Family members go from weekly contact to occasional family sessions that are held only if needed. Thus this phase of treatment is set up not only to reinforce and strengthen what was learned, but also as a fading process. As mentioned earlier, this fading to a group modality without parental involvement, with greater self-teaching and greater peer coaching, parallels an adolescent's normal developmental process. This graduate group mode may thus be uniquely important for adolescents, as they simultaneously strive not only to maintain their treatment gains and prevent relapse, but to master the developmental tasks of separating and individuating from parents and authority figures—and thus preparing for the greater self-sufficiency of adulthood.

CONCLUSION

This chapter is intended to help therapists gauge progress in treatment, to run a graduate or advanced group, to prepare clients for the transition to the next phase of therapy, and to handle the completion of therapy. Thus far, this volume has described the implementation of DBT with adolescents, from setting up a program and assessing client progress to terminating treatment. In the next and final chapter, we address program issues and practice barriers that can pose challenges to setting up and running effective DBT programs for adolescents.

CHAPTER 12

Program Issues

Various program issues can arise in efforts to implement and run an adolescent DBT program, particularly in settings unfamiliar with the treatment. Once a program has successfully gotten underway, issues may still arise that challenge effective delivery of the treatment. In surveying a variety of adolescent DBT programs nationwide, we and our colleagues found that several areas of difficulty were reported repeatedly (Miller, Rathus, et al., in press). These areas fell into two main categories: barriers to getting a program started, and challenges to carrying out effective treatment. The issues we discuss below pertain to both starting and running DBT programs, although we emphasize the former. After describing a general approach to addressing barriers to program implementation, we present each set of programmatic issues and provide suggestions for handling them. In particular, we address issues of administrative support, issues of financial support/feasibility, issues of limited staff resources, problems with getting staff to "buy into" DBT, and training issues.

ADDRESSING BARRIERS TO PROGRAM IMPLEMENTATION: A GENERAL APPROACH

Barriers to implementing a DBT program can be addressed in general by using the same DBT strategies that therapists use with individuals, groups, and families coming for treatment. Framing problems as "program-interfering behaviors" can organize thinking about what to do next. We recommend looking to the DBT tool kit of strategies to see what might be needed when problems are encountered in getting a program up or keeping one running. Questions to consider in assessing implementation problems are listed in Table 12.1.

ISSUES OF ADMINISTRATIVE SUPPORT

Some clinicians face reluctance from the administrators in their setting to support a DBT-focused adolescent program. There are several reasons for this. First, the nature of the population targeted by DBT may be of concern. Adolescents in general are considered a difficult group to treat, and multiproblem suicidal adolescents are considered even more difficult. When the setting is not already serving this population, some administrators may feel reluctant to start a program for clients who typically exhibit suicidal and self-injurious behaviors, high levels of attrition, poor treatment compliance, and frequent emergency room or inpatient visits. Site managers may worry that highly distressed clients will be aversive to other clients or staff. For example, we know of one clinic where therapists were told that their suicidal and

TABLE 12.1. Questions to Consider in Assessing Program Implementation Problems

Behavioral assessment

- Is there a need for DBT in my area or agency?
- Are financial resources available to pay for treatment?
- Can I find at least one other person willing to form a DBT team?
- If opposition or reluctance to a DBT team exists, are we clear about what factors are influencing the opposition? Who will gain from a DBT program, and who will lose?

Solution analysis

- Have we taken seriously others' opposition or reluctance, and devised ways either to solve their problems or to counteract them with information and/or data?

Contingency management

- Are we very skillful in reinforcing all pro-DBT program behaviors in others?
- Are we willing to shape the behavior we want rather than demand it now?

Exposure strategies

- Have we considered a desensitization procedure, starting with a very small DBT program and gradually expanding as administrators and coworkers get more comfortable?

Skills training

- Have we developed ways to solve staff training needs?
- Have we been interpersonally skillful in the process of implementing a change in the status quo?

Cognitive modification

- Have we assessed and then challenged erroneous or extreme beliefs about DBT, suicidal behavior, and/or adolescents?

Orienting

- Have we made clear to administrators and coworkers exactly what to expect, and what would be required of them if a DBT program is started?
- Have we clearly related the starting or implementing of a DBT program to the goals and needs of our administrators and coworkers? Can we show them how this can benefit them?

Didactic materials

- Have we assembled a presentation or set of materials describing what a DBT program is, what its outcomes can be expected to be, and who does what in a DBT program?

Commitment

- Once the DBT program is on board, have we used all of DBT's commitment strategies to strengthen the commitment of our administrators and coworkers to the program?
- Have we attended to troubleshooting problems that might arise before they come up?

Validation

- Do we take care to validate at every turn the thoughts, feelings, and actions of administrators, coworkers, and insurers?

Dialectics

- Are we willing to find a synthesis to get our DBT program going or keep it running once it is started?

drug-using clients had to use a separate waiting room so as not to upset other clients. Administrators may be concerned that attracting more high-risk, suicidal clients to the clinic might displace clients with other problems and place additional strain on therapists. Such concerns were the initial reactions at of one facility when the idea was raised of beginning a DBT program in a clinic staffed by graduate students. Other concerns included the ability of student trainees to handle such cases, and issues of risk and liability in the context of the broader institutional community. These concerns were taken seriously, considered, and addressed by using several approaches discussed below.

Most settings that consider starting a DBT program already have such clients. Still, an administration may be reluctant to support a DBT program because of the perception that it is a highly time-intensive program (e.g., including therapist consultation team, phone consultation); that it requires many resources in terms of training and staffing; and that it may be not feasible to provide comprehensive services under managed care billing. Some community mental health center staff members see 40–50 clients per week, and cannot imagine spending the kind of time DBT devotes to discussing therapists' problems in delivering treatments, team issues, and phone calls. Regarding insurance reimbursement, DBT programs are often constrained by "billing hours" in terms of the frequency of services and type of care provided. Managed care reimbursement for services rendered may be less than the cost of provision. For example, billing restrictions might place a financial strain on group therapy, making it difficult to recover the cost of services when a group runs for 2 hours or when fewer than a specified number of clients attend a group. Finally, some administrators may simply be resistant to an orientation change in their current milieu.

An administration's reluctance to implement DBT can be analyzed as therapy-interfering or program-interfering behavior; a team can work to understand the contingencies operating and can then apply DBT strategies. These strategies might include acceptance of the current reality of unsupportive administrative decisions, as well as measures for changing those administrative decisions in the future.

There are several possible responses to administrators' concerns about attracting a more high-risk, suicidal adolescent population by starting a DBT program. First, it's essential to provide information about DBT, its efficacy, and the populations it serves. It is also helpful to orient administrators to how a DBT program might fit within their own goals for the organization. Many administrators positively respond to the information that starting a DBT program is likely to generate more referrals (and consequently more income). It can also potentially enhance the reputation of the setting. Information about DBT's cost savings and published efficacy data can be particularly useful in persuading insurers and government agencies to pay for the treatment. Furthermore, the case can be made that learning DBT provides an excellent training experience for staff members, which may result in improved morale, less burnout, and more effective treatment in general. Providing workshops to educate the administrative staff about the population (i.e., suicidal clients with BPD or borderline features) and the treatment can help dispel myths and increase comfort level.

Overall, listening to administrators' concerns and making a serious effort to address them thoughtfully is critical. These steps not only will help increase the chances of gaining administrative support, but are likely to improve the quality of the program. For example, DBT advocates can respond to concerns about ability to handle suicidal crises in a particular setting by developing and then presenting a detailed plan for handling such crises.

As noted above, the majority of settings considering a DBT program will already be treating multiproblem suicidal adolescents. In such settings, the goal for clinicians who hope to implement DBT is to point out, "We are not likely to get rid of these challenging clients—so how can we best treat them?" Then the clinicians should use their best interpersonal effectiveness skills to explain their rationale, ask for what they need, reinforce others ahead of time, and negotiate. Although perceived barriers placed by the administration might lead the advocates of DBT to respond with anger or frustration (i.e., punishing the administration), it is more effective to reinforce the administration through validation, skillful communication, and providing managers with what they need. For example, therapists can start by using DBT with some suicidal multiproblem clients and holding the DBT team meetings on their own time to demonstrate the benefits of such a program. They can also provide the administrators with a plan showing how they won't lose money, since the costs of not doing DBT (e.g., hospitaliza-tion) are often greater than the costs of doing DBT. If the unit clinicians are working for does not bear the added costs of emergency care, then the clinicians can note that cutting down on such care will increase the unit's value to the insurance or government agencies that are pay-ing for this care. It can also be pointed out that DBT provides a useful training opportunity for staff members. Training in this approach not only may improve client outcomes, but may re-duce therapist burnout as well.

Orienting the administration through workshops and trainings can also be helpful. As a result of such an orientation, the client population is less likely to be seen as "manipulative," and administrators are more likely to understand that the treatment specifically targets the emotional and behavioral dysregulation that can seem so challenging. Moreover, adaptations to the treatment targeting the particular needs of adolescents can help make the treatment more manageable. These include interventions such as direct consultation to families and schools, and inclusion of family members in treatment. The engagement of school personnel and especially family members can provide a sense of partnership in treating the adolescents that can help ease administrators' concerns.

In addressing a skeptical administration, DBT program advocates will need to practice radical acceptance that they will have to do the work of selling and demonstrating the treat-ment, make some sacrifices, and address concerns. If the administration wants certain con-cerns addressed, the advocates must address them and validate them one by one. If adminis-trators are concerned about time (because of the multiple modes of treatment), the advocates can point out that it will probably take more time to deal with crises, noncompliance, suicide attempts, and other behaviors that the DBT format addresses. Also, they can point out that the time devoted to team meetings tends to help staff members manage high caseloads and re-duce burnout. Moreover, when there are concerns about time taken from other responsibili-ties, clinicians can start a team that meets during lunch or after work, as noted above. Then, when the administration sees improvement in the clients and begins to advocate for DBT, the practitioners can argue for moving these meetings into a regularly scheduled part of their work day. If administrators are concerned about money, the advocates can point out the ulti-mate savings in money by using DBT (largely because of reduced emergency room visits and inpatient days), also as noted above. If others are concerned about effectiveness of the model, the advocates can direct them to the data and offer to provide outcome data in their setting. This effort should begin with the collection of pre- and posttreatment measures; ideally, in-struments that are already in place as part of standard clinic assessments should be used. If administrators are simply not familiar with the DBT approach, advocates can familiarize them with the treatment by offering workshops and directing them to websites that offer detailed information about the treatment and outcomes (e.g., www.behavioraltech.org).

The need for administrative support and recognition is clear. In order for any interven-tion to succeed, internal administrative advocates for the DBT program are essential. Pro-moting the adoption of an empirically supported treatment for high-risk adolescents (i.e., those with BPD and/or related traits) requires a recognition of the benefits that this treatment will provide, both to the clients themselves and to the clinic setting as a whole. Installation of outcome measures offers the opportunity for ongoing evaluation of the program. Clear guidelines for all clinicians and treatment strategies will allow for a general understanding of who will assume what role in the intervention and how each professional fits within the larger system. Ideally, these steps will also allow the administration to develop a more receptive attitude toward the adoption of DBT as an adolescent treatment.[1] Finally, advocates can remember to use DBT commitment strategies to gain support, such as reviewing the pros and cons of implementing the program, using the foot-in-the-door technique (i.e., asking for just a small thing to begin with, such as a therapist consultation team or a skills training group only), and shaping commitment (reinforcing small steps toward support of the program).

ISSUES OF FINANCIAL SUPPORT/FEASIBILITY

Financial support for DBT and thus the fiscal feasibility of implementing the treatment, are crucial issues for administration, staff, and individual clients and their families. For administrative bodies and insurance companies, the most helpful strategy is to show the data demonstrating the efficacy of the treatment and its cost-effectiveness. Many sites are already admitting such teens, but are using a "treatment-as-usual" approach rather than DBT, and the data indicate that this will result in a relatively greater number of crises, suicidal behaviors, and hospitalizations (Rathus & Miller, 2002; H. Fellows, personal communication, December 11, 1998). These poorer outcomes ultimately not only create more stress and demand more time of the staff, but also make the treatment more costly. Once insurance companies become familiar with these sets of data, they often themselves solicit treaters who can provide DBT.

For a self-paying client, a therapist can work to find a way to get the treatment covered, through a combination of coaching the client (or the client's parents) on how to request DBT from the insurance company and speaking directly to the insurance company. Because of the now widely known replicated efficacy data supporting DBT, most insurance companies will now pay for Stage 1 of treatment. A common problem, however, is that when a client becomes nonsuicidal, the insurance company stops paying. In such a case, the therapist (and client) must argue skillfully for continuation of coverage. If coverage for the full treatment still cannot be obtained, one possibility is to structure the treatment according to what the insurance will cover. For example, if the insurance will cover 6 months of treatment per year, the therapist can offer intensive DBT for 4 or 5 months and then offer a titrated version (e.g., monthly sessions plus skills training group and phone coaching) for the following 6 months until benefits start again. But the therapist can continue attempting to get full coverage for treatment from the insurance company, by making use of DBT skills when communicating with them. The practitioner can lay out the alternatives to DBT and the likely consequences of these alternatives, including pointing out that not supplying proper and adequate treatment for a suicidal client may result in a death.

ISSUES OF LIMITED STAFF RESOURCES

Sometimes limited staff resources present a barrier to starting a DBT program. For example, few staff members in a faculty may be knowledgeable in DBT. Or a clinician may work in a rural area, with few mental health professionals scattered over a large geographic distance. Or a private practice setting may have too small a staff to provide comprehensive DBT services. When staff members are available but few are knowledgeable about DBT, training becomes the top priority; we discuss training issues below. In rural areas with few other mental health

---

[1]Some of these ideas are delineated in Webster-Stratton and Taylor (1998).

professionals near by, a clinician can create a team through weekly scheduled phone or online team meetings. Clients might travel to different sites for different modes of treatment (e.g., individual therapy and group skills training), while practitioners meet over the phone to discuss various difficulties in delivering the treatment. Or therapists may deliver all treatment modes at one site, but hold phone or online team meetings with therapists seeing similar clients at another site. In a private practice setting, there are several options. A clinician can connect with other practitioners in private practice who wish to form a DBT team. The clinician can also start small, with the aim of gradually developing a more comprehensive program by adding more trained professionals to the practice. As long as there is at least one other person with whom a therapist regularly discusses his or her clinical work in order to increase motivation, fidelity, and competence in DBT, the team modality is considered to be occurring (and the function of increasing therapists' capabilities and motivation is met).

Staff resources can also limit the comprehensiveness with which DBT is offered. One group of therapists may be willing and able to offer group skills training, while an individual practitioner may be able and willing to offer individual DBT but not skills training. Note that the data to date showing DBT's effectiveness are based on programs that include all four DBT components (skills training, individual therapy, phone consultation, therapist consultation team). However, nowhere does it say that all DBT treatment modes must be offered in the same setting. The University of Washington clinic often provides DBT skills training to individuals seeing community psychotherapists for individual therapy. In these cases, we require written contracts with the individual therapists saying that they are the primary therapists (and thus will take phone calls and manage crises) and will coach the clients in the application of the DBT skills. In short, although we do not always require that the individual therapists be "card-carrying" DBT therapists, we do require that they agree to focus on generalizing and strengthening clients' use of skills.

In public community mental health, the provision of DBT skills coaching is often the province of after-hours teams. In these cases, it is imperative for the after-hours team members to require that the clients' individual therapists also take phone calls. However, in some settings this may not be possible, due to administrative requirements that staff members not take after-hours phone calls from clients. Although we believe that this policy reduces the quality of care available to clients, in these instances the individual DBT therapists should provide after-hours coaches with treatment and crisis management plans, and the skills group leaders should keep the after-hours team up to date on what skills module is currently being taught. If the after-hours team members are providing DBT coaching, there is no reason why they should not be included on the DBT treatment team.

PROBLEMS WITH GETTING STAFF TO MEMBERS "BUY INTO" DBT

Problems with getting the staff or one segment of the staff to "buy into" DBT may be encountered even when an administration favors DBT. In some settings, team members report difficulty with other team members' not accepting the full treatment approach. The assumptions about patients, the orientation (e.g., understanding of or willingness to use learning principles), the hierarchy of targets, or the team agreements may be rejected. In other settings, team members have trouble accepting that team meetings are a critical component of therapy, requiring their full attendance (i.e., they cannot come for only part of meetings), undivided attention (e.g., pagers and cell phones must be turned off), willingness to disclose inadequacies, and efforts to help fellow group members. At times, such problems may occur because teams admit members with little orientation and training in DBT. At other times, they may occur because particular hospital or clinic departments are restructured to use DBT, and staff members who previously used other treatments get assigned to the DBT team, rather than joining of their own volition.

It is important to remember that DBT can be provided in any setting where two or more DBT therapists decide to form a team and provide the treatment. Thus, although DBT is programmatic, not all clients and not all therapists in a clinic have to be in the program. The easiest way to start a DBT team in a nonsupportive or ambivalent environment is to start small. A clinician can get together with at least one other person and begin a team. They can take the clients no one else wants (the most difficult, the most interpersonally distressing, etc.) and put in the effort required to maximize the chances of a positive outcome. They should ask for as few resources as possible, talk about the positive aspects of the team, and be sure to communicate to others the successes of the DBT program. Little by little, the team will build a reputation of getting good results and having fun doing it. At this point, others will probably want to join the team.

The team members should not make the mistake of letting people join "just to see how it goes." They should also not ask people to join the team as a method of recruitment, hoping that being on the team will persuade them to choose to do DBT. They should resist any attempts by the administration to assign individuals to the DBT team whether they like it or not. Instead, they should require voluntary commitments to learn and apply DBT and to abide by the DBT team agreements before joining the team. Remember, a DBT consultation team is a group of professionals who come together with the stated goal of using DBT to get clients better. The biggest problems occur when people who are not doing DBT get on the team.

The bottom line should be that clinicians cannot get on the DBT team if they do not want to be on it. Potential DBT therapists need to realize that by joining a team, they are in effect taking on responsibility for the welfare of all clients being treated by team members. At the University of Washington, we require a commitment session with potential therapists similar to that with clients before allowing them to join the team. We use all the commitment strategies used with clients, particularly the devil's advocate strategy. A small team is better than a larger team with ambivalent members.

If a DBT program is taking care of clients' egregious behaviors, the clinic staff and administration will be pleased. The team members should make it clear that DBT treats difficult behaviors and handles hard-to-treat clients. They can tell colleagues to call on *them* for handling their clients' egregious behaviors. In fact, they can offer to take all of the clinic's "trouble" clients, as suggested above. Ultimately, the program is likely to come across as integral to the sites—as one that the administrators cannot bear to lose. When this occurs, the team members can start asserting what they need to support the program better.

In essence, to get staff members to support DBT, the people who start a DBT program need to be effective, have fun, reinforce people, do miniworkshops, and (importantly) be nonjudgmental about those who still don't buy in. In fact, the team should also reinforce the people who are *not* doing DBT. Team members should radically accept that they will not "convert" everyone, and should not get religious about the treatment! Rather, they should listen, teach, and be open and nondefensive about problems others bring up.

ISSUES OF TRAINING

Getting Staff Members Trained

Program directors may face barriers because DBT training among their staff members is limited. Ordinarily it is not difficult to train someone in DBT who is already well trained in evidence-based forms of CBT. However, there may be few or no staff members trained in these treatments; program directors who have received in-depth training in DBT may find themselves the only ones or among only a few with such training. The challenge is even greater if a program director and his or her team have limited training themselves in forms of CBT. And a particular liability exists if the DBT-trained individuals have not had DBT supervision. With or without adequate DBT skills, the person with the most DBT training is likely to be counted on by the entire staff to implement the treatment and provide supervision. Although ongoing education and training for staff members could address this problem, lack of administrative support and lack of funding often make this unavailable.

Adequate staff training both in DBT and in a variety of evidence-based CBT interventions must be a high priority. There are a number of ways to accomplish this. The most important first step is to start a self-study group and be sure that everyone on the DBT team is reading the DBT treatment manual and skills training manual (Linehan, 1993a, 1993b). These should be read in small chunks, with adequate time set aside to discuss the manuals and ways they might apply to team members' own cases. Although a person can learn specific DBT skills by reading only the DBT skills training manual, neither that book nor the present book are sufficient for learning how to apply the treatment. Once the main manual (i.e., Linehan, 1993a) is read and understood, then both other books (Linehan, 1993b, and the present book) are necessary for applying the treatment in the specific cases of skills training and adolescent clients.

Once the three books have been digested, formal training via an intensive workshop in DBT is the optimal next step. If this is not possible or is possible only for a few members of a team, bringing in an expert DBT consultant to train staff members in a facility is the next best option. If this is not possible (or even if it is), getting the most experienced behavior therapist in the facility to be on the DBT team is the next best option. If no in-person trainer is available, finding an expert DBT therapist who can consult via phone during team meetings is an option worth exploring. Although a number of 1- and 2-day DBT workshops are available, none of these are aimed at actually teaching DBT to individuals who do not know the treatment. They can, however, be useful as an overview of what is most important to learn. They can also be helpful in learning such intangible elements as attitude and style, which are hard to learn out of a book. It is important to remember that DBT is a version of CBT; therefore, one needs training in CBT as a base. For staff members who are already trained in CBT, DBT is an easy leap. For those who are not, such training should occur either prior to or as an adjunct to training in DBT.

If comprehensive staff training is not available at the outset, the program goals might be modified to be more modest. For example, many programs start with just a DBT team and skills training group. After this becomes routinized, perhaps after a year, another mode might be added (e.g., phone coaching). It is preferable for programs to start with DBT skills training or individual therapy; starting small rather than big allows the staff to master one mode of DBT while additional training is sought to broaden skills. One model we would recommend for implementing a program would be the following: Study group → team → skills group + phone coaching → individual therapy (added slowly).

Handling Settings in Which Most Staff Members Are Trainees

The rotation of clinicians within training settings can be a barrier to effective treatment, especially when coupled with a lack of resources for training new staff. Psychiatry residents, psychology residents, psychology interns and externs, and social work interns typically enter settings with less training and experience than the regular staff members. And, to make matters worse, the nature of the training positions means that they have a high rate of turnover. Rotation throughout settings means that trainees leave their clients, often prematurely; in fact, this is the single biggest problem with trainees. But the turnover provides a problem for supervisory staff as well. For example, if supervisors are running a brief training program (1 year or less) with students who are new both to DBT and to clinical work itself, intensive DBT training—particularly with high-risk, highly disturbed individuals—is not practical. Even in an optimal training period such as a 2- or 3-year practicum, engaging high-risk clients in a setting with relatively inexperienced therapists requires both intensive supervision and adequate supervisory backup. In posttraining settings, such as residencies and internships, the limited training of many staff members may leave only a few persons to oversee all modes of DBT (i.e., individual therapy sessions, skills training group, team meetings, phone consultation) in many settings. This places a limitation on their available time and potential for additional activities (e.g., providing individual therapy to clients). And by the time trainees are trained and gain some experience with the treatment model, new trainees replace them. Therefore, supervisor burnout is another obstacle often experienced.

In order to address the problem of rapid turnover and all of its consequences, a DBT team should allow trainees to join the team only if they can stay for a certain length of time, determined by the team members. In graduate training programs, a period of at least 2 years is ordinarily required. In programs where trainees already have substantial clinical training as well as previous or ongoing CBT training, a minimum of 1 year may be sufficient. Training clinics generally provoke two main concerns: the engagement of high-risk clients in settings with relatively inexperienced therapists, and staff turnover that leaves supervisors continually training new clinicians. Ongoing training, supervision, and therapist consultation team meetings can all help to ensure that the trainees are delivering the best treatment possible. At the same time, it is essential to have novice clinicians working with high-risk patients, as they are the next generation of first-line care providers and must learn to treat such clients.

It is essential in such settings that the supervisors be available at all hours to provide consultation. A most important thing here is for the supervisors to communicate a welcoming attitude about calls. It should also be kept in mind that other team members can be excellent consultants, both during and between team meetings. At the University of Washington, it is not unusual for student therapists to call several team members as well as their supervisors to discuss very high-risk situations. Student therapists are required to page their supervisors after calls requiring suicide risk assessment, and all therapists must alert the clinic director after any medically serious suicide attempt or self-injury. At the Montefiore program, we require all student therapists to page their supervisors after they are paged by their clients. This requires 24-hours-a-day availability of the supervisors, since therapists in training are offering the same to their clients. In settings heavily staffed by trainees, the potential exists for supervisor burnout, as noted above. A 2-year commitment from trainees, when possible, is one way to handle this issue. This means that there are always more experienced trainees present, and program directors are not repeatedly losing most of their staff at once.

Another strategy for such settings is to make efforts to attract more seasoned clinicians to the team, to balance the ratio of trained staff members to trainees. When this is not possible, forging connections to external community supports can be helpful. For instance, outside consultation can be arranged for handling therapy, staff, or programmatic issues (such as crisis plans), and ample use of community resources can be made. It is particularly important that emergency referral and consultation information be readily available. At the University of Washington, for example, all therapists on a team are required to have access at all times to crisis information forms that are updated weekly. These provide contact information for all team clients, their individual and group therapists, and their emergency contact people; each client's emergency treatment plan; admission policies of all hospitals with inpatient units and/

or emergency rooms, together with requisite phone numbers; and phone numbers for the local crisis clinic. All therapy rooms have telephones, so that calls can be made without leaving clients alone.

Still another solution might be to develop contact with a similar setting, so that senior supervising staff members can support one another across programs. Program directors might also seek out more advanced training for their staffs and for themselves, since more experience and higher level of expertise can make the work more manageable. Telephone coaching supervision might be shared by multiple supervisors familiar with DBT skills and with each site's (and client's) suicide protocol, in order to reduce burnout as much as possible. Finally, training teams can start small and can gradually grow as a base of supervisors develops. So, rather than starting with a large, fully functioning program, staff members can accept that it may take 5 years to get a full program up and running. Part of the process would include training team members and getting the staffers capable of doing so to grow into supervisory roles. So that the staff does not have to do all of the training, team members can be sent for behavior therapy training and other related training through workshops and professional conferences, such as the Association for Behavioral and Cognitive Therapies (formerly the Association for Advancement of Behavior Therapy).

In summary, practitioners can face many barriers to starting or carrying out an adolescent DBT program. If not addressed, these can interfere with delivering effective treatment. But whether clinicians are just beginning a DBT program or running one, they can address challenges by applying the same DBT strategies used with clients.

CONCLUSION

Our aim in writing this book has been to provide practitioners with the tools and strategies they need to treat suicidal multiproblem adolescents and their families. Linehan et al.'s (1991) original randomized controlled trial included a proportion of older adolescents, and additional research has lent promising support for the use of DBT with adolescents (Rathus & Miller, 2002; Katz et al., 2004; Wood et al., 2001). We hope that this book has demonstrated how DBT can be applied to the particular issues of this younger but still quite troubled population. For example, DBT is readily adaptable to adolescent developmental considerations and to ongoing family interactions.

Research on using DBT with adolescents continues. A multicenter randomized trial is underway in Norway, and further work is underway regarding measurement of core problem areas in adolescents receiving DBT (Rathus et al., 2005). Yet further research is needed. For example, in addition to randomized controlled trials on adolescent DBT with traditional targets (e.g., suicidal behaviors and NSIB), the field could benefit from further research in a number of areas—such as investigating the impact of the Walking the Middle Path module; studying the effects of treatment on family members' adjustment and perceptions; measuring family interactions following treatment; and comparing treatment conditions (e.g., with family vs. without family present) and parameters (e.g., shortened length of treatment vs. standard length). Thus, in addition to aiding clinicians in applying this treatment, we hope that this book will encourage researchers to study the treatment with adolescents and help them define treatment conditions. Together, the efforts of the clinical and research communities will increase this treatment's ability to help suicidal multiproblem adolescents build lives worth living.

Mindfulness Exercises for Adolescents

This appendix presents a sampling of mindfulness exercises that work well with adolescents. Some of these were taken or adapted from standard DBT; we have developed others for this population. Therapists can use still other mindfulness exercises as well, as we do at times. These exercises often allow for practice in all components of mindfulness; thus the descriptions of which aspects of mindfulness are taught refer to those aspects that are particularly emphasized in each exercise.

GENERAL TIPS FOR CONDUCTING EXERCISES

- The group leaders should briefly orient the members to each exercise, including making a link between the exercise and a treatment goal (e.g., "helping us notice our experience more fully," "helping us reduce judgments, so that we can minimize emotion mind," etc.).

- All group members should participate, including family members.

- For most exercises, members can either close their eyes or focus on a point in front of them that will not be distracting.

- Cell phones and other potential distractors should be turned off, and objects group members are holding (e.g., pens, notebooks) should be put down.

- Most exercises can run for between 2 and 5 minutes. As group members gain more experience with doing exercises, they can run longer.

- Participants can be instructed that if their thinking or attention drifts, they should nonjudgmentally notice the drifting and bring attention back to the exercise.

- Group leaders should allow several minutes for participants to share observations regarding the exercise.

- Leaders can conclude by stating one purpose of the exercise (learning to participate without judgment; observing and describing emotions as the first steps for getting into wise mind; getting more information about a situation by taking the time to stop and notice our experiences; etc.).

EXERCISE 1. What's Different about Me?

Two group members pair off and mindfully observe each other. Then they turn their backs, change three things (e.g., glasses, watch, and hair), and turn back toward each other. Can they notice the changes?

Variant: Whose penny? Every group member takes a penny from a bowl, holds it a moment, and puts it back in the bowl. Then each member takes one again, and *really* studies it (staying focused, doing one thing at a time), and puts it back in the a bowl. Finally, each member tries to pick out his or her own penny. Discussion follows: Could they have identified their own pennies the first time? Why not?

Aspect of mindfulness taught: Observing one-mindfully

EXERCISE 2. Sound Ball

One group member "throws" a sound across the room to another group member. That member then "catches" the same sound by repeating it exactly and then "throws" a new sound to someone else—and so on, with a new sound each time.

Variant: Word ball. Same as above, using words instead of sounds.

Aspect of mindfulness taught: Observing and participating one-mindfully

EXERCISE 3. Snap, Crackle, and Pop

All group members are instructed to say "snap" when they cross their chests with their left or right arms and point either immediately left or right; to say "crackle" when they raise their left or right arms over their heads and point immediately left or right; and to say "pop" when they point at anyone around the circle (who does not need to be immediately left or right). Any one person starts by saying "snap" while simultaneously pointing either immediately left or right. Whoever receives the point says "crackle" while simultaneously pointing immediately left or right. Whoever receives the point says "pop" while pointing at anyone in the circle. That person then starts with "snap" and begins the sequence again. Anyone who misspeaks or misgestures, while trying to maintain a reasonably fast pace, is out of this portion of the exercise. These people then become "distractors" and stand outside of the circle trying to distract their peers (verbally, without physical contact). The "snap–crackle–pop" sequence continues until there are only two people remaining in the circle.

Aspect of mindfulness taught: Observing and participating one-mindfully

EXERCISE 4. Observation of Music

Leaders play a piece of music that is typically not a teen favorite and ask group members, while listening quietly, to observe and describe nonjudgmentally while fully letting the experience surround them (their thoughts, emotions, physiological changes, urges). Variants include playing segments of two or three very different pieces (in terms of style, tempo, etc.) and having group members observe changes in the music and in their internal reactions.

Aspect of mindfulness taught: Observing, describing, and participating without judgment

EXERCISE 5. Egg Balancing

Several members try to balance an egg upright on a table for 2 minutes.

Aspect of mindfulness taught: Observing one-mindfully, nonjudgmentally, and with effectiveness

EXERCISE 6. Hand Exercise

Group members stand around an oval or rectangular table. Each member is instructed to place his or her left hand on the table. Then each member places his or her right hand underneath the left hand of the person to the right. One person starts the sequence by picking the right hand off the table and quickly placing it back down. The person to the right quickly lifts up his or her right hand. The hand movements continue around the circle in sequence—until someone does a double tap. This move reverses the direction of the hand movements, and these continue in the reverse direction until someone does a double tap again. Anyone who picks up a hand too early or too late removes that one hand and leaves the other hand on the table (if the other hand was doing what it was supposed to do). The exercise continues until only a couple of hands are left.

Aspect of mindfulness taught: Observing one-mindfully and nonjudgmentally

EXERCISE 7. Mindfully Unwrapping a Hershey's Kiss

Each group member sits in a comfortable position with a Hershey's Kiss in front of him or her. A leader says:

"After I ring the bell the third time, observe and describe the outside of the Hershey's Kiss to yourself. Feel the differences in the texture between the paper tag and the foil. As you begin to unwrap the chocolate, note how the shape and texture of the foil change in comparison to the paper tag as well as the chocolate. Feel the chocolate and how it changes in your hand. If your mind wanders from the exercise, note the distraction without judgment, and then return your attention to the chocolate."

Aspect of mindfulness taught: Observing and describing one-mindfully

EXERCISE 8. Mindfulness PB&J

A leader says:

"Often when we are engaged in a monotonous activity—something we find boring, unengaging, or even unpleasant (but required)—we find that our minds wander. Rather than attending to what we are doing, our heads fill with thoughts of what we wish we were doing, how we can't stand what we are doing now, how unfair and stupid it is that we have to do this, and so on. Instead of being aware of our thoughts, feelings, and sensations in the present moment, without judging them, we cloud our minds with negative thoughts, feelings, and judgments. By using "wise mind," we are able to participate fully in the moment, without worry about future concerns or feelings of self-consciousness.

"Imagine that you are on the social committee for a group picnic. Your task is to make peanut butter and jelly sandwiches. Your supplies are arrayed on the table in front of you. I want you to pretend you are making a peanut butter and jelly sandwich. Go through each of the actions that you would need to do in order to make the sandwich. Take two pieces of bread, pick up your knife, and so on. Don't leave out any steps. As you are making your sandwich, concentrate fully on the act of making the sandwich—think about how creamy the peanut butter is, how the consistency of the jelly is different, how you have to handle the bread so as not to damage it. When you are done making your sandwich, put it aside and begin making the next sandwich. Your goal is to concentrate on the act of making the sandwich. If your mind starts to start to wander, bring your attention back to participating fully in the task."

Aspect of mindfulness taught: Observing, describing, and participating one-mindfully and nonjudgmentally

EXERCISE 9. Repeating an Activity

A leader says:

"When the bell rings, sit at the table with your arms resting on the table. Very slowly, reach several inches to pick up a pen. Raise it a few inches and then set it down. Move your hand back to its original position of rest. While you repeat this action throughout the time period, experience each repetition with freshness, as though you have never done it before. You can allow your attention to wander toward different aspects of the movement: watching your hand or feeling the muscles contracting. You can even notice your sense of touch, being aware of the different textures and pressures. Let go of any distractions or judgments you may have. This activity will help you to become mindful of a simple activity that you perform often throughout the day."

Aspect of mindfulness taught: Observing and describing one-mindfully, nonjudgmentally

EXERCISE 10. Focusing on Scent

Leaders bring in scented candles. Group members are instructed: "Choose a candle. When the bell rings, sit back in your chair and find a comfortable and relaxed position. Close your eyes and begin to focus on the smell of the candle. Let go of any distractions or judgments. Notice how the smell makes you feel and what images it evokes." Afterward, leaders and participants discuss observations, emotions, thoughts, feelings, and sensations: "How did the scent make you feel? What images came to your mind? Did the smell remind you of anything in particular?"

Aspect of mindfulness taught: Observing one-mindfully and nonjudgmentally

EXERCISE 11. Mindfully Eating a Raisin

Group leaders distribute raisins. Group members are each asked to hold a raisin; observe its appearance, texture, and scent; then put it in their mouths and slowly, with awareness, begin eating—noticing the tastes, sensations, and even the sounds of eating. This can also be done with candies (sweet tarts, caramels, fruit chews, fireballs, etc.)

Aspect of mindfulness taught: Observing and describing one-mindfully and nonjudgmentally

EXERCISE 12. Switched-Candy Exercise

Leaders bring in a box of assorted chocolates or bag of assorted treats, and ask group members to carefully select the item they think they would enjoy the most and place it in front of them. Leaders remind the group members to be fully present and nonjudgmental of the experience. Just before they begin, each member is asked to pass the chosen item to the person on his or her left. Members observe their reactions. Now members place their new piece of candy in their mouths; close their eyes; and use all of their senses to observe the smell, texture, and taste of their candy. Leaders remind them to bring their attention back to the selected focus if their minds wander. After a few minutes, group members are instructed to open their eyes, and leaders elicit observations about the experience.

Aspect of mindfulness taught: Radical acceptance; observing and describing one-mindfully and nonjudgmentally

EXERCISE 13. Ice Cube Exercise

Each group member holds an ice cube in a hand, lets it melt, and observes/describes the experience.

Aspect of mindfulness taught: Observing and describing, one-mindfully and nonjudgmentally

EXERCISE 14. Texture Exercise

Group members feel different-textured objects in a bag, and observe/describe these.

Aspect of mindfulness taught: Observing and describing one-mindfully

EXERCISE 15. Banging the Drum

Group members are asked to drum a beat on the table. One person starts, then the adjacent person adds to it, and so on, until all are drumming and keeping their beat.

Aspect of mindfulness taught: Participating one-mindfully

EXERCISE 16. Walking the Line

Leaders put a line of tape on the floor. Each group member in turn walks on the line, placing one foot directly in front of the other, with full attention to the activity. The members share observations about it (e.g., losing their balance, etc.).

Variant: Balancing on one foot. Group members stand up and get behind their chairs. With one hand on the chair to steady themselves, each member lifts one foot and attempts to balance on the other. When able, each person can remove the hand from the chair and balance on the one foot, with full attention to the activity.

Aspect of mindfulness taught: Observing and describing one-mindfully and nonjudgmentally; also, experiential metaphor for maintaining "balance" of emotion and reasonable mind, and of thoughts and actions

EXERCISE 17. Wise Mind Charades

Group leaders act out each of three states of mind, one at a time, while role-playing a scenario (e.g., argument with a relative over curfew). Group members try to guess their state of mind. They then discuss how they came to the answer (tone of voice, body language, word choice, etc.). Finally, leaders ask for two group member volunteers to act out a state of mind in their own role play.

Aspect of mindfulness taught: Observing and describing states of mind: reasonable mind, emotion mind, and wise mind

EXERCISE 18. Row Your Boat

Group members are divided into two or three groups, and are asked to sing "Row, Row, Row Your Boat" in rounds, starting with the first group. Leaders gesture when each group should start. Members then describe their experiences, including self-consciousness and judgments. Leaders discuss the notion of nonjudgmental participation, and now ask members to try again—this time really "hamming it up" with hand gestures and booming voices, throwing themselves into the experience. Leaders and participants discuss the difference between the first and second times.

Aspect of mindfulness taught: Participating without judgment

EXERCISE 19. Mindful Listening

Leaders ask group members to break into pairs and discuss a topic of importance to them. The listeners are asked *not* to be mindful, and instead to act distracted or bored. Leaders then ask the speakers what it was like to talk to someone who was not being mindful. Now the pairs practice again, with the listeners being mindful, putting all attention into the interaction. Leaders and speakers discuss the difference: What was it like?

Variant: Mindful listening and speaking. Same as above, except that the first time, speakers act distracted as well. Then, in the second practice, both speakers and listeners are mindful in the interaction. Both then discuss what it was like to interact with someone who was distracted versus mindful.

Aspect of mindfulness taught: Observing one-mindfully; also, interpersonal effectiveness and Level 1 validation (see Chapter 3)

EXERCISE 20. What's in a Face?

A leader says:

> "Be mindful of your face. Notice the different parts of your face from your forehead to your chin. Are they relaxed or tensed? Are there other sensations? What is your facial expression? Try to notice without changing your expression or experience." Afterward, leaders and participants discuss observations.

Variant: Body sensations. Leaders ask group members to be mindful of sensations, tension, position, and so forth within their bodies, since paying attention to physical sensations is important for learning to identify emotions. Discussion follows.

Aspect of mindfulness taught: Observing and describing one-mindfully

EXERCISE 21. Focusing on the Breath

A leader says:

> "Get into a comfortable position and just notice the experience of your breath going in and out. Pay attention to what each breath feels like coming in through your nose or mouth, and notice how your lungs expand like a balloon. Then notice how it feels when you exhale."

Aspect of mindfulness taught: Observing and describing one-mindfully

EXERCISE 22. Observing Emotions

A leader says:

> "Notice the emotions you are experiencing, and try to note how you know you are having those emotions. That is, what labels do you have in mind? What thoughts, what body sensations, and so on give you information about the emotions? Describe to yourself where you feel the sensations."

Aspect of mindfulness taught: Observing and describing

EXERCISE 23. What's My Experience?

A leader says:

> "Focus your mind on your experience this very moment. Be mindful of any thoughts feelings, body sensations, urges, or anything else you become aware of. Don't judge your ex-

perience, or try to push it away or hold onto it. Just let experiences come and go like clouds moving across the sky."

Aspect of mindfulness taught: Observing and describe one-mindfully and nonjudgmentally

EXERCISE 24. Noticing Urges

A leader says:

"Sit very straight in your chair. Throughout this exercise, notice any urges—whether to move, shift positions, scratch an itch, or do something else. Instead of acting on the urge, simply notice it."

Leaders and participants then discuss the experience. Was it possible to have an urge and not act on it?

Aspect of mindfulness taught: Observing and describing one-mindfully; also, distress tolerance (not acting on urges, even when not acting is uncomfortable)

EXERCISE 25. Observing Thoughts

A leader says:

"Notice your thoughts as they come and go, as if they were scrolling by on a message board on a marquee, or on the bottom of the screen on CNN. Truly notice your thoughts, as opposed to thinking them, dwelling on them, pushing them away, or changing them. Try not to get stuck on a thought or get caught up in believing or reacting to them. Notice what they are, which are just ... thoughts."

Aspect of mindfulness taught: Observing one-mindfully and nonjudgmentally

EXERCISE 26. Blowing Bubbles

Leaders pass out containers of bubble solution to group members. Members are asked to dip their wands and begin blowing bubbles—focusing all of their attention on this one moment, on the bubbles; noticing their shapes, textures, colors, and so on. If they get distracted by other thoughts, they should gently bring their attention back to the process of bubble blowing.

Aspect of mindfulness taught: Observing one mindfully and nonjudgmentally

EXERCISE 27. Imagery of a Recent Experience

A leader says:

"Think of a time you were upset recently with a boyfriend, girlfriend, or family member. Take a moment and try to conjure up the experience as though it were happening now— notice your thoughts, feelings, urges, body sensations, and so forth. Observe your experiences, let yourself experience them fully without judging them, and then silently put words on these experiences (e.g., 'Tears are welling up in my eyes,' 'My shoulders feel tense,' 'My thoughts are racing'). Your goal is to practice getting into wise mind as if you were in the situation this moment."

Variant: Doing what works. Same as above, except that after 2 minutes of observing experiencse, the leader says: "Think of one goal of yours in this situation. Think of something you could do or say to 'do what works.' That is, focus on effectiveness."

Aspect of mindfulness taught: Wise mind, observing and describing nonjudgmentally and effectively

EXERCISE 28. Changing One Letter

Group members sit in a comfortable position. When a group leader rings the bell the third time, he or she will start the exercise by saying a three-letter (or four-letter, if leaders would like to make it a bit more complex) word. Then the next person changes any one letter in the word just said by the leader to make a new word, and says it out loud. After that, the next person takes this new word and changes one letter to make a completely new word, and so on. (Sample sequence: "dog," "dig," "pig," etc.)

Aspect of mindfulness taught: Attending one-mindfully (staying focused)

EXERCISE 29. Last Letter, First Letter

To begin this exercise, group members sit in a circle. The first person begins by saying a word. Then the individual to the right must say a word that starts with the last letter of the word the first person says. (Sample sequence: "bus," "steak," "key," "yellow," etc.) "As you continue around the circle, let go of any distractions. Notice any judgments you may have regarding your ability to think of a word quickly." Afterward, leaders and participants discuss observations.

Aspect of mindfulness taught: Attending one-mindfully and nonjudgmentally

EXERCISE 30. Formal Walking Meditation

A leader says:

"To do the walking meditation, you need a place with enough space for at least 5–10 paces in a straight line. Select an unobstructed area and start at one end. Stand for a moment in an attentive position. Your arms can be held in any way that is comfortable. Then, while breathing in, lift one foot and bring it forward. While breathing out, bring the foot down and touch the floor. Repeat this for the other foot. Walk slowly to the opposite end, then turn around slowly, and stand there for a moment before you walk back. Then repeat the process. Keep your eyes open to maintain balance, but don't look at anything in particular. Walk naturally. Place your full attention on this experience of walking.

Watch for tensions building in the body; put all of your attention on the sensations coming from the feet and legs. Experience every tiny change in tactile sensation as the feet press against the floor and then lift again, so that the feet become your whole universe. If your mind wanders, note the distraction in the usual way, then return your attention to walking. Don't look at your feet while you are doing all of this, and don't walk back and forth watching a mental picture of your feet and legs."

Aspect of mindfulness taught: Observing one-mindfully

Walking the Middle Path Skills:
Lecture and Discussion Points

As we have noted in Chapter 4, we found that after several years of working with teens and families, several topic areas arose repeatedly that were not elaborated in the standard DBT skills training manual (Linehan, 1993b). These topic areas included the polarities in behavioral patterns experienced by families with suicidal adolescents; the definition of, rationale for, and application of validation; and the explicit application of learning principles to self and others. We have discovered that these topics fit well together as a unique skills module.

The Walking the Middle Path Skills module is about learning to recognize truths such as the following: Two things that seem like opposites can both be true, and there is more than one way to see a situation or solve a problem. By recognizing such truths, group members can work on changing painful or difficult thoughts, feelings, or circumstances, while at the same time accepting themselves, others, and circumstances as they are in the moment.

Note that the material on dialectics may exceed the length of a typical skills training group session. Leaders can select which points to expand on and which points to acknowledge only briefly, based on the needs and comprehension of group members. As in teaching all DBT skills, remember to make lecture points succinct. Provide frequent examples, and elicit examples from group members.

GOALS OF THE MODULE

The goals of this new module are to help group members effectively manage adolescent–family dilemmas by means of the following:

- *Dialectics:* Balancing acceptance and change, and "walking the middle path."
- *Validation:* Working on acceptance.
- *Behaviorism:* Working on change.

DIALECTICS

Clients Are Oriented to the Skills to Be Learned and the Rationale for Their Importance

Leaders first draw a deep canyon on the blackboard, with an adolescent at the top on one side and a parent at the top on the other. A skills trainer poses the question to the group:

> "On what issues do teenagers and parents find themselves polarized—that is, on opposite sides? How about curfew? How about grades? How about sex, body piercings, smoking cigarettes, drinking alcohol, and so on? Do you find yourselves getting stuck and unable to find a middle path between you? And on what issues do you find *yourself* flipping back and forth from one position to another? For example, do you ever feel you have been too lax with yourself for a time, and so then jump over to the other side and become overly strict?"

Emotion Mind Pushes Us toward Extremes

LECTURE POINT: The problem is that when people are in emotion mind, they tend to act in extreme "black-or-white," "all-or-nothing" ways.

Example: A teenage boy comes home repeatedly after curfew, and his father tells him, "You're grounded for the rest of the school year!" Or a teenage girl screams at her mother, "You never think about me! You only care about yourself!" because the mother has forgotten to buy the teen's favorite cereal. Get other examples of extreme behavioral responses from participants at this point.

What's Being Left Out?

DISCUSSION POINT: Ask group members to consider what's being left out when the second adolescent above says, "You never think about me! You only care about yourself!" Generate alternative explanations for the parent's oversight that are more balanced. If the group fails to generate any examples, leaders may choose to give the following: The teen considers the possibility that her mother was preoccupied with work while food shopping, *and* at the same time realizes that her mother does love her. This "both–and" perspective synthesizes the "either–or" stance so commonly held by emotionally dysregulated individuals.

> *Introduce and Review Handout C.1, "Dialectics: What Is It?"*

When We Get Stuck in Our Own Viewpoint, How Do We Get Unstuck?

LECTURE POINT: A dialectical approach can help us get unstuck. The skills in this module help people learn how to "walk the middle path" in what they think and how they act. This approach takes into account our current viewpoint *and* an opposing viewpoint, which leads to a synthesis of both perspectives; this is how we get unstuck and change occurs.

Example: One mother of a teenage girl was extremely concerned about her daughter's romantic relationship with an older boy. She was afraid they were having sex and that her daughter would get pregnant. The first thing she thought to do was to try and break up the relationship. But doing that would alienate her daughter, and that increased her distress. Then she started to ignore the topic of the relationship completely, in order to avoid her emotional distress—the opposite extreme of trying to break up the relationship. Rather than opting for either one of these two extreme positions, she learned to consider both. This led her to find a third option, a "middle path" synthesis: to speak calmly to her daughter about appropriate birth control methods.

LECTURE POINTS: Dialectics teaches the following:

1. **There is always more than one way to see a situation, and more than one way to solve a problem.**
   The idea here is that there is no absolute truth (at the one extreme) and truth is not completely relative (at the other extreme). Instead, truth evolves over time. Use as examples rules that used to be correct when an adolescent was a child, or when the parents were not divorced or were less experienced as parents, but are no longer true. This is consistent with the DBT assumption "There is no absolute truth" presented in the orientation to the skills training group (see Chapter 10).

2. **All people have unique qualities and different points of view.**
   This point normalizes and accepts differences among people's attitudes and behaviors, rather than seeing these differences as cause for conflict. Some people believe that anything deviating from their own point of view is wrong.
   Example: A parent insists that a teenage boy begin his homework immediately upon returning from school. The teen insists on watching TV to help him unwind from a long day. The truth from the parent's perspective is that the teen does not begin his homework until after dinner and then stays up past his bedtime in order to complete the work. This results in his being overtired and less focused the next day. The truth from the adolescent's perspective is that he is mentally fatigued and requires a break before beginning his homework.

3. **It is important not to see the world in "black-or-white," "all-or-nothing" ways.**
   Truths do not have to fall into one extreme or another.

4. **Two things that seem like opposites can both be true.**
   There is wisdom to be gained from examining the truth in both perspectives. See the examples on Handout C.1: "You are doing the best you can, *and* you need to do better, try harder, and be more motivated to change," "You are tough, *and* you are gentle."

5. **Change is the only constant.**
   This idea derives from the dialectical world view (see Linehan, 1993a) and has two major applications to teens and their families. When both teens and adults feel hopeless and think that nothing will ever change, a dialectical philosophy argues that change occurs continually. The world is one large system with many interfacing parts. The sun, the trees, the water, the fruit, the farmer, the grocer, the teacher, the friend, the parent, the sibling—these things are all interconnected and influence one another.

So on any given day, things are never the same as the moment before or the moment after.

6. **Meaning and truth evolve over time.**

What was true in the past may no longer be true, simply because of changes in the environment and in the person. Thus truth evolves transactionally over time. Parents often look back on the hard work and sacrifices they made to get ahead or succeed when they were young adults, and then impose the same demands on their own children now. However, the meaning of hard work for the parents was learned over time; thus meaning and truth for the teenagers will also evolve over time and are unlikely to be gained from being forced upon them.

7. **Change is transactional.**

Each individual influences his or her environment, just as each environment influences the individual. Reciprocity is the key word here. *A* affects *B* which alters *B*, which in turn alters *A*, and so forth. Each adolescent has a completely different "family" that has a unique impact on his or her life. The "family" can consist of parents, grandparents, siblings, teachers, peers, therapists, coaches, and others. The impact that these people in the environment have on the individual is just as varied as the impact the individual has on those in the environment. The bottom line here is that it takes at least two to tango.

LECTURE POINTS: The points above all help pave the way toward the middle path by helping us do the following:

- Expand our thoughts and ways of considering life situations.
- "Unstick" standoffs and conflicts.
- Be more flexible and approachable.
- Avoid assumptions and blaming.

DISCUSSION POINTS: Elicit from the group one or two examples of when people were operating from a nondialectical perspective—that is, when they were "stuck" in an extreme way of seeing things. Why was that a problem? Can anyone generate an alternative position?

> *Review Dialectics Handout C.2, "Walking the Middle Path: 'How To' Guide"*

1. Move away from "either–or" thinking to "both–and" thinking. Avoid extreme words: "always," "never," "you make me." Be descriptive.
   Example: Instead of saying, "Everyone always treats me unfairly," say, "Sometimes I am treated fairly, and at other times I am treated unfairly."
2. Practice looking at all sides of a situation/all points of view. Find the kernel of truth in every side.
3. Remember: *No one* has the absolute truth. Be open to alternatives.
4. Use "I feel ..." statements, instead of "You are ... ," "You should ... ," "or "That's just the way it is" statements.
5. Accept that different opinions can be valid, even if you do not agree with them ("I can see your point of view, even though I do not agree with it").

6. Do not assume that you know what others are thinking; check your assumptions ("What did you mean when you said ... ?").

7. Do not expect others to know what you are thinking ("What I am trying to say is ...").

Practice Exercises

DISCUSSION POINT: Have group members read the "Practice" examples at the bottom of Handout C.2. Then ask them to circle the statement that reflects a dialectical viewpoint. Next, discuss members' answers and confirm their understanding of the "both–and" concept.

Example: A parent says to an adolescent, "I want you to rely more on yourself and less on me when it comes to figuring out what you think and feel, *and* you must ask me before you make plans to go to the city with your friends." Discuss how the preceding "both–and" statement makes sense and may promote change.

> *Introduce and Review Handout C.3, "Dialectical Dilemmas"*

In discussing this handout, make it clear that these dialectical behavioral patterns operate within teens as well as between teens and family members, between parents (e.g., parent vs. parent), and between therapists and teens.

Understanding Dialectical Dilemmas

LECTURE POINT: A skills trainer says to the group:

> "Do you ever find that you're going along with a certain way of thinking and acting, and then something hits you and you swing to the other extreme? For example, for the parents in the group, you let your kids do what they want to do, like coming in late, slacking off on homework, or being disrespectful—and then one day, you say, 'That's it!' You then switch to the other extreme and say, 'I've had it! You're grounded—no going out and no TV for the rest of the school year!' Do you think that works? Is that usually an effective way of changing your teen's behavior? From our experience, and from the research literature, the answer is no. And as you may know from your personal experience, your teens do not respond, and then you revert to your old ways. Teenagers can also swing from one extreme to the other in trying to manage their own emotions and behaviors. Lastly, have you noticed that parents and their teenagers often get stuck in polarized positions? For instance, parents say, 'Come home early!' and teens say, 'I'm coming home late!' One of the goals of this module is to help you find the middle path within yourself and in your relationships in order to achieve your goals. If you find yourself landing at one extreme pole or another, you are unlikely to be able to maintain that position. Even if you are, it is likely to be ineffective."

LECTURE POINT: When these polarized positions occur, we call them "dialectical dilemmas." These behavior patterns can take place within a person (e.g., within a teen or parent) or between two people (e.g., between a teenager and a parent). Three dialectical dilemmas are commonly observed in working with families:

1. Being too loose versus being too strict.
2. Making light of problem behaviors versus making too much of typical adolescent behaviors.
3. Forcing independence too soon versus holding on too tight.

Review Dialectical Dilemmas Handout C.4, "Walking the Middle Path"

Offer brief definitions and examples of each dialectical dilemma as follows: Excessive leniency versus authoritarian control; normalizing pathological behaviors versus pathologizing normative behaviors; forcing autonomy versus fostering dependence (Rathus & Miller, 2000). Note that for use in skills training, these have been reworded respectively as the three dilemmas listed in the previous Lecture Point.

Too Loose vs. Too Strict

LECTURE POINT: The first dialectical dilemma is called "being too lose versus being too strict." "Being too loose" refers to having too few demands and limits. The other extreme, "being too strict," refers to imposing too many demands and limits while being inflexible.
   Examples:

• A 15-year-old girl insists on getting body piercings, staying up past midnight instant-messaging friends, and sleeping at a boy's house without permission. The parents insist that she not have a boyfriend or any body piercings until she turns 18, and that she has to be in bed with lights out by 10 P.M.

• A high-achieving, perfectionistic teenage boy has been avoiding doing homework for the past several weeks, for a variety of reasons. The teen then gets a poor report card, which propels him into an overly strict response—dismissing all social engagements and leisure-time activities, and focusing exclusively on schoolwork.

Note to Leaders: Some group members might think that one of the responses in either of these examples is an appropriate response. Ask group members whether this is so, and whether this is the most effective long-term strategy.

Does the Dilemma Apply to Group Members?

DISCUSSION POINT: A skills trainer says:

"Now let's get some examples of these and determine where we all fall along these behavior patterns. Place an *X* on the line in Handout C.4 that notes where you are *right now*, and a *Y* where your family member is *right now*.
   "Can any of you share with the group if you found yourself on one pole or the other? Is there a middle path between these poles that might be a more effective solution?"

What Is a Middle Path?

Is it your goal to walk the middle path? If so, the following dialectical synthesis could help you achieve your goal: **Have clear rules and enforce them consistently,** *and at the same time* **be willing to negotiate on some issues.**

> "For instance, in the example where the 15-year-old girl is insisting on body piercings, sleeping over at a boy's house, and instant-messaging friends past midnight, the parent could negotiate on some issues while not bending on others. For example, sleeping over at a boy's house would not be permissible, but she could spend time with a boy (and even boyfriend) during the day. Furthermore, she could earn the privilege of staying up until 11 P.M. (and instant-messaging friends) if she completes her homework and abides by her weekend curfew. However, for this parent, the body piercings would not be negotiable."

DISCUSSION POINT: Elicit other examples from teens and parents.

Making Too Light vs. Making Too Much of Problem Behaviors

LECTURE POINT: The second dialectical dilemma is called **"making light of problem behaviors versus making too much of typical adolescent behaviors."** "Making light of problem behaviors" refers to minimizing the seriousness of behaviors that could be maladaptive or harmful. "Making too much of typical adolescent behaviors" refers to overreacting to behaviors that would generally be considered normal.

Example: A well-meaning parent might ignore, for a long period, an adolescent's increasingly maladaptive behaviors, such as failing grades, spending more time with a drug-using peer group, and greater irritability at home. The parent might give the adolescent the benefit of the doubt, believing that this stage would pass. Then, after the adolescent makes a suicide attempt, the parent begins watching the adolescent like a hawk and interpreting even minor mood changes or request for privacy as signs of impending danger.

Does the Dilemma Apply to the Group?

DISCUSSION POINT: A skills trainer says:

> "Now let's get some examples of these and determine where we all fall along these behavior patterns. Place an *X* on the line in Handout C.4 that notes where you are *right now*, and a *Y* where your family member is *right now*.
>
> "Can any of you share with the group if you found yourself on one pole or the other? Is there a middle path between these poles that might be a more effective solution?"

What Is a Middle Path?

Is it your goal to walk the middle path? If so, the following dialectical synthesis could help you achieve your goal:

Recognize when a behavior 'crosses the line' and try to get help for that behavior, *and at the same time* **recognize which behaviors are part of typical adolescent development.**

"For instance, the synthesis in the example just given could be for the parent to recognize the pattern of deteriorating behaviors and proactively intervening, while inquiring about but not overreacting to the teen's requests for privacy and minor moodiness."

DISCUSSION POINT: Elicit other examples from teens and parents.

> *Introduce and Review Handout C.5, "What's Typical for Adolescents and What's Not"*

Note to Leaders: To help group members recognize which behaviors cross the line and which are typical adolescent behaviors, introduce What's Typical for Adolescents and What's Not (Handout C.5). This handout offers some examples of normative adolescent behaviors, as well as those adolescent behaviors that should raise a flag for concern. Not every possible behavior of concern is listed here. When parents are unsure whether a behavior crosses the line, they should consult with a professional or with an objective friend or family member.

DISCUSSION POINT: Elicit examples from teens and parents, using Handout C.5 as a starting point.

Forcing Independence Too Soon vs. Holding on Too Tight

LECTURE POINT: The third dialectical dilemma is called "**Forcing independence too soon versus holding on too tight.**" "Forcing independence too soon" refers to cutting the strings prematurely. "Holding on too tight" refers to restricting moves toward independence.

Example: The parents of a 17-year-old daughter have spent the past several years rescuing and protecting her from any negative consequences of her actions (e.g., problems with school, peers, after-school jobs). Then, when the daughter becomes pregnant, they switch to the other extreme and demand that she move out of the house immediately and find a way to support herself.

Does the Dilemma Apply to Group Members?

DISCUSSION POINT: A skills trainer says:

"Now let's get some examples of these and determine where we all fall along these behavior patterns. Place an *X* on the line in Handout C.4 that notes where you are *right now*, and a *Y* where your family member is *right now*.

"Can any of you share with the group if you found yourself on one pole or the other? Is there a middle path between these poles that might be a more effective solution?"

What Is a Middle Path?

Is it your goal to walk the middle path? If so, the following dialectical synthesis could help you achieve your goal: **Give your adolescent guidance, support, and rules to help the teen figure out how to be responsible for his or her life,** *and at the same time* **slowly give your** adolescent greater amounts of freedom and independence while continuing to allow an appropriate amount of reliance on others.

> "For instance, a synthesis for the example just given could be for the parents to have held the teen more accountable for her actions earlier in her life. At the same time, now that she is pregnant, they could begin to wean her from their care more slowly and encourage her to take on greater responsibility for herself."

DISCUSSION POINT: Elicit other examples from teens and parents.

Other Types of Dialectical Dilemmas

Note to Leaders: Other types of dialectical dilemmas may arise in your interactions with families, such as overindulging versus withholding/depriving, being overly intrusive versus overly distant, and others. Should you note such patterns in discussions with clients, you can similarly point out the extremes in each position and ask group members to help generate a synthesis.

Handout C.6, "Homework Practice Exercise 1: Dialectical Dilemmas"

There is a take-home practice exercise for the dialectics segment of this module (Handout C.6). This handout asks group members to identify one personal example of not thinking or acting dialectically (i.e., getting stuck at one pole of a dialectical dilemma) and one personal example of not-thinking or not-acting dialectically. This assignment requires therapists to help participants by employing the secondary treatment targets described in Chapter 5 (and included in simplified form in Handout C.4).

Example: For being too loose versus being too strict, the secondary targets include (1) increasing authoritative discipline and decreasing excessive leniency, and (2) increasing adolescent self-determination and decreasing authoritarian control. In practical terms, the parents are encouraged to employ an authoritative parenting style rather than a laissez-faire or authoritarian style, which involves discussing and possibly negotiating house rules with their teenagers and being firm yet flexible. In so doing, the parents are more easily respected (neither feared nor ignored), and the adolescents feel a greater sense of self-determination in that they have some input (neither all nor none) into their lives.

VALIDATION

The Group Is Oriented to the Skill of Validation and the Rationale for Its Importance

Introduce the topic of validation with a vignette illustrating invalidation, such as the following:

> "Johnny is sitting in class, trying to pay attention, and he accidentally knocks his notebook off his desk, making a loud noise on the floor. The peers next to him chuckle. The

teacher stops in her tracks and says, 'There you go again, Johnny, disrupting the class, trying to get attention ... I am really getting tired of this behavior!' Johnny feels extremely embarrassed, hurt, and angry, since he'd been making a true effort to focus and behave more skillfully. He later goes home and recounts the story to his mother, who replies, 'Why do you keep doing this to yourself? You're never going to get into college at this rate. You'd better shape up!' "

Ask group members what they think Johnny must have felt after his teacher's and mother's responses. Why were these responses so hurtful? What was missing from their responses?

> *Introduce and Review Handout C.7, "Validation: What Is It?"*

Note to Leaders: At this point, introduce Validation—What Is It? (Handout C.7). Invite a group member to read the definition of validation there. "Validation communicates to another person that his or her feelings, thoughts, and actions make sense and are understandable to you in a particular situation."

How Could the Teacher/Mother Have Validated Johnny?

DISCUSSION POINT: Now ask group members: "What would be a validating thing the teacher could have done?" A reasonable response here would be for the teacher to have simply ignored the dropping of the notebook, since ignoring it would have implied that it was insignificant and nondeliberate. Next, ask: "What would be a validating response the mother could have given?" If group members have trouble generating a validating response, then offer an example of one, such as "Oh, Johnny, that must have been so upsetting and frustrating for you, especially since you were really trying your best to pay attention and behave appropriately." If teens say that this sounds too "sappy," encourage them to put into words a validating response they would welcome from their own parents.

Validation Is Not Agreement

LECTURE POINT: Remember, validation does not equal agreement. Validation does not necessarily mean liking or agreeing with what the other person is doing, saying, or feeling. It means understanding where the other person is coming from. A therapist might validate an adolescent client's desire to get high with friends by saying, "I do understand that it makes you feel good to spend time with your friends, including when you are getting high. Frankly, however, I think it is a bad idea for you to get high right now, given your depression and recent suicidal urges."

How Do You Validate without Agreeing?

DISCUSSION POINT: Many people get this point confused.
Example: Most parents struggle in the attempt to validate their teen who asks for a later curfew, because they don't agree with a later time—so they simply say "No!" Is there a way to

validate the desire for the later curfew without *agreeing* with the teen? If group members cannot generate examples, leaders can provide one, such as saying, "I *get* that you want to stay out later, since you're having fun with your friends. Yet we agreed this would be your curfew time until you got back on track with your schoolwork."

Trouble Shooting Parent Difficulties with Validation

DISCUSSION POINT: Some people may raise the point that they do not see how they can validate when they simply do not understand the other person's point of view. That is, the other person's feelings or behaviors make no sense to them at all.

Example: Some parents might say that they cannot in the least understand their adolescents' suicidal behaviors. A leader might then say to such a parent, "I can understand how that might be difficult for you to understand." (The point is, as a leader, to model the concept being taught at any point—in this case, validation.) The leader can then say that because the adolescent is in tremendous pain and cannot see any other way out, suicidal behavior is logical and valid to the teen in that moment. If a parent still does not "get" the suicidality, a leader can respond: "Could you say to your teenager, as a first step, 'I can see that you are obviously in a lot of pain,' even though you don't understand the choice of suicide as a solution?" In this case, leaders can explain, the parent is validating the emotion, though not the behavior. This is important, because the teen will feel as if the parent understands at least one aspect of the teen's experience. An alternative strategy that can be very effective is to say "I know you want me to understand this, and, believe me, I *want* to understand this, but I just can't get it. Let's keep talking. Tell me again." The parent might want to get the adolescent to think of times he or she has had a lot of trouble understanding something in school that everyone else seemingly understood (such as algebra), but with persistence finally "got it."

This type of communication, presented in a nonjudgmental way, communicates that the parent's lack of understanding is the problem in this conversation, not the invalidity of the adolescent's emotions or behavior. It also communicates deep interest in the adolescent's difficulties. This leads logically to the next two sections of Handout C.7, on what and why we should validate.

What Should We Validate?

LECTURE POINT: Ask someone to read the **"What should we validate?"** section of Handout C.7 aloud. As stated there, we should validate:

- Feelings, thoughts, and behaviors in ourselves and in other people.

Leaders or group members can give examples of each, or can refer back to the example of Johnny, above.

Suggested Exercise

Note to Leaders: One exercise that can be used to emphasize "What should we validate?" is the following: Invite group members to practice talking about something, and have the rest of the group first pay close attention. Then, on cue from the leaders, the group members should act completely uninterested. What happens is that people can speak coherently when being listened to and then become incoherent when ignored.

Why Should We Validate?

LECTURE POINT: Ask someone to read the "Why should we validate?" section of Handout C.7 aloud. As stated there, validation improves relationships. Specifically, it can show that:

- We are listening.
- We understand.
- We are being nonjudgmental.
- We care about the relationship.
- Conflict is possible with decreased intensity.

In addition, validation can result in a communication partner who is:

- More calm.
- Less angry.
- More receptive to what we have to say.

Ask for Examples of Feeling Invalidated and Validated

DISCUSSION POINT: Can group members think of a time when they felt invalidated and contrast that to another time when they did? How were the two times different? How did they feel each time? How did it affect their behavior each time?

Introduce and Review Handout C.8, "A 'How To' Guide to Verbal and Nonverbal Validation"

Now introduce "A 'How To' Guide to Verbal and Nonverbal Validation" (Handout C.8). Emphasize that these points are not listed in order of importance or in order of how types of validation should be carried out. Rather, when people are familiar with various forms of validation, they have a choice of which they can use in each situation. Read through the "How can we validate others?" points.

1. **Actively listen. Make eye contact and stay focused.**
   After reading this point, a leader might pause and leave a moment of silence, which will result in group members' looking up expectantly at the leader. The leader can say, "This is Step 1 in validation—you are doing it. I can tell you are looking and listening right now." Note that culture has to be considered with regard to this point, as in some cultures (e.g., certain Hispanic subgroups and Asian cultures), maintaining eye contact may be considered disrespectful and thus invalidating.
2. **Be mindful of both nonverbal and verbal reactions in order to avoid invalidation (e.g., rolling eyes; sucking teeth; walking away; saying, "That's stupid, don't be sad" or "I don't care what you say").**
   Leaders can illustrate this point by sighing and rolling their eyes while a participant is reading, and then asking what this experience was like. The main point here is that

a person who is trying to validate someone must be careful to avoid *in*validating with both verbal and nonverbal behaviors.

3. **Observe what the other person is feeling in the moment. Look for a word that describes the feeling.**

    For example, as a start, a person can say, "I can see that you are really disappointed."

4. **Reflect the feeling back without judgment. The goal is to communicate that you understand how the other person feels (e.g., "It makes sense that you are angry," "I understand that you are having a tough time right now;" for self, "I have a right to feel sad.").**

    Take an example from one of the participants' earlier comments or homework reviews in which they had expressed distress (e.g., a teen's earlier expression of being in "a bad mood" today because of a conflict with a peer), and then ask each group member to make one validating comment to this group member. This illustrates that there are many possible validating responses.

5. (a) **Show tolerance! Look for how the feelings, thoughts, and actions make sense, given the other person's (or your) history and current situation, even if you don't approve of the behaviors, emotions, or actions themselves.** For example, a teenager might report her unwillingness to attend this treatment, due to the fact that none of her prior therapy experiences were helpful. Ask each member of the group to offer a validating statement, taking history and current situation into account. For example, one validating response might be "I don't blame you for feeling hopeless about this, given your past experience." (Leaders should use a relevant example generated from within the group whenever possible.)

    (b) **Look for how the feelings, thoughts, and actions make sense given the current situation.** This type of validation is at the heart of DBT. Validating in terms of the current situation means looking for how the person's behavior makes sense because it is a reasonable or normative response to a current situation. For example, Sharon is sometimes shy in groups. Now she is attending the DBT multifamily skills training group with her mother, and when she occasionally speaks up in group, another girl on the other side of the table gives her an angry, threatening look. On the way home, Sharon says to her mom: "That kid across the table was really mean to me. I don't want to sit near her next time." A response that would validate Sharon in terms of what actually happened would be "Boy, I really understand, and I wouldn't want to sit near her either. She gave you quite a look when you spoke up," A perhaps equally honest but invalidating response would be Sharon's mother saying to her, "I know you're shy, and it's hard for you to speak up in group." When a behavior is supported by current events, implying that it is caused by past events can be invalidating.

6. **Respond in a way that shows you are taking the other person seriously (with or without words).**

    Sometimes words are not necessary to convey validation. For example, if someone is crying, a validating response is to give a tissue or a hug. Or if a person says "I'm thirsty," giving him or her a glass of water communicates validation. Or if a friend or family member says, "I have a serious problem," it may be validating to dive in with efforts at problem solving without saying, "Wow, it sounds like you're having some serious problems and you're upset." Be careful in this latter case, however; depending on what the person wants in the moment, problem solving can be experienced as invalidating. Sometimes merely listening is sufficient validation. It may pay to ask, "Do you want me to help solve this problem, or do you just want to talk about it?"

Validating Ourselves

LECTURE POINT: Leaders now shift gears and begin talking about how to apply validation skills to oneself. **What is self-validation, and why is it important?** Self-validation involves perceiving one's *own* feelings, thoughts, and actions as accurate and acceptable in a particular situation. This is important, because many suicidal adolescents have the tendency to invalidate themselves. Examples of self-invalidation are "I shouldn't feel sad about this," or "it's stupid that I got that upset." The important point is the unaccepting or judgmental stance toward one's own experience. Self-validation relates to other-validation. It is important for parents to help their adolescents self-validate, particularly if their adolescents are constantly asking their parents for reassurance. Sometimes the self-invalidation comes from modeling the responses of an invalidating environment. Sometimes it comes from looking at the world through the lens of a person who is depressed. Regardless, it is important to learn how to validate oneself, because self-validation:

- Helps reduce emotional and physical arousal (i.e., it is calming).
- Reduces vulnerability to emotion mind.
- Helps in the processing of new information, which in turn permits more effective responses.

To return to the earlier example of Johnny, after the teacher accuses him of deliberately causing a distraction and trying to get attention, he second-guesses his own good intention to pay attention and behave well. He also thinks to himself, as he feels his eyes well up with tears, "This isn't such a big deal—why am I getting so upset?" This dual self-invalidation results in an intensification of his negative emotions, and impairs his ability to stay focused during the remaining class time.

How Could Johnny Have Validated Himself?

DISCUSSION POINT: What could Johnny have said to validate himself? How would that affect his thinking, feeling, and behavior? If group members have trouble generating responses, leaders can give the following alternative outcome: Johnny could have said to himself, "I know this was not intentional. I know I am trying to pay attention to what the teacher is teaching, and I'm doing the best I can. But she didn't see that—no wonder I feel so upset! I'll just keep paying attention, and talk to the teacher after class to explain this." Then group members can be asked to offer one quick example of self-validation, based on events of the past day.

> *Assign Handout C.9, "Practice Exercise 2: Self-Validation and Validation of Others"*
> *as a homework practice exercise*

BEHAVIORISM

> *Introduce and Review Handout C.10, "Behaviorism: What Is It?*
> *Ways to Increase Behaviors"*

Note to Leaders: Begin by introducing Behaviorism—What Is It/Ways to Increase Behaviors (Handout C.10). Ask a group member to read the definition of behaviorism there: "Strategies or principles used to *increase* behaviors we *do* want and *reduce* behaviors we *don't* want (in ourselves or others)."

Are There Behaviors You Want to Change in Yourself or Others?

DISCUSSION POINT: Ask the group, "Are there behaviors you would like to change in yourself or other people? If so, what are some of these?" Elicit brief examples from two or three group members. For others, these behaviors might include getting someone else to nag less, listen more, clean up his or her room more, obey curfew more, give more privileges, or do homework more often. For oneself, these might include exercising more, eating less, yelling less, listening more, engaging in more pleasurable activities (music, sports, etc.), or procrastinating less.

DISCUSSION POINT: Now ask the group, "Can all of us identify and share one behavior we would like to increase in ourselves?" Go around the room and elicit examples.

Reinforcers Increase Behaviors

LECTURE POINT: A skills trainer says:

> "An important way to increase a behavior is to provide 'reinforcers'—that is, consequences that result in more of the behavior. Reinforcers provide information to a person (or yourself) about what you want that person to do.
>
> "*Remember, timing is very important*: The reinforcer should follow the desired behavior immediately. If you wait too long, the reinforcer won't be connected with the behavior. For example, you are trying to improve your backhand in tennis, and your coach is observing 30 swings. Would you prefer your coach to tell you, 'That's the swing! Nice job!' immediately after you use the right form, or would you prefer the coach to wait until you are done and then say, 'Your 14th swing—I liked that one'?
>
> "*Also remember to choose motivating reinforcers, for yourself and others.* A fresh plate of broccoli normally won't do it for most people. Some examples of motivating reinforcers might include a nice dinner in a special restaurant, or downloading some new music after the completion of a major project."

Two Types of Reinforcement

LECTURE POINT: There are two different types of reinforcement: **"positive reinforcement"** and **"negative reinforcement."** *Positive reinforcement* increases the frequency of behavior by providing a *rewarding* consequence (e.g., praise, a privilege, an A on an exam, a satisfying outcome to an interpersonal situation).

Positive Reinforcers

DISCUSSION POINT: Ask group members, "What would be a positive reinforcer for the behavior you identified that you would like to increase? What would make you likely to do it?"

Note to Leaders: Guide group members in their responses to keep reinforcers small, realistic, safe, and age-appropriate (e.g., teens should not choose cars, large amounts of money, drinking alcohol, or staying out all night with friends). Also encourage participants to search for meaningful reinforcers beyond just money, such as time spent with a parent. In addition, discuss the concept of *satiation*: Something that is reinforcing may not be a reinforcer and may even be aversive when given too much.
  Examples: Food is not a reinforcer after a really big meal; affection is not a reinforcer if one receives plenty of that; and so on. Something is only a reinforcer if it is given in appropriate doses. This is also true with praise. Elicit examples, particularly from adolescents.

Negative Reinforcers

LECTURE POINT: The best way to remember the principle of negative reinforcement is to associate it with the word "relief." A more technical way to understand it is that *negative reinforcement increases the frequency of a behavior by removing an aversive condition.*
  Examples: Taking aspirin to get rid of a headache, doing homework to get Mom to stop nagging, or cutting oneself to decrease negative feelings (although the skills taught in group are better ways of managing such feelings). First, leaders can share an example, such as having back pain that gets relieved by receiving a massage. This reduction in pain increases the likelihood of seeking another massage in the future.

Ask for Examples of Negative Reinforcers in Group Members' Lives

DISCUSSION POINT: Next, leaders ask group members to identify a negative consequence or source of discomfort that they would like relieved or removed.
  Example: A teenage girl might mention a parent's nagging her to clean her room. What new behavior might help reduce this discomfort? For instance, if the teen's cleaning her room led to a reduction in the parent's nagging, the adolescent might be more likely to pick up after herself in the future. Elicit one or two other examples from the group.

Note to Leaders: Emphasize that positive and negative reinforcement can be applied in adaptive or maladaptive ways. For example, one can positively reinforce oneself for a desirable behavior by buying a new CD versus getting drunk. Or one can negatively reinforce oneself (e.g., get relief from emotional pain) by taking a long bath versus cutting oneself.

"Shaping"

LECTURE POINT: **"Shaping"** is a special form of reinforcement. It means reinforcing small steps that lead toward a bigger goal
  Example: One can take small, reinforced steps toward overcoming school anxiety (by at-

tending for 1 hour on Monday, 2 hours on Tuesday, etc., until attendance all day every day is achieved) or toward increasing abstinence from self-harm behavior.

Sometimes our expectations of ourselves and others set us up for disappointment and potential failure.

Example: If teens think, or their parents think, that the teens can achieve abstinence from self-cutting instantly, they are probably going to be disappointed with themselves, each other, and the treatment. So the principles of shaping need to be brought into the discussion of all new goals.

What Does "Shaping" Look Like?

DISCUSSION POINT: Note that each successive approximation or step toward a larger goal needs to be reinforced, to increase the chances of continuing to work toward the goal.

Example: Has a parent ever been frustrated with a child for not starting a large school project until the night before? How would shaping apply? Discuss. Group members' examples might include approaches such as saying, "Why don't you sit down and outline the paper the week before the due date? Once that's done, you can go watch TV." Step 2 would be to write the introduction and provide a small reinforcement for that, and so on.

> *Introduce and Review Handout C.11, "Ways to Decrease or Stop Behaviors"*

"Extinction"

LECTURE POINT: Two learning principles that can be used to decrease or stop behaviors are "extinction" and "punishment." A skills trainer says:

> "*Extinction is the reduction of a behavior because reinforcement is withheld.* That is, you might ignore the unwanted behavior when attention to it will cause it to continue to happen. However, make sure you reinforce other, adaptive behaviors in the process.
>
> "For example, if a little boy begins to throw a tantrum in the supermarket because he wants a candy bar, a parent is likely to give in to stop the escalation of the tantrum. This giving in, however, reinforces the tantrum behavior and makes it more likely to occur during the next visit to the supermarket. By contrast, if the parent withholds reinforcement—that is, does not buy the candy bar—the tantrum is likely to escalate in the moment (making everyone unhappy!). However, if the parent holds the line during this and subsequent shopping trips—that is, tolerates the 'behavioral burst' (escalating tantrum) by not giving in, while positively reinforcing any efforts to walk calmly through the store—the tantrum behavior is likely to extinguish over time.
>
> "Note that if the parent says no the first three times, but the fourth time gives in and buys the candy bar, thinking, 'It's just this one time,' the parent now has a *real* problem. This is called '**intermittent reinforcement**,' and an intermittently reinforced behavior is the most difficult to extinguish. So don't give up in the face of a behavioral burst—you have to ride it out. Also, don't forget to orient the person that you are beginning to work to extinguish the behavior, so that it does not seem arbitrary or punitive. And, again, don't forget to reinforce alternative, adaptive behaviors."

What Behaviors Might Group Members Reduce through Extinction?

DISCUSSION POINT: Elicit some examples from group members of behaviors that might be reduced or eliminated through extinction. For each example, note also what alternative behaviors might be reinforced and how behavioral bursts might be handled.

"Punishment"

LECTURE POINT: A skills trainer says:

> "The difference between extinction and punishment is that extinction involves taking away a reinforcer for a behavior, but punishment involves adding something that is negative or aversive. That is, punishment means giving a consequence that results in a decrease in behavior. It tells another person what you don't want that person to do.
>
> "For example, let's say that you're a parent and your teenage daughter harasses you to let her stay up later at night by nagging, criticizing, or 'guilt–tripping' you. Extinction of this harassment would involve defining this behavior for the girl as harassment and then never, ever giving in to it. Punishment of it might involve sending the girl to her room even earlier than usual.
>
> "Punishment can be either effective or ineffective. One type of effective punishment is just to let natural consequences happen. For example, let's say you're a teenager who stays up all night. As a result, you may be too tired to focus in school, may fail a test, and may get in trouble for failing. If a behavior doesn't have natural consequences, the punishment should be specific and time–limited, and it should fit the 'crime.' For instance, if you're a teen who misses curfew, you might be punished by losing the chance to go out the next day. In contrast, an ineffective punishment is one that isn't specific, lasts too long, and/or doesn't fit the behavior. For instance, if you miss curfew, your parents might ground you for 2 months, take away your cell phone, and remind you of the mistake constantly."

Note to Leaders: Emphasize that punishment may make a person stay away from the person who punishes, hide a behavior, or suppress the behavior when the punisher is around. Punishment may at times be necessary, but it is essential to keep it specific, time-limited, and appropriate to the "crime," as well as to reinforce an alternative behavior. Otherwise, punishment will not work. Punishment by itself does not teach new behavior, and it may even lead to self-punishment.

DISCUSSION POINT: Elicit some examples from teens and parents of behaviors that appear necessary to punish rather than extinguish. For each example, debate the possible advantages versus disadvantages of punishment.

> *Assign Handout C.12, "Practice Exercise 3–Behaviorism: Positive Reinforcement"*
> *as a homework practice exercise*

Handouts for Walking the Middle Path Skills

Dialectics

What Is It?

Dialectics teaches us that:

- There is always more than one way to see a situation, and more than one way to solve a problem.
- All people have unique qualities and different points of view.
- It is important not to see the world in "black-and-white," "all-or-nothing" ways.
- Two things that seem like (or are) opposites can both be true.
- Change is the only constant.
- Meaning and truth evolve over time.
- Change is transactional.

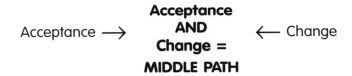

Examples:
- You are doing the best you can, *and* you need to do better, try harder, and be more motivated to change.
- You are tough *and* you are gentle.

This perspective helps pave the way toward the middle path by helping you:

- Expand your thoughts and ways of considering life situations.
- "Unstick" standoffs and conflicts.
- Be more flexible and approachable.
- Avoid assumptions and blaming.

Other examples of dialectics:
- Balancing validation with change
- Balancing reward with punishment
- Others: _____

Dialectics

Walking the Middle Path: "How to" Guide

Hints for thinking and acting dialectically

1. Move away from "either-or" thinking to "both-and" thinking. Avoid extreme words: "always," "never," "you make me." Be descriptive.

   Example:
   - Instead of saying, "Everyone always treats me unfairly," say, "Sometimes I am treated fairly and at other times I am treated unfairly."

2. Practice looking at all sides of a situation/all points of view. Find the kernel of truth in every side.

3. Remember: *No one* has the absolute truth. Be open to alternatives.

4. Use "I feel ... " statements, instead of "You are ... ," "You should ... ," or "That's just the way it is" statements.

5. Accept that different opinions can be valid, even if you do not agree with them ("I can see your point of view, even though I do not agree with it").

6. Do not assume that you know what others are thinking; check your assumptions ("What did you mean when you said ... ?").

7. Do not expect others to know what you are thinking ("What I am trying to say is ...").

Practice:

Circle the dialectical statements:

1. a. "It is hopeless. I just cannot do it."
   b. "This is a breeze. I got no problems."
   c. "This is really hard for me, and I am going to keep trying."

2. a. "I know I am right about this."
   b. "The way you are thinking doesn't sound right to me."
   c. "Well, I can see it this way, and you can see it that way."

Dialectical Dilemmas

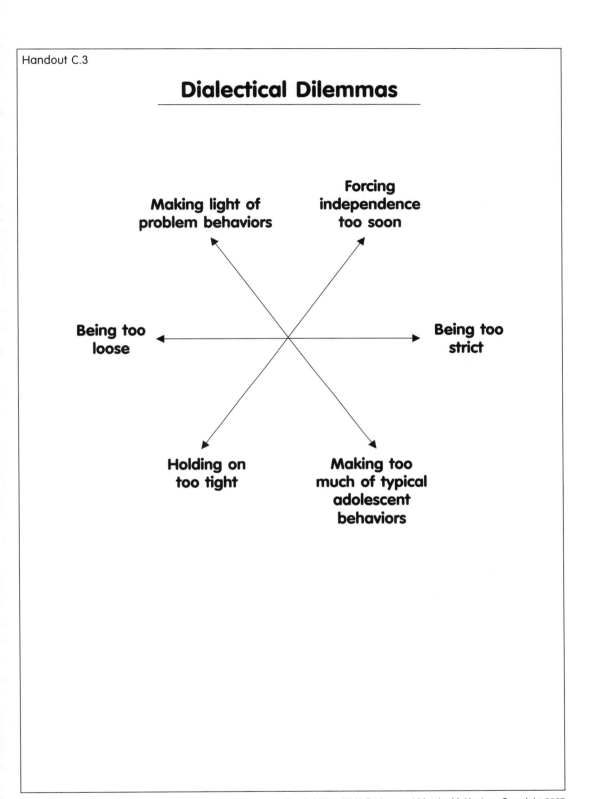

Dialectical Dilemmas

Walking the Middle Path

(Note: These apply to everyone, including yourself.)

| **Being too loose** | 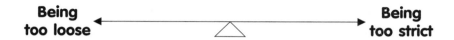 | **Being too strict** |

Have clear rules and enforce them consistently, *and at the same time* be willing to negotiate on some issues.

| **Making light of problem behaviors** | 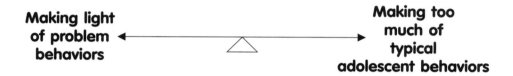 | **Making too much of typical adolescent behaviors** |

Recognize when a behavior "crosses the line" and try to get help for that behavior, *and at the same time* recognize which behaviors are part of typical adolescent development.

| **Holding on too tight** | 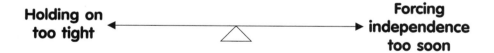 | **Forcing independence too soon** |

Give your adolescent guidance, support, and rules to help the teen figure out how to be responsible with his or her life, *and at the same time* slowly give your adolescent greater amounts of freedom and independence, while continuing to allow an appropriate amount of reliance on others.

Place an X on each continuum that notes where you are, and a Y where your family member is.

What's Typical for Adolescents and What's Not

Typical	Not typical; cause for concern
➤ Increased sexual maturation; increased focus on body image and self-consciousness	➤ Sexual promiscuity; bingeing, purging, or restricting eating, social withdrawal
➤ Sexual experimentation	➤ Multiple partners; unsafe sexual practices; pregnancy
➤ Increased parent–adolescent conflict	➤ Verbal or physical aggression; running away
➤ Experimentation with drugs, alcohol, and cigarettes	➤ Substance abuse; selling drugs; heavily substance-using peer group
➤ Increased sensation seeking and risk taking	➤ Multiple accidents; encounters with firearms; excessive risk taking (e.g., "subway surfing")
➤ Stressful transitions to middle and high school	➤ Lack of connection to school or peers; school truancy, failure, or dropout
➤ Increased argumentativeness, idealism, and criticism	➤ Rebellious questioning of social rules and conventions; causing trouble with family members, teachers, or others who attempt to exert control over the adolescent
➤ Becoming overwhelmed with everyday decision making	➤ Becoming paralyzed with indecision

Walking the Middle Path

Practice Exercise 1
Dialectical Dilemmas

Identify a time this week when you DID NOT think or act dialectically.

Example 1: Briefly describe the situation (who, what, when) _____

_____

_____

How did you think or act in this situation? _____

_____

Are you making any thinking mistakes? If so, what are they? _____

_____

What is another dialectical belief about the situation? _____

_____

What was the outcome?_____

_____

Identify a time this week when you DID think or act dialectically.

Example 2: Briefly describe the situation (who, what, when) _____

_____

_____

How did you think or act in this situation? _____

_____

Are you making any thinking mistakes? If so, what are they? _____

_____

What was the outcome? _____

_____

Validation

What Is It?

Validation communicates to another person that his or her feelings, thoughts, and actions make sense and are understandable to you in a particular situation.

Self-validation involves perceiving your *own* feelings, thoughts, and actions as accurate and acceptable in a particular situation.

> **Remember: Validation ≠ Agreement**

Validation *does not* necessarily mean that you like or agree with what the other person is doing, saying, or feeling. It means that you understand where the other person is coming from.

WHAT should we validate?

- Feelings, thoughts, and behaviors in:
  - Ourselves
  - Other people

WHY should we validate?

- It improves relationships!
- Validation can show that:
  - We are listening.
  - We understand.
  - We are being nonjudgmental.
  - We care about the relationship.
  - Conflict is possible with decreased intensity.

Validation

A "How To" Guide to Verbal and Nonverbal Validation

How can we validate **others**?

1. Actively listen. Make eye contact and stay focused.

2. Be mindful of both nonverbal and verbal reactions in order to avoid invalidation (e.g., rolling eyes; sucking teeth; walking away; saying, "That's stupid, don't be sad", or "I don't care what you say").

3. Observe what the other person is feeling in the moment. Look for a word that describes the feeling.

4. Reflect the feeling back without judgment. The goal is to communicate that you understand how the other person feels (e.g., "It makes sense that you're angry," "I understand that you are having a tough time right now") (for self, "I have a right to feel sad").

5. Show tolerance! Look for how the feelings, thoughts, and actions make sense, given the other person's (or your) history and current situation, even if you don't approve of the behaviors, emotions, or actions themselves.

6. Respond in a way that shows you are taking the other person seriously (with or without words). If someone is crying, give a tissue or a hug. If someone is presenting a problem, start problem solving immediately (unless the person wishes merely to be heard).

How can we validate **ourselves**?

Use Steps 3, 4, and 5.

Examples of validation of others _____

_____

Examples of self-validation _____

_____

Practice Exercise 2

Self-Validation and Validation of Others

List <u>one</u> self-invalidating statement and <u>two</u> self-validating statements:

1. _____

2. _____

3. _____

List <u>one</u> invalidating statement to others and <u>two</u> validating statements to others:

1. _____

2. _____

3. _____

Choose a situation during the week in which you used validation skills with someone else or yourself.

Situation: _____

_____

Who was the person you validated? _____

What *exactly* did you do or say to validate yourself or that person? _____

_____

What was the outcome? _____

_____

_____

How did you feel afterward? _____

_____

Would you say or do something differently next time? If so, what? _____

_____

_____

Behaviorism
What Is It?/Ways to Increase Behaviors

What Is Behaviorism?

Behaviorism is a set of strategies or principles used to *increase* behaviors we *do* want and *reduce* behaviors we *don't* want (in ourselves and others).

Are there behaviors you would like to change in yourself or other people? If so, what are some of these? _____

Ways to Increase Behaviors

- **Reinforcers:** *Consequences* that result in more of a behavior. Reinforcers provide information to a person about what you want that person to do. Remember: Timing is very important, and you should choose motivating reinforcers!

  Examples: _____

  - **Positive reinforcement:** *Increases* the frequency of a behavior by providing a *rewarding* consequence (e.g., praise, a compliment, or an A on an exam).

  - **Negative reinforcement:** *Increases* the frequency of a behavior by removing a *negative* consequence. Examples of negative reinforcement include taking aspirin to get rid of a headache, doing homework to get Mom to stop nagging, or self-cutting to decrease or avoid negative feelings (although you are learning skills to manage this better).

  #### Negative reinforcer = RELIEF

  - **Self-reinforcement:** Don't forget to reinforce yourself as well as others!

- **Shaping:** Reinforcing small steps that lead toward the ultimate goal. (For example, If a teenager is anxious about going to school and doesn't usually go, she might be encouraged to go for 1 hour on Monday, 2 hours on Tuesday, and so on until she is able to stay for a whole day, ultimately leading up to staying every day all week long.) Reinforce each step!

Behaviorism
Ways to Decrease or Stop Behaviors

- **Extinction:** Reducing the likelihood of a behavior because reinforcement is not given. For example, you ignore the unwanted behavior when attention to it will cause it to continue to happen. However, make sure you reinforce other, adaptive behaviors in the process.
  - If a little boy begins to throw a tantrum in the supermarket because he doesn't get what he wants, and the parent ignores it, he will eventually (over time) stop having tantrums.
  - Remember: Extinguishing a behavior that has been reinforced in the past may cause a "behavioral burst" (a temporary increase) of the very behavior you are trying to extinguish. *Don't give up* because of this! Also, don't forget to orient the person that you are beginning to extinguish the behavior. And remember to reinforce other adaptive behaviors during the extinction process.

- **Punishment:** *Consequence* that results in a *decrease* in behavior. It tells another person what you don't want the person to do.
  - **Effective punishment:**
    - Actions used to *decrease* behaviors that don't have natural consequences. These actions should be specific and time-limited, and the punishment should fit the "crime" (e.g., if you're out past curfew, you lose the chance to go out the next day).
    - Natural consequences (e.g., if you stay up all night, you will be too tired to focus in school, may fail a test, and may get in trouble for failing).
  - **Ineffective punishment:** Actions used to *decrease* behaviors that are not specific, time-limited, or appropriate for the crime (e.g., you break curfew and your parents forbid you to leave the house for 2 months, take away your cell phone, and remind you of the mistake constantly).

Remember:
- Punishment does not teach new behavior.
- Punishment may lead to self-punishment.

Practice Exercise 3

Behaviorism: Positive Reinforcement

Look for opportunities (since they are occurring all the time) to provide positive reinforcement to yourself or someone else.

1. In advance, identify the behavior you want to increase and the reinforcer you will use.

   a. For yourself:
      Behavior: _____
      Reinforcer: _____

   b. Someone else: _____
      Behavior: _____
      Reinforcer: _____

2. Describe the situation(s) when you used positive reinforcement.

   a. For yourself: _____

   b. Someone else: _____

3. What was the outcome? What did you observe?

   a. For yourself: _____
      _____
      _____
      _____

   b. Someone else: _____
      _____
      _____
      _____

References

Adams, D. A., Overholser, J. C., & Lehnert, K. L. (1994). Perceived family functioning and adolescent suicidal behavior. *Journal of the American Academy of Child and Adolescent Psychiatry, 33,* 498–507.

Agerbo, E., Nordentoft, M., & Mortensen, P. B. (2002). Familial, psychiatric, and socioeconomic risk factors for suicide in young people: Nested case–control study. *British Medical Journal, 325,* 74–77.

Aitken, R. (2003). *The morning star: New and selected zen writings.* Emeryville, CA: Shoemaker, & Hoard.

Allard, R., Marshall, M., & Plante, M. C. (1992). Intensive follow-up does not decrease the risk of repeat suicide attempts. *Suicide and Life-Threatening Behavior, 22,* 303–314.

Ambrosini, J. (2000). Historical development and present status of the Schedule for Affective Disorders and Schizophrenia for School-Age Children (K-SADS). *Journal of the American Academy of Child and Adolescent Psychiatry, 39,* 49–58.

American Association of Suicidology. (2003). *Suicide in the U.S.A.: Based on current (2003) statistics.* Retrieved from www.suicidology.org/associations/1045/files/SuicideInTheUS.pdf

American Psychiatric Association (APA). (2000). *Diagnostic and statistical manual of mental disorders* (4th ed., text rev.). Washington, DC: Author.

American Psychiatric Association (APA). (2001). *Practice guidelines for the treatment of patients with borderline personality disorder.* Washington, DC: Author.

Anderson, R. N. (2002). Deaths: Leading causes for 2000. *National Vital Statistics Reports, 50*(16) [Electronic version]. Retrieved from www.cdc.gov/nchs/data/nvsr/nvsr50/nvsr50_16.pdf

Andrews, J. A., & Lewinsohn, P. M. (1992). Suicidal attempts among older adolescents: *Academy of Child and Adolescent Psychiatry, 31,* 655–662.

Appleby, L., Shaw, J., Amos, T., McDonnell, R., Harris, C., McKann, K. et al. (1999). Suicide within 12 months of contact with mental health services: National clinical survey. *British Medical Journal, 318,* 1235–1239.

Apter, A., Bleich, A., Plutchik, R., Mendelsohn, S., & Tyano, S. (1988). Suicidal behavior, depression, and conduct disorder in hospitalized adolescents. *Journal of the American Academy of Child and Adolescent Psychiatry, 27,* 696–699.

Apter, A., Gothelf, D., Orbach, I., Weizman, R., Ratzoni, G., Har-even, D., et al. (1995). Correlation of suicidal and violent behavior in different diagnostic categories in hospitalized adolescent patients. *Journal of the American Academy of Child and Adolescent Psychiatry, 34,* 912–918.

Arnett, J. J. (1999). Adolescent storm and stress, reconsidered. *American Psychologist, 54,* 317–326.

Azerrad, M. (2004, January 4). Punk's earnest new mission. *The New York Times,* Arts, p. 1.

Baldessarini, R. J., & Jamison, K. R. (1999). Effects of medical interventions of suicidal behavior. *Journal of Clinical Psychiatry, 60*(Suppl. 2), 117–122.

Barenboim, C. (1977). Developmental changes in the interpersonal cognitive system from middle childhood to adolescence. *Child Development, 48,* 1467–1474.

Bateman, A., & Fonagy, P. (1999). Effectiveness of partial hospitalization in the treatment of borderline personality disorder: A randomized controlled trial. *American Journal of Psychiatry, 156,* 1563–1569.

Baumrind, D. (1991a). The influence of parenting style on adolescent competence and substance use. *Journal of Early Adolescence, 11,* 56–95.

Baumrind, D. (1991b). Parenting styles and adolescent development. In R. Lerner, A. C. Petersen, & J. Brooks-Gunn (Eds.), *Encyclopedia of adolescence.* New York: Garland.

Beasley, C. M., Dornseif, B. E., Bosomworth, J. C., Sayler, M. E., Rampey, A. H., Heiligenstein, J. H., et al. (1992). Fluoxetine and suicide: A meta-analysis of controlled trials of treatment for depression. *International Clinical Psychopharmacology, 6,* 35–57.

Beasley, C. M., Sayler, M. E., Bosomworth, J. C., & Wernicke, J. F. (1991). High-dose fluoxetine: Efficacy and activating–sedating effects in agitated and retarded depression. *Journal of Clinical Psychopharmacology, 11,* 166–174.

Beautrais, A. L. (2001). Child and young adolescent suicide in New Zealand. *Australian and New Zealand Journal of Psychiatry, 35,* 647–653.

Beautrais, A. L., Joyce, P. R., & Mulder, R. T. (1996). Risk factors for serious suicide attempts among youth aged 13 through 24 years. *Journal of the American Academy of Child and Adolescent Psychiatry, 35,* 1174–1182.

Beck, A. T., Freeman, A., Davis, D. D., & Associates. (2003). *Cognitive therapy of personality disorders* (2nd ed.). New York: Guilford Press.

Beck, A. T., Herman, I., & Schuyler, D. (1974). Development of suicidal intent scales. In A. T. Beck, H. L. P. Resnik, & D. Lettieri (Eds.), *The prediction of suicide* (pp. 45–56), Bowie, MD: Charles Press.

Beck, A. T., Rush, A. J., Shaw, B. F., & Emery, G. (1979). *Cognitive therapy of depression.* New York: Guilford Press.

Beck, A. T., Steer, R. A., & Brown, G. K. (1996). *Beck Depression Inventory–II.* San Antonio, TX: Psychological Corporation.

Beck, A. T., Steer, R. A., & Ranieri, W. F. (1988). Scale for Suicide Ideation: Psychometric properties of a self-report version. *Journal of Clinical Psychology, 44(4),* 499–505.

Behavioral Tech. (2002). Retrieved from www.behavioraltech.com

Behavioral Tech (Producer). (2004). *The wise movement* [Recorded by Mind & South] [CD]. Seattle, WA: Producer.

Berk, L. E. (2004). *Infants, children and adolescents* (5th ed.). Boston: Allyn & Bacon.

Berman, A. L., & Jobes, D. A. (1991). *Adolescent suicide: Assessment and intervention.* Washington, DC: American Psychological Association.

Berman, A. L., Jobes, D.A., & Silverman, M.M. (2006). *Adolescent suicide: Assessment and intervention* (2nd ed.). Washington, DC: American Psychological Association.

Berman, A. L., & Schwartz, R. (1990). Suicide attempts among adolescent drug users. *American Journal of Diseases of Children, 144,* 310–314.

Bernstein, D. P., Cohen, P., Velez, C. N., Schwab-Stone, M., Siever, L. J., & Shinsato, L. (1993). Prevalence and stability of the DSM-III-R personality disorders in a community-based survey of adolescents. *American Journal of Psychiatry, 150,* 1237–1243.

Bille-Brahe, U., Kerkhor, A., DeLeo, D., & Schmidtke, A. (2004). Definitions and terminology used in the WHO/EURO Multicentre Study. In A. Schmidtke, D. Wasserman, U. Bille-Brahe, & W. Rutz (Eds.), *Suicidal behaviour in Europe: Results from the WHO/EURO Multicentre Study on Suicidal Behaviour* (pp. 11–14). Cambridge, MA: Hogrefe & Huber.

Birmaher, B., Brent, D. A., Kolko, D., Baugher, M., Bridge, J., Holder, D., et al. (2000). Clinical outcome after short-term psychotherapy for adolescents with major depressive disorder. *Archives of General Psychiatry, 57,* 29–36.

Blake, S. M., Ledsky, R., Lehman, T., Goodenow, C., Sawyer, R., & Hack, T. (2001). Preventing sexual risk behaviors among gay, lesbian, and bisexual adolescents: The benefits of gay-sensitive HIV instruction in schools. *American Journal of Public Health, 91(6),* 940–946.

Blumenthal, S. J., & Kupfer, D. J. (1986). Generalizable treatment strategies for suicidal behavior. *Annals of the New York Academy of Sciences, 487,* 327–340.

Boergers, J., Spirito, A., & Donaldson, D. (1998). Reasons for adolescent suicide attempts: Associations with psychological functioning. *Journal of the American Academy of Child and Adolescent Psychiatry, 37*(12), 1287–1293.

Bradley, R., Jenei, J., & Westen, D. (2005). Etiology of borderline personality disorder: Disentangling the contributions of intercorrelated antecedents. *Journal of Nervous and Mental Disease, 193*(1), 24–31.

Brady, E. U., & Kendall, P. C. (1992). Comorbidity of anxiety and depression in children and adolescents. *Psychological Bulletin, 111*, 244–255.

Brent, D.A. (1999). *Age, sex, and adolescent suicide*. Unpublished manuscript.

Brent, D. A., Bridge, J., Johnson, B. A., & Connolly, J. (1996a). Suicidal behavior runs in families: A controlled family study of adolescent suicide victims. *Archives of General Psychiatry, 53*(12), 1145–1152.

Brent, D. A., Baugher, M., Bridge, J., Chen, T., & Chiappetta, L. (1999a). Age- and sex-related risk factors for adolescent suicide. *Journal of the American Academy of Child and Adolescent Psychiatry, 38*, 1497–1505.

Brent, D. A., Johnson, B., Bartle, S., Bridge, J., Rather, C., Matta, J., et al (1993a). Personality disorder, tendency to impulsive violence, and suicidal behavior in adolescents. *Journal of the American Academy of Child and Adolescent Psychiatry, 32*, 69–75.

Brent, D. A., Johnson, B. A., Perper, J. A., Connolly, J., Bridge, J., Bartle, S., et al. (1994). Personality disorder, personality traits, impulsive violence, and completed suicide in adolescents. *Journal of the American Academy of Child and Adolescent Psychiatry, 33*, 1080–1086.

Brent, D. A., Kerr, M. M., Goldstein, C., Bozigar, J., Wartella, M. E., & Allan, M. J. (1989). An outbreak of suicide and suicidal behavior in high school. *Journal of the American Academy of Child and Adolescent Psychiatry, 28*, 918–924.

Brent, D. A., Kolko, D. J., Birmaher, B., Baugher, M., & Bridge, J. (1999b). A clinical trial for adolescent depression: Predictors of additional treatment in the acute and follow-up phases of the trial. *Journal of the American Academy of Child and Adolescent Psychiatry, 38*, 263–271.

Brent, D. A., Moritz, G., Bridge, J., Perper, J., & Canobbio, R. (1996b). The impact of adolescent suicide on siblings and parents: A longitudinal follow-up. *Suicide and Life-Threatening Behavior, 26*(3), 253–259.

Brent, D. A., Perper, J. A., & Allman, C. J. (1987). Alcohol, firearms, and suicide among youth. *Journal of the American Medical Association, 257*, 3369–3372.

Brent, D. A., Perper, J. A., Allman, C. J., Moritz, G. M., Wartella, M. E., & Zelenak, J. P. (1991). The presence and accessibility of firearms in the homes of adolescent suicides. *Journal of the American Medical Association, 266*, 2989–2995.

Brent, D. A., Perper, J. A., Goldstein, C. E., Kolko, D. J., Allan, M. J., Allman, C. J., et al. (1988). Risk factors for adolescent suicide: A comparison of adolescent suicide victims with suicidal inpatients. *Archives of General Psychiatry, 445*, 581–588.

Brent, D. A., Perper, J. A., Moritz, G., Allman, C., Friend, A., Roth, C., et al. (1993b). Psychiatric risk factors for adolescent suicide: A case–control study. *Journal of the American Academy of Child and Adolescent Psychiatry, 35*, 521–529.

Brent, D. A., Perper, J. A., Moritz, G., Baugher, M., Schweers, J., & Roth, C. (1993c). Stressful life events, psychopathology, and adolescent suicide: A case–control study. *Suicide and Life-Threatening Behavior, 23*, 179–187.

Bridge, J. A., Brent, D. A., Johnson, B. A., & Connolly, J. (1997). Familial aggregation of psychiatric disorders in a community sample of adolescents. *Journal of the American Academy of Child and Adolescent Psychiatry, 36*(5), 628–636.

Brooks-Gunn, J., & Petersen, A. C. (1991). Studying the emergence of depression and depressive symptoms during adolescence. *Journal of Youth and Adolescence, 20*, 115–119.

Brown, B. B. (1990). Peer groups. In S. Feldman & G. Elliot (Eds.), *At the threshold: The developing adolescent* (pp. 171–196). Cambridge, UK: Cambridge University Press.

Brown, G. K., Have, T. T., Henriques, G. R., Xie, S. X., Hollander, J. E., & Beck, A. T. (2005). Cognitive therapy for the prevention of suicide attempts: A randomized controlled trial. *Journal of the American Medical Association, 294*, 563–570.

Brown, M., & Linehan, M. M. (1996, November). *The relationship of negative emotions and parasuicidal behavior in borderline personality disorder.* Poster presented at the meeting of the Association for Advancement of Behavior Therapy, New York, NY.

Brown, M. Z., Comtois, K. A., & Linehan, M. M. (2002). Reasons for suicide attempts and nonsuicidal self-injury in women with borderline personality disorder. *Journal of Abnormal Psychology, 111*(1), 198–202.

Buchanan, C. M., Eccles, J. S., & Becker, J. B. (1992). Are adolescents the victims of raging hormones?: Evidence for activational effects of hormones on moods and behavior at adolescence. *Psychological Bulletin, 111,* 62–107.

Buchholtz-Hansen, P. E., Wang, A. G., & Kragh-Sorensen, P. (1993). Mortality in major affective disorder: Relationship to subtype of depression. *Acta Psychiatrica Scandinavica, 87,* 329–335.

Bukstein, O. G., Brent, D. A., Perper, J. A., Moritz, G., Baugher, M., Schweers, J., et al. (1993). Risk factors for completed suicide among adolescents with a lifetime history of substance abuse: A case–control study. *Acta Psychiatrica Scandinavica, 88*(6), 403–408.

Bukstein, O. G., Glancy, L. J., & Kaminer, Y. (1992). Patterns of affective comorbidity in a clinical population of dually diagnosed substance abusers. *Journal of the American Academy of Child and Adolescent Psychiatry, 6,* 1041–1045.

Burns, D. D. (1989). *The feeling good handbook: Using the new mood therapy in everyday life.* New York: HarperCollins.

Campbell, N. B., Milling, L., Laughlin, A., & Bush, E. (1993). The psychosocial climate of families with suicidal, pre-adolescent children. *American Journal of Orthopsychiatry, 63,* 142–145.

Canetto, S. S. (1997a). Meanings of gender and suicidal behavior during adolescence. *Suicide and Life-Threatening Behavior, 27,* 339–351.

Canetto, S. S. (1997b). Gender and suicidal behavior: Theories and evidence. In R. W. Maris, M. M. Silverman, & S. S. Canetto (Eds.), *Review of suicidology, 1997* (pp. 138–167). New York: Guilford Press.

Cedereke, M., Monti, K., & Öjehagen, A. (2002). Telephone contact with patients in the year after a suicide attempt: Does it affect treatment attendance and outcome? A randomised controlled study. *European Psychiatry, 17*(2), 82–91.

Centers for Disease Control (CDC). (1988). Recommendations for a community plan for the prevention and containment of suicide clusters. *Morbidity and Mortality Weekly Report, 37,* 1–11.

Centers for Disease Control (CDC. (1992). Physical fighting among high school students—United States, 1990. *Morbidity and Mortality Weekly Report, 41,* 91.

Centers for Disease Control and Prevention (CDC). (1995, March 24). Youth Risk Behavior Surveillance—United States, 1993. *Morbidity and Mortality Weekly Report, 44* (SS-1).

Centers for Disease Control and Prevention (CDC). (2004). Youth Risk Behavior Surveillance—United States, 2003. *Morbidity and Mortality Weekly Report, 53*(SS-2), 1–96.

Chanen, A. M., Jackson, H. J., McGorry, P. D., Allot, K. A., Clarkson, V., & Yuen, H. P. (2004). Two-year stability of personality disorder in older adolescent outpatients. *Journal of Personality Disorders, 18*(6), 526–541.

Chowdhury, N., Hicks, R. C., & Kreitman, N. (1973). Evaluation of an after-care service for parasuicide (attempted suicide) patients. *Social Psychiatry, 8,* 67–81.

Cialdini, R. B., Vincent, J. E., Lewis, S. K., Catalan, J., Wheeler, D., & Darby, B. L. (1975). Reciprocal concessions procedure for inducing compliance: The door-in-the-face technique. *Journal of Personality and Social Psychology, 31,* 206–215.

Clarkin, J. F., Friedman, R. C., Hurt, S. W., Corn, R., & Aronoff, M. (1984). Affective and character pathology of suicidal adolescent and young adult inpatients. *Journal of Clinical Psychiatry, 45,* 19–22.

Clarkin, J. F., Glick, I. D., Haas, G. L., Spencer, J. H., Lewis, A. B., Peyser, J., et al. (1990). A randomized clinical trial of inpatient family intervention: V. Results for affective disorders. *Journal of Affective Disorders, 18,* 17–28.

Conners, C. K., Sitarenios, G., Parker, J. D., & Epstein, J. N. (1998a). The revised Conners Parent Rating Scale (CPRS-R): Factor structure, reliability, and criterion validity. *Journal of Abnormal Child Psychology, 26,* 257–268.

Conners, C. K., Sitarenios, G., Parker, J. D., & Epstein, J. N. (1998b). Revision and restandardization of the Conners Teacher Rating Scale (CTRS-R): Factor structure, reliability, and criterion validity. *Journal of Abnormal Child Psychology, 26*, 279–291.

Cooper, J., Kapur, N., Webb, R., Lawlor, M., Guthrie, E. Mackway-Jones, K., & Appleby, L. (2005). Suicide after deliberate self-harm: A 4–year cohort study. *American Journal of Psychiatry, 162*, 297–303.

Cote, T. R., Biggar, R. J., & Dannenberg, A. L. (1992). Risk of suicide among persons with AIDS: A national assessment. *Journal of the American Medical Association, 268*, 2066–2068.

Cotgrove, A. J., Zirinsky, L., Black, D., & Weston, D. (1995). Secondary prevention of attempted suicide in adolescence. *Journal of Adolescence, 18*, 569–577.

Cowmeadow, P. (1995). Very brief psychotherapeutic interventions with deliberate self-harmers. In A. Ryle (Ed.), *Cognitive analytic therapy: Developments in theory and practice* (pp. 55–66). Chichester, UK: John Wiley.

Crawford, T. N., Cohen, P., & Brook, J. S. (2001). Dramatic–erratic personality disorder symptoms: I. Continuity from early adolescence into adulthood. *Journal of Personality Disorders, 15*, 319–335.

Crumley, F. E. (1979). Adolescent suicide attempts. *Journal of the American Medical Association, 241*, 2404–2407.

Csikszentmihalyi, M., & Larson, R. (1984). *Being adolescent.* New York: Basic Books.

Cummings, E. M., & Davies, P. (1994). *Children and marital conflict: The impact of family dispute and resolution.* New York: Guilford Press.

Dannenberg, A. L., McNeil, J. G., Brundage, J. F., & Brookmeyer, R. (1996). Mortality follow-up of 4147 HIV-seropositive military applicants. *Journal of the American Medical Association, 276*, 1743–1746.

Delate, T., Gelenberg, A. J., Simmons, V. A., & Motheral, B. R. (2004). Trends in the use of antidepressants in a national sample of commercially insured pediatric patients, 1998 to 2002. *Psychiatric Services, 55*, 387–391.

DeKovic, M., & Janssens, J. (1992). Parents' child-rearing style and child's sociometric status. *Developmental Psychology, 28*, 925–932.

Derogatis, L. R. (1994). Symptom Checklist-90—Revised *(SCL-90-R): Administration, scoring and procedures manual* (3rd ed.). Minneapolis, MN: National Computer Systems.

DeRosa, R., Habib, M., Pelcovitz, D., Rathus, J. H., Sonnenklar, J., Ford, J., et al. (2006). *Structured psychotherapy for adolescents responding to chronic trauma (SPARCS): A trauma focused guide.* Manhasset, NY: North Shore University Hospital.

Dishion, T. J., McCord, J., & Poulin, F. (1999). When interventions harm: Peer groups and problem behavior. *American Psychologist, 54*(9), 755–764.

Donaldson, D., Spirito, A., & Esposito-Smythers, C. (2005). Treatment for adolescents following a suicide attempt: Results of a pilot trial. *Journal of the American Academy of Child and Adolescent Psychiatry, 44*(2), 113–120.

Downey, J. I. (1994). Sexual orientation issues in adolescent girls. *Women's Health Issues, 4*, 117–121.

Dumas, J. E., & La Freniere, P. J. (1993). Mother-child relationships as sources of support or stress: A comparison of competent, average, aggressive, and anxious dyads. *Child Development, 64*, 1732–1754.

Eccles, J. S., Midgley, C., Wigfield, A., Buchanan, C. M., Reuman, D., Flanagan, C., et al. (1993). Development during adolescence: The impact of stage–environment fit on young adolescents' experiences in schools and in families. *American Psychologist, 48*, 90–101.

Eddleston, M., & Phillips, M. R. (2004). Self-poisoning with pesticides. *British Medical Journal, 328*, 42–44.

Elkind, D. (1984). *All grown up and no place to go: Teenagers in crisis.* Reading, MA: Addison-Wesley.

Ellis, A. (1962). *Reason and emotion in psychotherapy.* New York: Lyle Stuart.

Ellis, A. (1973). *Humanistic psychotherapy: The rational–emotive approach.* New York: Julian Press.

Essau, C., & Dobson, K. (1999). Epidemiology of depressive disorders. In C. Essau & F. Petermann (Eds.), *Depressive disorders in children and adolescents: Epidemiology, course and treatment* (pp. 69–103). Northvale, NJ: Aronson.

Epstein, N. B., Baldwin, L. M., & Bishop, D. S. (1983). The McMaster Family Assessment Device. *Journal of Marital and Family Therapy, 9,* 171–180.

Erikson, E. H. (1968). *Identity, Youth, and Crisis.* New York: Norton.

Evans, M. O., Morgan, H. G., Hayward, A., & Gunnell, D. J. (1999). Crisis telephone consultation for deliberate self-harm patients: Effects on repetition. *British Journal of Psychiatry, 175,* 23–27.

Farberow, N. L., & Shneidman, E. S. (1961). *The cry for help.* New York: McGraw-Hill.

Farmer, R. D. (1988). Assessing the epidemiology of suicide and parasuicide. *British Journal of Psychiatry, 153,* 16–20.

Favazza, A. (1998). The coming of age of self-mutilation. *Journal of Nervous and Mental Disease, 186*(5), 259–268.

Favazza, A., & Rosenthal, R. (1990). Varieties of pathological self-mutilation. *Behavioral Neurology, 3,* 77–85.

Fawcett, J. (1990). Targeting treatment in patients with mixed symptoms of anxiety and depression. *Journal of Clinical Psychiatry, 51,* 40–43.

Fawcett, J. (1997). Suicide: The consequences of anxiety in clinical depression. *Primary Psychiatry, 4,* 35–42.

Feindler, E. L., Rathus, J. H., & Silver, L. B. (2003). *Assessment of family violence: A handbook for researchers and practitioners.* Washington, DC: American Psychiatric Association.

Fergusson, D. M., Horwood, L. J., & Lynskey, M. T. (1996). Childhood sexual abuse and psychiatric disorder in young adulthood, II: Psychiatric outcomes of childhood sexual abuse. *Journal of the American Academy of Child and Adolescent Psychiatry, 35,* 1365–1374.

Fergusson, D. M., & Lynskey, M. T. (1995). Suicide attempts and suicidal ideation in a birth cohort of 16-year-old New Zealanders. *Journal of the American Academy of Child and Adolescent Psychiatry, 34,* 1308–1317.

Fergusson, D. M., Woodward, L. J., & Horwood, L. J. (2000). Risk factors and life processes associated with the onset of suicidal behaviour during adolescence and early adulthood. *Psychological Medicine 30,* 23–39.

First, M. B., Gibbon, M., Spitzer, R. L., Williams, J. B. W., & Benjamin, L. S. (1997). User's guide for the *Structured Clinical Interview for DSM-IV Axis II Personality Disorders (SCID-II).* Washington, DC: American Psychiatric Press.

Foa, E. B., Johnson, K. M., Feeny, N. C., & Treadwell, K. R. H. (2001). The Child PTSD Symptom Scale: A preliminary examination of its psychometric properties. *Journal of Clinical Child Psychology, 30*(3), 376–384.

Foa, E. B., & Kozak, M. J. (1986). Emotional processing of fear: Exposure to corrective information. *Psychological Bulletin, 99,* 20–35.

Foa, E. B., Steketee, G., & Grayson, J. B. (1985). Imaginal and *in vivo* exposure: A comparison with obsessive–compulsive checkers. *Behavior Therapy, 16*(3), 292–302.

Fossati, A., Madeddu, F., & Maffei, C. (1999). Borderline personality and childhood sexual abuse: A meta-analytic study. *Journal of Personality Disorders, 13,* 268–280.

Frances, A., & Blumenthal, S. J. (1989). Personality as a predictor of youth suicide. In L. Davidson & M. Linnoila (Eds.), *Report of the Secretary's Task Force on Youth Suicide: Vol. 2. Risk factors for youth suicide* (pp. 160–171). Rockville, MD: U.S. Department of Health and Human Services.

Freedman, J. L., & Fraser, S. C. (1966). Compliance without pressure: The foot-in-the-door technique. *Journal of Personality and Social Psychology, 57,* 212–228.

Friedman, R. C., Clarkin, J. F., Corn, R., Aronoff, M. S., Hurt, S. W., & Murphy, M. C. (1982). DSM-III and affective pathology in hospitalized adolescents. *Journal of Nervous and Mental Disease, 170,* 511–521.

Galambos, N. L., & Almeida, D. M. (1992). Does parent–adolescent conflict increase in early adolescence? *Journal of Marriage and the Family, 54,* 737–747.

Garber, J., Little, S., Hilsman, R., & Weaver, K. R. (1998). Family predictors of suicidal symptoms in youth adolescents. *Journal of Adolescence, 21*(4), 445–447.

Garfinkel, B. D., Froese, A., & Hood, J. (1982). Suicide attempts in children and adolescents. American Journal of Psychiatry, *138,* 35–40.

Garner, D. M. (1993). Pathogenesis of anorexia nervosa. *Lancet, 341,* 1631–1635.

Garofalo, R., Wolf, R. C., Wissow, L. S., Woods, E. R., & Goodman, E. (1999). Sexual orientation and risk of suicide attempts among a representative sample of youth. *Archives of Pediatrics and Adolescent Medicine, 153,* 487–493.

Giaconia, R. M., Reinherz, H. Z., Silverman, A. B., Pakiz, B., Frost, A. K., & Cohen, E. (1995). Traumas and post-traumatic stress disorder in a community population of older adolescents. *Journal of the American Academy of Child and Adolescent Psychiatry, 34,* 1369–1380.

Gibbons, J. S., Butler, J., Urwin, P., & Gibbons, J. L. (1978). Evaluation of a social work service for self-poisoning patients. *British Journal of Psychiatry, 133,* 111–118.

Goldberg, C. (1980). The utilization and limitations of paradoxical intervention in group psychotherapy. *International Journal of Group Psychotherapy, 30,* 287–297.

Goldston, D. B., Daniel, S. S., Reboussin, D. M., Reboussin, B. A., Frazier, P. H., & Kelley, A. E. (1999). Suicide attempts among formerly hospitalized adolescents: A prospective naturalistic study of risk during the first 5 years after discharge. *Journal of the American Academy of Child and Adolescent Psychiatry, 38,* 660–671.

Goodstein, J. L. (1982). Cognitive characteristics of suicide attempters. *Dissertation Abstracts International, 43*(05), 1613B. (UMI No. AAT8223846)

Gould, M. S. (2001). Suicide and the media. *Annals of the New York Academy of Sciences, 932,* 200–224.

Gould, M. S., Fisher, P., Parides, M., Flory, M., & Shaffer, D. (1996). Psychosocial risk factors of child and adolescent completed suicide. *Archives of General Psychiatry, 53,* 1155–1162.

Gould, M. S., Greenberg, T., Velting, D. M., & Shaffer, D. (2003). Youth suicide risk and preventive interventions: A review of the past 10 years. *Journal of the American Academy of Child and Adolescent Psychiatry, 42,* 386–405.

Gould, M. S., King, R., Greewald, S., Fisher, P., Schwabstone, M., Kramer, R., et al. (1998). Psychopathology associated with suicidal ideation and attempts among children and adolescents. *Journal of the American Academy of Child and Adolescent Psychiatry, 37,* 915–923.

Gould, M. S., Wallenstein, S., Kleinman, M., O'Carroll, P., & Mercy, J. (1990). Suicide clusters: An examination of age-specific effects. *American Journal of Public Health, 80,* 211–212.

Gratz, K. L. (2001). Measurement of deliberate self-harm: Preliminary data on the Deliberate Self-Harm Inventory. *Journal of Psychopathology and Behavioral Assessment, 23*(4), 253–263.

Gratz, K. L. (2003). Risk factors for and functions of deliberate self-harm: An empirical and conceptual review. *Clinical Psychology: Science and Practice, 10,* 192–205.

Grilo, C. M., Sanislow, C., Fehon, D. C., Marino, S., & McGlashan, T. H. (1999). Psychological and behavioral functioning in adolescent psychiatric inpatients who report histories of childhood abuse. *American Journal of Psychiatry, 156*(4), 538–543.

Groholt, B., Ekeberg, O., Wichstrom, L., & Haldorsen, T. (1998). Suicide among children and younger and older adolescents in Norway: A comparative study. *Journal of the American Academy of Child & Adolescent Psychiatry, 37*(5), 473–481.

Groholt, B., Ekeberg, O., Wichstrom, L., & Haldorsen, T. (2000). Young suicide attempters: A comparison between a clinical and an epidemiological sample. *Journal of the American Academy of Child and Adolescent Psychiatry, 39*(7), 868–875.

Grosz, D. E., Lipschitz, D. S., Eldar, S., Finkelstein, G., Blackwood, N., Gerbino-Rosen, G., et al. (1994). Correlates of violence risk in hospitalized adolescents. *Comprehensive Psychiatry, 35,* 296–300.

Grunbaum, J. A., Kann, L., Kinchen, S. A., Williams, B., Ross, J. G., Lowry, R., & Kolbe, L. (2002). Youth Risk Behavior Surveillance—United States, 2001. *Morbidity and Mortality Weekly Report, 51*(SS-4), 1–64.

Guthrie, E., Kapur, N., Mackway-Jones, K., Chew-Graham, C., Moorey, J., Mendel, E., Marino-Francis, F., Sanderson, S., Turpin, C., Boddy, G., & Tomenson, B. (2001). Randomised control trial of brief psychological intervention after deliberate self poisoning. *British Medical Journal, 323*(7305).

Halaby, K. S. (2004). Variables predicting noncompliance with short-term dialectical behavior therapy for suicidal and parasuicidal adolescents. *Dissertation Abstracts International, 65*(06), 3160B. (UMI No. AAI3135769)

Harkavy-Friedman, J. M., & Asnis, G. M. (1989). Assessment of suicidal behavior: A new instrument. *Psychiatric Annals, 19,* 382–387.

Harkavy-Friedman, J. M., Asnis, G. M., Boeck, M., & Difiore, J. (1987). Prevalence of specific suicidal behaviors in a high school sample. *American Journal of Psychiatry, 144,* 1203–1206.

Harrington, R., Kerfoot, M., Dyer, E., McNiven, R., Gill, J., Harrington, V., et al. (1998). Randomized trial of a home-based family intervention for children who have deliberately poisoned themselves. *Journal of the American Academy of Child and Adolescent Psychiatry, 37,* 512–518.

Harris, H. E., & Myers, W. C. (1997). Adolescents' misperception of the dangerousness of acetaminophen in overdose. *Suicide and Life-Threatening Behavior, 27,* 274–277.

Harry, J. (1989). Sexual identity issues. In L. Davidson & M. Linnoila (Eds.), *Report of the Secretary's Task Force on Youth Suicide: Vol. 2. Risk factors for youth suicide* (pp. 131–142). Rockville, MD: U.S. Department of Health and Human Services.

Harter, S. (1990). Issues in the assessment of the self-concept of children and adolescents. In A. La Greca (Ed.), *Through the eyes of a child* (pp. 292–325). Boston: Allyn & Bacon.

Hawton, K., Bancroft, J., Catalan, J., Kingston, B., Stedeford, A., & Welch, N. (1981). Domiciliary and out-patient treatment of self-poisoning patients by medical and non-medical staff. *Psychological Medicine, 11,* 169–177.

Hawton, K., & Catalan, J. (1982). *Attempted suicide.* Oxford, UK: Oxford Medical.

Hawton, K., & Fagg, J. (1992). Deliberate self-poisoning and self-injury in adolescents: A study of characteristics and trends in Oxford, 1976–89. *British Journal of Psychiatry, 161,* 816–823.

Hawton, K., Fagg, J., & McKeown, S. P. (1989). Alcoholism, alcohol and attempted suicide. *Alcohol and Alcoholism, 24,* 3–9.

Hawton, K., Harriss, L., Simkin, S., Bale, E., & Bond, A. (2004). Self-cutting: Patient characteristics compared with self-poisoners. *Suicide and Life-Threatening Behavior, 34*(3), 199–208.

Hawton, K., McKeown, S., Day, A., Martin, P., et al. (1987). Evaluation of out-patient counselling compared with general practitioner care following overdoses. *Psychological Medicine, 17*(3), 751–761.

Hawton, L., Arensman, E., Townsend, E., Bremner, S., Feldman, E., et al. (1998). Deliberate self-harm: Systematic review of efficacy of psychosocial and pharmacological treatments in preventing repetition. *British Medical Journal, 317,* 441–447.

Henggeler, S. W., Schoenwald, S. K., Rowland, M. D., & Cunningham, P. B. (2002). *Serious emotional disturbance in children and adolescents: Multisystemic therapy.* New York: Guilford Press.

Herpertz, S. (1995). Self-injurious behavior: Psychopathological and nosological characteristics in subtypes of self-injurers. *Acta Psychiatrica Scandinavica, 91,* 57–68.

Hoberman, H. M., & Garfinkel, B. D. (1988). Completed suicide in children and adolescents. *Journal of the American Academy of Child and Adolescent Psychiatry, 27,* 689–695.

Hoffman, P. (2004, November). *Family connections: A pilot study of the effectiveness of a family program for relatives of persons with borderline personality disorder.* Paper presented at the annual meeting of the International Society for Improvement of and Training in Dialectical Behavior Therapy, New Orleans, LA.

Holinger, P. C., Offer, D., Barter, J. T., & Bell, C. C. (1994). *Suicide and homicide among adolescents.* New York: Guilford Press.

Huey, S. J., Henggeler, S. W., Rowland, M. D., Halliday-Boykins, C. A., Cunningham, P. B., Pickrel, S. G., et al. (2004). Multisystemic therapy effects on attempted suicide by youths presenting psychiatric emergencies. *Journal of the American Academy of Child and Adolescent Psychiatry, 43,* 183–190.

Inamdar, S. C., Lewis, D. O., Siomopoulos, G., Shanok, S. S., & Lamela, M. (1982). Violent and suicidal behavior in psychotic adolescents. *American Journal of Psychiatry, 139,* 932–935.

Jacobson, C.M., Muehlenkamp, J.J., & Miller, A.L. (2006). *Psychiatric impairment and deliberate self-harm in a clinical sample of adolescents.* Manuscript submitted for publication.

Jacobson, N. S., & Christensen, A. (1996). *Integrative couple therapy: Promoting acceptance and change.* New York: Norton.

Johnson, B. A., Brent, D. A., Bridge, J., & Connally, J. (1998). The family aggregation of adolescent suicide attempts. *Acta Psychiatrica Scandinavia, 97*(1), 18–24.

Johnson, J. G., Cohen, P., Gould, M. S., Kasen, S., Brown, J., & Brook, J. S. (2002). Childhood adversities, interpersonal difficulties, and risk for suicide attempts during late adolescence and early adulthood. *Archives of General Psychiatry, 59,* 741–749.

Kahlbaugh, P., & Haviland, J. M. (1991). Formal operational thinking and identity. In R. M. Lerner, A. C. Petersen, & J. Brooks-Gunn (Eds.), *Encyclopedia of adolescence* (pp. 369–372). New York: Garland.

Kann, L., Kinchen, S. A., Williams, B. I., & Ross, J. G. (2000). Youth risk behavior surveillance—United States, 1999. *Journal of School Health, 70,* 271–285.

Kaplan, M. L., Asnis, G. M., Sanderson, W. C., Keswani, L., De Lecuona, J.M., & Joseph, S. (1994). Suicide assessment: Clinical interview versus self-report. *Journal of Clinical Psychology, 50,* 294–298.

Kasen, S., Cohen, P., Skodol, A. E., Johnson, G., & Brook, J. S. (1999). Influence of child and adolescent psychiatric disorders on young adult personality disorder. *American Journal of Psychiatry, 156,* 1529–1535.

Kashani, J. H., Goddard, P., & Reid, J. C. (1989). Correlates of suicidal ideation in a community sample of children and adolescents. *Journal of the American Academy of Child and Adolescent Psychiatry, 28,* 912–917.

Katz, L. Y., & Cox, B. J. (2002). Dialectical behavior therapy for suicidal adolescent inpatients: A case study. *Clinical Case Studies, 1,* 81–92.

Katz, L. Y., Gunasekara, S., Cox, B. J., & Miller, A. L. (2004). Feasibility of dialectical behavior therapy for parasuicidal adolescent inpatients. *Journal of the American Academy of Child and Adolescent Psychiatry, 43,* 276–282.

Kaufman, J., Birmaher, B., Brent, D., Rao, U., Flynn, C., Moreci, P., et al. (1997). Schedule for Affective Disorders and Schizophrenia for School-Aged Children—Present and Lifetime Version (K-SADS-PL): Initial reliability and validity data. *Journal of the American Academy of Child and Adolescent Psychiatry, 36,* 980–988.

Keitner, G. I., Ryan, C. E., Miller, I. W., Epstein, N. B., Bishop, D. S., & Norman, W. H. (1990). Family functioning, social adjustment, and recurrence of suicidality. *Psychiatry, 53,* 17–30.

Kendall, P. C., & Sugarman, A. (1997). Attrition in the treatment of childhood anxiety disorders. *Journal of Consulting and Clinical Psychology, 65(5),* 883–888.

Kernberg, O. F., Weiner, A. S., & Bardenstein, K. K. (2000). *Personality disorders in children and adolescents.* New York: Basic Books.

Kessler, R. C., Borges, G., & Walters, E. E. (1999). Prevalence of and risk factors for lifetime suicide attempts in the National Comorbidity Study. *Archives of General Psychiatry, 36,* 617–626.

Kienhorst, C. W. M., DeWilde, E. J., van den Bout, J., Diekstra, R. F. W., & Wolters, W. H. G. (1990). Characteristics of suicide attempters in a population-based sample of Dutch adolescents. *British Journal of Psychiatry, 156,* 243–248.

King, C. A. (1997). Suicidal behavior in adolescence. In E. W. Maris, M. W. Silverman, & S. S. Canetto (Eds.), *Review of suicidology, 1997* (pp. 61–95). New York: Guilford Press.

King, C. A., Segal, H., Kaminski, K., Naylor, M., Ghaziuddin, N., & Radpour, L. (1995). A prospective study of adolescent suicidal behavior following hospitalization. *Suicide and Life-Threatening Behavior, 25,* 327–338.

King, C. A., Segal, H., Naylor, M., & Evans, T. (1993). Family functioning and suicidal behavior in adolescent inpatients with mood disorders. *Journal of the American Academy of Child and Adolescent Psychiatry, 32,* 1198–1206.

Kizer, K. W., Green, M., Perkins, C. I., Coebbert, G., & Hughes, M. J. (1988). AIDS and suicide in California. *Journal of the American Medical Association, 260,* 1881.

Koerner, K., & Linehan, M. M. (1997). Case formulation in dialectical behavior therapy for borderline personality disorder. In T. Eells (Ed.), *Handbook of psychotherapy case formulation.* New York: Guilford Press.

Kohlberg, L. (1984). *Essays on moral development: Vol. 2. The psychology of moral development.* San Francisco: Harper & Row.

Koons, C. R., Robins, C. J., Tweed, J. L., Lynch, T. R., Gonzalez, A. M., Morse, J. Q., et al. (2001). Efficacy of dialectical behavior therapy in women veterans with borderline personality disorder. *Behavior Therapy, 32,* 371–390.

Kotila, L. (1992). The outcome of attempted suicide in adolescence. *Journal of Adolescent Health, 13,* 415–417.

Kovacs, M., Goldston, D., & Gatsonis, C. (1993). Suicidal behaviors and childhood-onset depressive disorders: A longitudinal investigation. *Journal of the American Academy of Child and Adolescent Psychiatry, 32,* 8–20.

Kreitman, N. (1977). *Parasuicide.* Chichester, UK: Wiley.

Kyokai, B. D. (1966). *The teachings of Buddha.* Tokyo: Bukkyo Dendo Kyokai.

La Greca, A. M., & Prinstein, M. J. (1999). Peer group. In W. K. Silverman & T. H. Ollendick (Eds.), *Developmental issues in the clinical treatment of children* (pp. 171–198). Needham Heights, MA: Allyn & Bacon.

Lapsley, D. K. (1991). Egocentrism theory and the "new look" at the imaginary audience and personal life fable in adolescence. In R. M. Lerner, A. C. Petersen, & J. Brooks-Gunn (Eds.), *Encyclopedia of adolescence* (pp. 281–286). New York: Garland.

Larson, R., & Ham, M. (1993). Stress and "storm and stress" in early adolescence: The relationship of negative events with dysphoric affect. *Developmental Psychology, 29,* 130–140.

Larson, R., & Richards, M. H. (1991). Daily companionship in late childhood and early adolescence: Changing developmental contexts. *Child Development, 2,* 284–300.

Larson, R., & Richards, M. H. (1994). *Divergent realities: The emotional lives of mothers, fathers, and adolescents.* New York: Basic Books.

Leon, A. C., Friedman, R. A., Sweeney, J. A., Brown, R. P., & Mann, J. J. (1990). Statistical issues in the identification of risk factors for suicidal behavior: The application of survival analysis. *Psychiatry Research, 31,* 99–108.

Lesage, A. D., Boyer, R., Grunberg, F., Vanier, C., Morissette, R., Menard-Buteau, C., & Loyer, M. (1994). Suicide and mental disorders: A case-control study of young men. *American Journal of Psychiatry, 151,* 1063–1068.

Levenson, M., & Neuringer, C. (1971). Problem-solving behavior in suicidal adolescents. *Journal of Consulting and Clinical Psychology, 37,* 433–436.

Levenson, M., & Neuringer, C. (1972). Phenomenal environmental oppressiveness in suicidal adolescents. *Journal of Genetic Psychology, 120,* 253–256.

Levy, K. N., Becker, D. F., Grilo, C. M., Mattanah, J. J. F., Garnet, K. E., Quinlan, D. M., et al. (1999). Concurrent and predictive validity of the personality disorder diagnosis in adolescent inpatients. *American Journal of Psychiatry, 156,* 1522–1528.

Lewinsohn, P. M., Rohde, P., & Seeley, J. R. (1994). Psychosocial risk factors for future adolescent suicide attempts. *Journal of Consulting and Clinical Psychology, 62,* 297–305.

Lewinsohn, P. M., Rohde, P., & Seeley, J. R. (1996). Adolescent suicidal ideation and attempts: Prevalence, risk factors, and clinical implications. *Clinical Psychology Science and Practice, 3,* 25–46.

Lewinsohn, P. M., Rohde, P., Seeley, J. R., & Baldwin, C. L. (2001). Gender differences in suicide attempts from adolescence to young adulthood. *Journal of the American Academy of Child and Adolescent Psychiatry, 40,* 427–434.

Lewinsohn, P. M., Rohde, P., Seeley, J. R., & Klein, D. N. (1997). Axis II psychopathology as a function of Axis I disorders in childhood and adolescence. *Journal of the American Academy of Child and Adolescent Psychiatry, 36,* 1752–1759.

Liberman, R. P., & Eckman, T. (1981). Behavior therapy versus insight-oriented therapy for repeated suicide attempters. *Archives of General Psychiatry, 38*(10), 1126–1130.

Lieb, K., Zanarini, M. C., Schmahl, C., Linehan, M. M., & Bohus, M. (2004). Seminar Section: Borderline Personality Disorder. *Lancet, 364,* 453–461.

Linehan, M. M. (1973). Suicide and attempted suicide: Study of perceived sex differences. *Perceptual and Motor Skills, 37,* 31–34.

Linehan, M. M. (1981). A social–behavioral analysis of suicide and parasuicide: Implications for clinical assessment and treatment. In H. Glaezer & J. F. Clarkin (Eds.), *Depression: Behavioral and directive intervention strategies* (pp. 229–294). New York: Garland.

Linehan, M. M. (1986). Suicidal people: One population or two? *Annals of the New York Academy of Sciences, 487,* 16–33.

Linehan, M. M. (1987a). Dialectical behavior therapy: A cognitive behavioral approach to parasuicide. *Journal of Personality Disorders, 1*, 328–333.

Linehan, M. M. (1987b). Dialectical behavior therapy for borderline personality disorder: Theory and method. *Bulletin of the Menninger Clinic, 51*, 261–276.

Linehan, M. M. (1989). Cognitive and behavior therapy for borderline personality disorder. In A. Tasman, R. E. Hales, & A. J. Frances (Eds.), *Review of psychiatry* (pp. 84–102). Washington, DC: American Psychiatric Press.

Linehan, M. M. (1993a). *Cognitive-behavioral treatment of borderline personality disorder.* New York: Guilford Press.

Linehan, M. M. (1993b). *Skills training manual for treating borderline personality disorder.* New York: Guilford Press.

Linehan, M. M. (1995). *Essential steps for targeting in-session dysfunctional behavior.* Unpublished manuscript, University of Washington, Seattle, WA.

Linehan, M. M. (1997). Validation and psychotherapy. In A. Bohart & L. Greenberg (Eds.), *Empathy reconsidered: New directions in psychotherapy* (pp. 353–392). Washington, DC: American Psychological Association.

Linehan, M. M. (1998). Dialectical behavior therapy. In J. Todd & A. C. Bohart (Eds.), *Foundations of clinical and counseling psychology* (3rd ed., pp. 298–299). Long Grove, IL: Waveland Press.

Linehan, M. M. (1999). Development, evaluation, and dissemination of effective psychosocial treatments: Levels of disorder, stages of care, and stages of treatment research. In M. D. Glantz & C. R. Hartel (Eds.), *Drug abuse: Origins and interventions* (pp. 367–394). Washington, DC: American Psychological Association.

Linehan, M. M. (2006). Foreword. In T. E. Ellis, (Ed.), *Cognition and suicide: Theory, research, and therapy* (pp. 757–766). Washington, DC: American Psychological Association.

Linehan, M. M., Armstrong, H. E., Suarez, A., Allmon, D., & Heard, H. L. (1991). Cognitive-behavioral treatment of chronically parasuicidal borderline patients. *Archives of General Psychiatry, 48*, 1060–1064.

Linehan, M. M., Camper, P., Chiles, J. A., Strosahl, K., & Shearin, E. (1987). Interpersonal problem solving and parasuicide. *Cognitive Therapy and Research, 11*, 1–12.

Linehan, M. M., Cochran, B. N., & Kehrer, C. A. (2001). Dialectical behavior therapy for borderline personality disorder. In D. H. Barlow (Ed.), *Clinical handbook of psychological disorders* (3rd ed., pp. 470–552). New York: Guilford Press.

Linehan, M. M., & Comtois, K. (1996). *Lifetime parasuicide history.* Unpublished manuscript, University of Washington.

Linehan, M. M., Comtois, K. A., Brown, M. Z., Heard, H. L., & Wagner, A. W. (2006a). *Suicide Attempt Self-Injury Interview (SASII): Development, reliability, and validity of a scale to assess suicide attempts and intentional self-injury.* Manuscript submitted for publication.

Linehan, M. M., Comtois, K. A., Murray, A. M., Brown, M. Z., Gallop, R. J., Heard, H. L., et al. (2006b). Two year randomized trial and follow-up of dialectical behavior therapy vs. therapy by experts for suicidal behaviors and borderline personality disorder. *Archives of General Psychiatry, 63*, 757–766.

Linehan, M. M., & Heard, H. (1999). Borderline personality disorder: Costs, course, and treatment outcomes. In N. Miller & K. Magruder (Eds.), *The cost-effectiveness of psychotherapy: A guide for practitioners, researchers and policy-makers* (pp. 291–305). New York: Oxford Press.

Linehan, M. M., Heard, H. L., & Armstrong, H. E. (1993a). Naturalistic follow-up of a behavioral treatment for chronically parasuicidal borderline patients. *Archives of General Psychiatry, 50*, 971–974.

Linehan, M. M., Heard, H. L., & Armstrong, H. E. (1993b). *Standard dialectical behavior therapy compared to psychotherapy in the community for chronically parasuicidal borderline patients.* Unpublished manuscript, University of Washington, Seattle, WA.

Linehan, M. M., Rizvi, S. L., Welch, S. S., & Page, B. (in press). Suicide and personality disorders. In K. Hawton & K. van Heeringen (Eds.), *International handbook of suicide and attempted suicide.* Chichester, UK: Wiley.

Linehan, M. M., & Shearin, E. N. (1988). Lethal stress: A social–behavioral model of suicidal behavior.

In S. Fisher & J. Reason (Eds.), *Handbook of life stress, cognition and health* (pp. 265–285). Chichester, UK: Wiley.

Lipschitz, D. S., Winegar, R. K., Nicolaou, A. L., Hartnick, E., Wolfson, M., & Southwick, S. M. (1999). Perceived abuse and neglect as risk factors for suicidal behavior in adolescent inpatients. *Journal of Nervous and Mental Disease, 187*(1), 32–39.

Lyketsos, C. G., & Federman, E. B. (1995). Psychiatric disorders and HIV infection: Impact on one another. *Epidemiology Review, 17,* 152–164.

Lynch, T. R., Chapman, A. L., Rosenthal, M. Z., Kuo, J. R., Linehan, M. M. (2006). Mechanisms of change in dialectical behavior therapy: Theoretical and empirical observations. *Journal of Clinical Psychology, 62,* 459–480.

Malone, K. M., Szanto, K., Corbitt, E. M., & Mann, J. J. (1995). Clinical assessment versus research methods in the assessment of suicidal behavior. *American Journal of Psychiatry, 152,* 1601–1607.

Mann, J. J., Waternauz, C., Haas, G. L., & Malone, K. M. (1999). Toward a clinical model of suicidal behavior in psychiatric patients. *American Journal of Psychiatry, 156*(2), 181–189.

Marlatt, G. A., & Donovan, D. M. (Eds.), (2005). *Relapse prevention: Maintenance strategies in the treatment of addictive behaviors* (2nd ed.). New York: Guilford Press.

Martin, G., & Waite, M. (1994). Parental bonding and vulnerability to adolescent suicide. *Acta Psychiatrica Scandinavica, 89,* 246–254.

Marton, P., Korenblum, M., Kutcher, S., Stein, B., Kennedy, B., & Pakes, J. (1989). Personality dysfunction in depressed adolescents. *Canadian Journal of Psychiatry, 34,* 810–813.

Marttunen, M. J., Aro, H. M., Henriksson, M. M., & Lönnqvist, J. K. (1991). Antisocial behavior in adolescent suicide. *Acta Psychiatrica Scandinavica, 89,* 167–173.

Marttunen, M. J., Aro, H. M., Henriksson, M. M., & Lönnqvist, J. K. (1994). Psychosocial stressors more common in adolescent suicides with alcohol abuse compared with depressive adolescent suicides. *Journal of the American Academy of Child and Adolescent Psychiatry, 33,* 490–497.

Marttunen, M. J., Aro, H. M., & Lönnqvist, J. K. (1992). Adolescent suicide: Endpoint of long-term difficulties. *Journal of the American Academy of Child and Adolescent Psychiatry, 31,* 649–654.

Marttunen, M. J., Aro, H. M., & Lönnqvist, J. K. (1993). Precipitant stressors in adolescent suicide. *Journal of the American Academy of Child and Adolescent Psychiatry, 32,* 1178–1183.

Marttunen, M. J., Henriksson, M. M., Aro, H. M., Heikkinen, M. E., Isometsa, E. T., & Lönnqvist, J. K. (1995). Suicide among female adolescents: Characteristics and comparison with males in the age group 13 to 22 years. *Journal of the American Academy of Child and Adolescent Psychiatry, 34,* 1297–1307.

Mazza, J. J. (2000). The relationship between posttraumatic stress symptomatology and suicidal behavior in school-based adolescents. *Suicide and Life-Threatening Behavior, 30,* 91–103.

McKegney, F. P., & O'Dowd, M. A. (1992). Suicidality and HIV status. *American Journal of Psychiatry, 149,* 396–398.

McKenry, P. C., Tishler, C. L., & Kelley, C. (1982). Adolescent suicide: A comparison of attempters and nonattempters in an emergency room population. *Clinical Pediatrics, 21*(5), 266–270.

McLeavey, B. C., Daly, R. J., Ludgate, J. W., & Murray, C. M. (1994). Interpersonal problem-solving skills training in the treatment of self-poisoning patients. *Suicide and Life-Threatening Behavior, 24*(4), 382–394.

McManus, M., Lerner, H., Robbins, D., & Barbour, C. (1984). Assessment of borderline symptomatology in hospitalized adolescents. *Journal of the American Academy of Child and Adolescent Psychiatry, 23,* 685–694.

Meltzer, H. Y., & Okayli, G. (1995). Reduction of suicidality during clozapine treatment of neuroleptic-resistant schizophrenia: Impact on risk-benefit assessment. *American Journal of Psychiatry, 152*(2), 183–190.

Middlebrook, D. L., LeMaster, P. L., Beals, J., Novins, D. K., & Manson, S. M. (2001). Suicide prevention in American Indian and Alaska Native communities: A critical review of programs. *Suicide and Life-Threatening Behavior, 31*(Suppl. 1), 132–149.

Miller, A. L., & Glinski, J. (2000). Youth suicidal behavior: Assessment and intervention. *Journal of Clinical Psychology, 56*(9), 1131–1152.

Miller, A. L., Glinski, J., Woodberry, K., Mitchell, A., & Indik, J. (2002). Family therapy and dialectical behavior therapy with adolescents: Part 1. Proposing a clinical synthesis. *American Journal of Psychotherapy, 56,* 568–584.

Miller, A. L., Muehlenkamp, J. J., & Jacobson, C. M. (2006). *A review of borderline personality disorder in adolescents.* Manuscript submitted for publication.

Miller, A. L., Nathan, J. S., & Wagner, E. E. (in press). Engaging suicidal multi-problem adolescents with DBT. In D. Castro-Blanco (Ed.), *Treatment engagement with high-risk adolescents: Empirically-based treatments.* Washington, DC: American Psychological Association.

Miller, A. L., & Rathus, J. H. (2000). Dialectical behavior therapy: Adaptations and new applications. *Cognitive and Behavioral Practice, 7,* 420–425.

Miller, A. L., Rathus, J. H., Dubose, T., Dexter-Mazza, E., & Goldklang, A. (in press). Adaptations and applications of DBT with adolescents. In L. A. Dimeff, K. Koerner, C. Sanderson, & M. Byars (Eds.), *Adaptations of dialectical behavior therapy.* New York: Guilford Press.

Miller, A. L., Rathus, J. H., & Linehan, M. M. (1999). *DBT with adolescents: Multi-family group skills training manual.* Unpublished treatment manual, Montefiore Medical Center/Albert Einstein College of Medicine, Bronx, NY.

Miller, A. L., Rathus, J. H., Linehan, M. M., Wetzler, S., & Leigh, E. (1997). Dialectical behavior therapy adapted for suicidal adolescents. *Journal of Practical Psychiatry and Behavioral Health, 3*(2), 78–86.

Miller, A. L., Wyman, S. E., Glassman, S. L., Huppert, J. D., & Rathus, J. H. (2000). Analysis of behavioral skills utilized by adolescents receiving dialectical behavior therapy. *Cognitive and Behavioral Practice, 7,* 183–187.

Miller, I. W., Epstein, N. B., Bishop, D. S., & Keitner, G. I. (1985). The McMaster Family Assessment Device: Reliability and validity. *Journal of Marital and Family Therapy, 11,* 345–356.

Miller, T. R., & Taylor, D. M. (2005). Adolescent suicidality: Who will ideate, who will act? *Suicide and Life-Threatening Behavior, 35*(4), 425–435.

Millon, T. (1987). On the genesis and prevalence of the borderline personality disorder: A social learning thesis. *Journal of Personality Disorders, 1,* 354–372.

Minino, A. M., Arias, E., Kochanek, K. D., Murphy, S. L., & Smith, B. L. (2002). Deaths: Final data for 2000. *National Vital Statistics Reports, 50*(15), p. 99.

Mintz, R. S. (1968). Psychotherapy of the suicidal patient. In H.L.P. Resnik (Ed.), *Suicidal behaviors: Diagnoses and management* (pp. 271–296). Boston: Little, Brown.

Möller, H-J. (1992). Attempted suicide: Efficacy of different aftercare strategies. *International Clinical Psychopharmacology, 6,* 58–69.

Morgan, H. G., Jones, E. M., & Owen, J. H. (1993). Secondary prevention of non-fatal deliberate self-harm: The green card study. *British Journal of Psychiatry, 163,* 111–112.

Motto, J. A. (1976). Suicide prevention for high-risk persons who refuse treatment. *Suicide and Life-Threatening Behavior, 6,* 223–230.

Motto, J. A. (1984). Suicide in male adolescents. In H. S. Sudak, A. B. Ford, & N. B. Rushforth (Eds.), *Suicide in the young* (pp. 227–244). Boston: John Wright–PSG.

Motto, J. A., & Bostrom, A. G. (2001). A randomized controlled trial of postcrisis suicide prevention. *Psychiatric Services, 52*(6), 828–833.

Muehlenkamp, J. J., & Gutierrez, P. M. (2004). An investigation of differences between self-injurious behavior and suicide attempts in a sample of adolescents. *Suicide and Life-Threatening Behavior, 34,* 12–23.

National Center for Health Statistics. (1996). Advance report of final mortality statistics, 1994. *NCHS Monthly Vital Statistics Report, 45,* 63.

National Clearinghouse on Child Abuse and Neglect Information. (2004, March). *Long-term consequences of child abuse and neglect.* Retrieved from http://nccanch.acf.hhs.gov/pubs/factsheets/long_term_consequences.cfm.

Nelson, S. H. & Grunebaum, H. (1971). A follow-up study of wrist slashers. *American Journal of Psychiatry, 127*(10), 1345–1349.

Neuringer, C. (1961). Dichotomous evaluations in suicidal individuals. *Journal of Consulting Psychology, 25,* 445–449.

Neuringer, C. (1964). Rigid thinking in suicidal individuals. *Journal of Consulting Psychology, 28*, 54–58.

Newcomb, M. D., & Bentler, P. M. (1988). Consequences of adolescent substance abuse on young adult health status and utilization of health services: A structural equation model over four years. *Social Science and Medicine, 24*, 71–82.

O'Conner, T. (1989). Cultural voices and strategies for multicultural education. *Journal of Education, 171*, 57–74.

O'Carroll, P. W., Berman, A. L., Maris, R., Moscicki, E., Tanney, B., & Silverman, M. (1996). Beyond the tower of Babel: A nomenclature for suicidology. *Suicide and Life-Threatening Behavior, 26*, 23–39.

Osman, A., Downs, W. R., Kopper, B. A., Barrios, F. X., Baker, M. T., Osman, J. R., et al. (1998). The Reasons for Living Inventory for Adolescents (RFL-A): Development and psychometric properties. *Journal of Clinical Psychology, 54*, 1063–1078.

Otto, O. (1972). Suicidal acts by children and adolescents. *Acta Psychiatrica Scandinavica*, 48(1, Suppl. 233),

Overton, W. F. (1991). Reasoning in the adolescent. In R. M. Lerner, A. C. Petersen, & J. Brooks-Gunn (Eds.), *Encyclopedia of adolescence* (pp. 912–916). New York: Garland.

Paris, J. (1997). Childhood trauma as an etiological factor in the personality disorders. *Journal of Personality Disorders, 11*, 34–49.

Paris, J., & Zweig-Frank, H. (2001). A 27-year follow-up of patients with borderline personality disorder. *Comprehensive Psychiatry, 43*, 103–107.

Patsiokas, A. T., & Clum, G. A. (1985). Effects of psychotherapeutic strategies in the treatment of suicide attempters. *Psychotherapy: Theory, Research, Practice, Training, 22*(2), 281–290.

Patsiokas, A. T., Clum, G. A., & Luscomb, R. L. (1979). Cognitive characteristics of suicide attempters. *Journal of Consulting and Clinical Psychology, 47*, 478–484.

Patterson, G. R. (1976). The aggressive child: Victim and architect of a coercive system. In E. J. Walsh, L. A. Hamerlynck, & L. C. Handy (Eds.), *Behavior modification and families* (pp. 267–316). New York: Brunner/Mazel.

Pattison, E. M., & Kahan, J. (1983). The deliberate self-harm syndrome. *American Journal of Psychiatry, 140*(7), 867–872.

Pfeffer, C. R. (1989). Family characteristics and support systems as risk factors for youth suicidal behavior. In L. Davidson & M. Linnola (Eds.), *Report of the Secretary's Task Force on Youth Suicide: Vol. 2. Risk factors for youth suicide* (pp. 71–87). Rockville, MD: U.S. Department of Health and Human Services.

Pfeffer, C. R., Klerman, G. L., Hurt, S. W., Lesser, M., Peskin, J. R., & Siefker, C. A. (1991). Suicidal children grow up: Demographic and clinical risk factors for adolescent suicide attempts. *Journal of the American Academy of Child and Adolescent Psychiatry, 30*, 609–616.

Pfeffer, C. R., Newcorn, J., Kaplan, G., Mizruchi, M. S., & Plutchik, R. (1988). Suicidal behavior in adolescent psychiatric inpatients. *Journal of the American Academy of Child and Adolescent Psychiatry, 27*, 357–361.

Phinney, J., & Rosenthal, D. A. (1992). Ethnic identity in adolescence: Process, context, and outcome. In G. R. Adams, T. P. Gullotta, & R. Montemayor (Eds.), *Adolescent identity formation* (pp. 145–172). Newbury Park, CA: Sage.

Pilowsky, D. J., Wu, L. T., & Anthony, J. C. (1999). Panic attacks and suicide attempts in mid-adolescence. *American Journal of Psychiatry, 156*(10), 1545–1549.

Plutchik, R., van Praag, H. M., & Conte, H. R. (1989). Correlates of suicide and violence risk: III. A two stage model of countervailing forces. *Psychiatry Research, 28*, 215–225.

Porr, V. (2004, November). *DBT skills training with family members.* Paper presented at the annual meeting of the International Society for Improvement of and Training in Dialectical Behavior Therapy, New Orleans, LA.

Potenza, D. (1998). Integrating dialectical behavior therapy into a community mental health program. *Psychiatric Services, 49*, 1338–1340.

Rathus, J. H., & Feindler, E. L. (2004). Assessment of partner violence: A handbook for researchers and practitioners. Washington, DC: American Psychological Association.

Rathus, J. H., & Miller, A. L. (1995a). *Life Problems Inventory.* Unpublished instrument, Bronx, NY.

Rathus, J. H., & Miller, A. L. (1995b). *DBT Skills Rating Scale for Adolescents*. Unpublished instrument, Bronx, NY.

Rathus, J. H., & Miller, A. L. (2000). DBT for adolescents: Dialectical dilemmas and secondary treatment targets. *Cognitive and Behavioral Practice, 7*, 425–434.

Rathus, J. H., & Miller, A. L. (2002). Dialectical behavior therapy adapted for suicidal adolescents. *Suicide and Life-Threatening Behavior, 32*, 146–157.

Rathus, J. H., Wagner, D., & Miller, A. L. (2005, November). *Measurement of emotion dysregulation, impulsivity, interpersonal chaos, and confusion about self: Psychometric evaluation of the Life Problems Inventory*. Paper presented at the annual meeting of the Association for Behavioral and Cognitive Therapies (ABCT), Washington, DC.

Razin, A. M., O'Dowd, M. A., Nathan, A., Rodriguez, I., Goldfield, A., Martin, C., et al. (1991). Suicidal behavior among inner-city Hispanic adolescent females. *General Hospital Psychiatry, 13*, 45–58.

Reiser, D. E., & Levenson, H. (1984). Abuses of the borderline diagnosis: A clinical problem with teaching opportunities. *American Journal of Psychiatry, 141*, 1528–1532.

Remafedi, G., Farrow, J. A., & Deisher, R. W. (1993). Risk factors for attempted suicide in gay and bisexual youth. In L. G. Garnets & D. C. Kimmel (Eds.), *Psychological perspectives on lesbian and gay male experiences*. (pp. 486–499). New York: Columbia University Press.

Remafedi, G., French, S., Story, M., Resnick, M. D., & Blum, R. (1998). The relationship between suicide risk and sexual orientation: Results of a population-based study. *American Journal of Public Health, 88*(1), 57–60.

Reynolds, W. M. (1987). *Suicidal Ideation Questionnaire: Professional manual*. Odessa, FL: Psychological Assessment Resources.

Reynolds, W. M., & Mazza, J. J. (1992, June). *Suicidal behavior in nonreferred adolescents*. Paper presented at the International Conference for Suicidal Behavior, Western Psychiatric Institute and Clinic, Pittsburgh, PA.

Reynolds, W. M., & Mazza, J. J. (1994). Suicide and suicidal behaviors in children and adolescents. In W. M. Reynolds & H. F. Johnston (Eds.), *Handbook of depression in children and adolescents* (pp. 525–580). New York: Plenum Press.

Rich, C. L., & Runeson, B. S. (1992). Similarities in diagnostic comorbidity between suicide among young people in Sweden and the United States. *Acta Psychiatrica Scandinavica, 86*, 335–339.

Rich, C. L., Young, D., & Fowler, R. C. (1986). San Diego suicide study: I. Young vs. old subjects. *Archives of General Psychiatry, 43*, 577–582.

Robbins, D. R., & Alessi, N. E. (1985). Depressive symptoms and suicidal behavior in adolescents. *American Journal of Psychiatry, 142*, 588–592.

Roberts, R. E., Chen, Y. R., & Roberts, C. R. (1997). Ethnocultural differences in prevalence of adolescent suicidal behaviors. *Suicide and Life-Threatening Behavior, 27*, 208–217.

Romaine, S. (1984). *The language of children and adolescents: The acquisition of communicative competence*. Oxford: Blackwell.

Rosenberg, M. L., Mercy, J. A., & Houk, V. N. (1991). Guns and adolescent suicides. *Journal of the American Medical Association, 266*, 3030.

Rosenthal, M. Z., Lynch, T. R., & Linehan, M. M. (2005). Dialectical behavior therapy for borderline personality disorder and substance use disorders. In R. Frances, S. Miller, & A. Mach (Eds.), *Clinical textbook of addictive disorders* (pp. 615–636.). New York: Guilford Press.

Runeson, B. S., & Beskow, J. (1991). Borderline personality disorder in young Swedish suicides. *Journal of Nervous and Mental Disease, 179*, 153–156.

Runeson, B. S., Beskow, J., & Waern, M. (1996). The suicidal process in suicides among young people. *Acta Psychiatrica Scandinavica, 93*(1), 35–42.

Russell, S. T., & Joyner, K. (2001). Adolescent sexual orientation and suicide risk: Evidence from a national survey. *American Journal of Public Health, 91*, 1276–1281.

Rutter, M. (1986). The developmental psychopathology of depression: Issues and perspectives. In M. Rutter, C. Izard, & P. Read (Eds.), *Depression in young people* (pp. 3–30). New York: Guilford Press.

Sabo, A. N. (1997). Etiological significance of associations between childhood trauma and borderline personality disorder: Conceptual and clinical implications. *Journal of Personality Disorders, 11*(1), 50–70.

Sakinofsky, I., Roberts, R. S., Brown, Y., Cumming, C., & James, P. (1990). Problem resolution and repetition of parasuicide: A prospective study. *British Journal of Psychiatry, 156*, 395–399.

Salkovskis, P. M., Atha, C., & Storer, D. (1990). Cognitive-behavioural problem solving in the treatment of patients who repeatedly attempt suicide: A controlled trial. *British Journal of Psychiatry, 157*, 871–876.

Sally, M., Jackson, L., Carney, J., Kevelson, J., & Miller, A. L. (November, 2002). *Implementing DBT skills training groups in an underperforming high school.* Poster session presented at the annual meeting of the International Society for the Improvement and Training of DBT, Reno, NV.

Santisteban, D. A., Muir, J. A., Mena, M. P., & Mitrani, V. B. (2003). Integrated borderline adolescent family therapy: Meeting the challenges of treating borderline adolescents. *Psychotherapy: Theory/ Research/Practice/Training, 40*(4), 251–264.

Schmidtke, A., & Hafner, H. (1988). The Werther effect after television films: New evidence for an old hypothesis. *Psychological Medicine, 18*, 665–676.

Schotte, D. E., & Clum, G. A. (1982). Suicide ideation in a college population: A test of a model. *Journal of Consulting and Clinical Psychology, 50*, 690–696.

Schroeder, S. R., Oster-Granite, M. L., & Thompson, T. (Eds.). (2002). *Self-injurious behavior: Gene–brain–behavior relationships.* Washington, DC: American Psychological Association.

Shaffer, D., Garland, A., Gould, M., Fisher, P., & Trautman, P. (1988). Preventing teenage suicide: A critical review. *Journal of the American Academy of Child and Adolescent Psychiatry, 27*, 675–687.

Shaffer, D., Gould, M. S., Brasic, J., Ambrosini, P., Fisher, P., Bird, H., et al. (1983). A Children's Global Assessment Scale (CGAS). *Archives of General Psychiatry, 40*, 1228–1231.

Shaffer, D., Gould, M., Fisher, P., Trautman, M. P., Moreau, D., Kleinman, M., et al. (1996). Psychiatric diagnosis in child and adolescent suicide. *Archives of General Psychiatry, 53*, 339–348.

Shaffer, D., Gould, M., & Hicks, R. (1994). Worsening suicide rate in black teenagers. *American Journal of Psychiatry, 151*, 1810–1812.

Shaffer, D., & Piacentini, J. (1994). Suicide and attempted suicide. In M. Rutter & E. Taylor (Eds.), *Child psychiatry: Modern approaches* (3rd ed., pp. 407–424). Oxford: Blackwell Scientific.

Shafii, M., Carrigan, S., Whittinghill, J. R., & Derrick, A. (1985). Psychological autopsy of completed suicide in children and adolescents. *American Journal of Psychiatry, 142*, 1061–1064.

Shafii, M., Steltz-Lenarsky, J., Derrick, A. M., Beckner, C., et al. (1988). Comorbidity of mental disorders in the post-mortem diagnosis of completed suicide in children and adolescents. *Journal of Affective Disorders, 15*(3), 227–233.

Shearer, S. L., Peter, C. P., Quaytman, M. S., & Wadman, B. E. (1988). Intent and lethality of suicide attempts among female borderline in-patients. *American Journal of Psychiatry, 145*, 1424–1427.

Shneidman, E. S. (1996). *The suicidal mind.* New York: Oxford University Press.

Sigurdson, E., Staley, D., Matas, M., Hildahl, K., & Squair, K. (1994). A five year review of youth suicide in Manitoba. *Canadian Journal of Psychiatry, 39*, 397–403.

Silk, K. R., Lee, S., Hill, E. M., & Lohr, N. E. (1995). Borderline personality disorder symptoms and severity of sexual abuse. *American Journal of Psychiatry, 152*, 1059–1064.

Simpson, J. A., & Weiner, E. S. (Eds.). (1989). *Oxford English dictionary* (2nd ed.) [Electronic version]. University of Washington Information Navigator.

Smith, K., & Crawford, S. (1986). Suicidal behavior among "normal" high school students. *Suicide and Life-Threatening Behavior, 16*, 313–325.

Smith, W. T., & Glaudin, V. (1992). A placebo-controlled trial of paroxetine in the treatment of major depression. *Journal of Clinical Psychiatry, 53*, 36–39.

Spencer, M. B., Dornbusch, S. M., & Mont-Reynaud, R. (1990). Challenges in studying minority youth. In S. S. Feldman & G. R. Elliot (Eds.), *At the threshold: The developing adolescent* (pp. 123–146). Cambridge, MA: Harvard University Press.

Spirito, A., Brown, L., Overholser, J., & Fritz, G. (1989). Attempted suicide in adolescence: A review and critique of the literature. *Clinical Psychology Review, 9*, 335–363.

Stanley, B., Gameroff, M. J., Michalsen, V., & Mann, J. J. (2001). Are suicide attempters who self-mutilate a unique population? *American Journal of Psychiatry, 158*(3), 427–432.

Substance Abuse and Mental Health Services Administration. (1996). *Preliminary estimates from the 1995 National Household Survey on Drug Abuse* (Advance Report No. 18). Rockville, MD: Author.

Suter, B. (1976). Suicide and women. In B. B. Wolman & K. H. Kraus (Eds.), *Between survival and suicide* (pp. 129–161). New York: Gardner Press.

Swann, W., Jr., Stein-Seroussi, A., & Giesler, B. (1992). Why people self-verify. *Journal of Personality and Social Psychology, 62,* 392–401.

Symons, F. S. (2002). Self-injury and pain: Models and mechanisms. In S. R. Schroeder, M. L. Oster-Granite, & T. Thompson (Eds.), *Self-injurious behavior: Gene–brain–behavior relationships* (pp. 223–234). Washington, DC: American Psychological Association.

Teicher, M. H. (2002, March). Scars that won't heal: The neurobiology of child abuse. *Scientific American,* pp. 68–75.

Termansen, P. E., & Bywater, C. (1975). S.A.F.E.R.: A follow-up service for attempted suicide in Vancouver. *Canadian Psychiatric Association Journal, 20,* 29–34.

Torhorst, A., Möller, H. J., Bürk, F., Kurz, A., et al. (1987). The psychiatric management of parasuicide patients: A controlled clinical study comparing different strategies of outpatient treatment. *Crisis: The Journal of Crisis Intervention and Suicide Prevention, 8*(1), 53–61.

Torhorst, A., Möller, H. J., & Schmid-Bode, K. W. (1988). Comparing a 3–month and a 12–month-outpatient aftercare program for parasuicide repeaters. In H. J. Moller, A. Schmidtke, & R. Welz (Eds.), *Current Issues of Suicidology* (pp. 19–24). Berlin, Germany: Springer-Verlag.

Tortolero, S. R., & Roberts, R. E. (2001). Differences in nonfatal suicide behaviors among Mexican and European American middle school children. *Suicide and Life-Threatening Behavior, 31,* 214–223.

Trautman, P. D., Stewart, N., & Morishima, A. (1993). Are adolescent suicide attempters noncompliant with outpatient care? *Journal of the American Academy of Child and Adolescent Psychiatry, 32,* 89–94.

Treatment for Adolescents with Depression Study (TADS) Team. (2004). Fluoxetine, cognitive-behavioral therapy, and their combination for adolescents with depression. *Journal of the American Medical Association, 292,* 807–820.

Trupin, E. W., Stewart, D. G., Beach, B., & Boesky, L. (2002). Effectiveness of a dialectical behavior therapy program for incarcerated juvenile offenders. *Child and Adolescent Mental Health, 7,* 121–127.

Turner, R. M. (2000). Naturalistic evaluation of dialectical behaviour therapy-oriented treatment for borderline personality disorder. *Cognitive and Behavioral Practice, 7,* 413–419.

Tyrer, P., Thompson, S., Schmidt, U., Jones, V., Knapp, M., Davidson, K., et al. (2003). Randomized controlled trial of brief cognitive behaviour therapy versus treatment as usual in recurrent deliberate self-harm: The POPMACT study. *Psychological Medicine, 33*(6), 969–976.

U.S. Department of Health and Human Services. (1994). *Vital Statistics of the United States, 1991.* Washington, DC: U.S. Government Printing Office.

U.S. Department of Justice. (1994). *Crime in the United States* Washington, DC: U.S. Government Printing Office.

van den Bosch, L. M. C., Koeter, M., Stijnen, T., Verheul, R., van den Brink, W. (2005). Sustained efficacy of dialectical behaviour therapy for borderline personality disorder. *Behaviour Research and Therapy, 43,* 1231–1241.

van der Sande, R., Buskens, E., Allart, E., van der Graaf, Y., & van Engeland, H. (1997). Psychosocial intervention following suicide attempt: A systematic review of treatment interventions. *Acta Psychiatrica Scandinavica, 96*(1), 43–50.

van der Sande, R., van Rooijen, L., Buskens, E., & Allart, E. (1997). Intensive in-patient and community intervention versus routine care after attempted suicide. A randomised controlled intervention study. *British Journal of Psychiatry, 171,* 35–41.

van Heeringen, C., Jannes, S., Buylaert, W., Henderick, H., De Bacquer, D., & van Remoortel, J. (1995). The management of non-compliance with referral to out-patient after-care among attempted suicide patient: A controlled intervention study. *Psychological Medicine, 25,* 963–970.

Velting, D. M., & Gould, M. S. (1997). Suicide contagion. In R. W. Maris, M. M. Silverman, & S. S. Canetto (Eds.), *Review of suicidology, 1997* (pp. 96–137). New York: Guilford Press.

Velting, D. M., & Miller, A. L. (1999, April). Diagnostic risk factors for adolescent parasuicidal behavior. In D. M. Velting (Chair), *Methodological advances in suicide assessment: The Lifetime Parasuicide Count Interview.* Symposium conducted at the 32nd annual meeting of the American Association of Suicidology, Houston, TX.

Velting, D. M., Rathus, J. H., & Asnis, G. M. (1998). Asking adolescents to explain discrepancies in self-reported suicidality. *Suicide and Life-Threatening Behavior, 28*(2), 187–196.

Velting, D. M., Rathus, J. H., & Miller, A. L. (2000). MACI personality scale profiles of depressed, adolescent suicide attempters: A pilot study. *Journal of Clinical Psychology, 56*(10), 1381–1385.

Verheul, R., van den Bosch, L. M., Koeter, M. W., de Ridder, M. A., Stijnen, T., & van den Brink, W. (2003). Dialectical behaviour therapy for women with borderline personality disorder: 12-month, randomised clinical trial in the Netherlands. *British Journal of Psychiatry, 182,* 135–140.

Vinoda, K. S. (1966). Personality characteristics of attempted suicides. *British Journal of Psychiatry, 112,* 1143–1150.

Volkmar, F. R., & Woolston, J. L. (1997). Comorbidity of psychiatric disorders in children and adolescents. In S. Wetzler & W. C. Sanderson (Eds.), *Treatment of patients with psychiatric comorbidity* (pp. 307–322). New York: Wiley.

Wagner, B. M. (1997). Family risk factors for child and adolescent suicidal behavior. *Psychological Bulletin, 121,* 246–298.

Waterhouse, J., & Platt, S. (1990). General hospital admission in the management of parasuicide: A randomised controlled trial. *British Journal of Psychiatry, 156,* 236–242.

Webster's, new universal unabridged dictionary. (1983). Cleveland, OH: Dorset & Barber.

Webster-Stratton, C., & Taylor, T. K. (1998). Adopting and implementing empirically supported interventions: A recipe for success. In A. Buchanan & B. L. Hudson (Eds.), *Parenting, schooling and children's behavior* (pp. 127–160). Aldershot, UK: Ashgate.

Weishaar, M. E., & Beck, A. T. (1992). Hopelessness and suicide. *International Review of Psychiatry, 4,* 177–184.

Weiss, R. L., & Tolman, A. O. (1990). The Marital Interaction Coding System—Global (MICS-G): A global companion to the MICS. *Behavioral Assessment, 12,* 271–294.

Wekerle, C., Miller, A. L., Wolfe, D. A., & Spindel, C. (2006). *Childhood maltreatment.* Hogrefe & Huber.

Welu, T. C. (1977). A follow-up program for suicide attempters: Evaluation of effectiveness. *Suicide and Life-Threatening Behavior, 7,* 17–30.

Whitaker, C. A. (1975). Psychotherapy of the absurd: With special emphasis on the psychotherapy of aggression. *Family Process, 14,* 1–16.

Wichstrom, L. (2000). Predictors of adolescent suicide attempts: A nationally representative longitudinal study of Norwegian adolescents. *Journal of the American Academy of Child and Adolescent Psychiatry, 39,* 603–610.

Williams, J. M. G. (1991). Autobiographical memory and emotional disorders. In S. A. Christianson (Ed.), *Handbook of emotion and memory* (pp. 451–477). Hillsdale, NJ: Erlbaum.

Williams, J. M. G. (1993). *The psychological treatment of depression: A guide to the theory and practice of cognitive behavior therapy* (2nd ed.). New York: Free Press.

Windle, M., Miller-Tutzauer, C., & Domenico, D. (1992). Alcohol use, suicidal behavior, and risky activities among adolescents. *Journal of Research on Adolescence, 2,* 317–330.

Wold, C. I., & Litman, R. E. (1973). Suicide after contact with a suicide prevention center. *Archives of General Psychiatry, 28*(5), 735–739.

Wonderlich, S. A., Crosby, R. D., Mitchell, J. E., Roberts, J. A., Haseltine, B., DeMuth, G., & Thompson, K. M. (2000). Relationship of childhood sexual abuse and eating disturbance in children. *Journal of the American Academy of Child and Adolescent Psychiatry, 39*(10), 1277–1283.

Wood, A., Trainor, G., Rothwell, J., Moore, A., & Harrington, R. (2001). Randomized trial of a group therapy for repeated deliberate self-harm in adolescents. *Journal of the American Academy of Child and Adolescent Psychiatry, 40,* 1246–1253.

Woodberry, K., Miller, A. L., Glinski, J., Indik, J., & Mitchell, A. (2002). Family therapy and dialectical behavior with adolescents: Part 2. A theoretical review. *American Journal of Psychotherapy, 56,* 585–602.

Worden, J. W. (1989). Methods as a risk factor in youth suicide. In L. Davidson & M. Linnoila (Eds.), *Report of the Secretary's Task Force on Youth Suicide: Vol. 2. Risk factors for youth suicide* (pp. 184–192). Rockville, MD: U.S. Department of Health and Human Services.

World Health Organization (WHO) (2002). Suicide rates and absolute numbers of suicide by country. Retrieved from www.who.int/mental_health

Wunderlich, U., Bronish, T., & Wiichen, H. U. (1998). Comorbidity patterns in adolescents and young adults with suicide attempts. *European Archives of Psychiatry and Clinical Neuroscience, 248,* 87–95.

Zanarini, M. C. (2003, October). *Update on borderline personality disorder.* Paper presented at the conference of the National Education Alliance for Borderline Personality Disorder, White Plains, NY.

Zanarini, M. C., Frankenburg, F. R., Hennen, J., & Silk, K. R. (2003). The longitudinal course of borderline psychopathology: 6-year prospective follow-up of the phenomenology of borderline personality disorder. *American Journal of Psychiatry, 160,* 274–283.

Zlotnick, C., Mattia, J. I., & Zimmerman, M. (1999). Clinical correlates of self-mutilation in a sample of general psychiatric patients. *Journal of Nervous and Mental Disease, 187,* 296–301.

Zuckerman, M. (1979). *Sensation seeking: Beyond the optimum level of arousal.* Hillsdale, NJ: Erlbaum.

Index